A Divine Dance
of Madness

by Mairi Colme

Published by:
Chipmunkapublishing
PO Box 6872
Brentwood
Essex
CM13 1ZT
United Kingdom

http://www.chipmunkapublishing.com

Copyright © 2006 Mairi Colme

ISBN: 978 1 84747 023 2

Cry of the Unworthy.

I am mentally ill; Oh hear me!

As my mind unfolds, as life is born to me
Let not the long white coats and the frantic syringe
And the binding of the straightjacket come near me.

I am mentally ill; Oh save me

From the ponderous minds that relegate to cage-like walls,
From the psychiatrist's hands that sign away my meaning,
From the faceless many who condemn an accidental illness in me
As blameworthy, as shameful, a lameness to be shunned.

I am mentally ill; Oh cure me

Of the irrational hatred aimed at my vulnerability,
Of the pitiless despising which refuses work's dignity,
Makes living redundant, dispossesses with self-righteousness
Me from my home, my loved-ones, the children I give birth to;
Of the contagion which is thought to attach to me.

I am mentally ill; Oh pity me!

I am existing in the prison of other people's minds;
I am given no choice, no destiny, no freedom;
I am a voice that is not heard, my tongue condemned
As forever irrational, symbol of the brute-born;
I am dying daily, till the prejudice and the dark fear
In the labyrinth of the human mind shall be extinguished.

I am mentally ill; Oh see my worth!

Chapter 1
My Story of Madness.

This story is about "madness"; about the suffering which may drive us into madness, what that madness is like, and how we may return from such madness. It is I hope an insight for others into the condition labelled as "manic depression." It is also about love; the universal love of God which was revealed to me in madness, and the love of one particular man, which was light to me in the darkness.

When I began this book two years ago it seemed to me it was primarily about the anguished scream of my motherhood, for I needed to express that scream. After explaining that for 7 years, from '88 to '95, I was permanently sectioned under the Mental Health act, robbed of my freedom, my integrity, my rights, I wrote at the time;-

"What they did to me was to take my young son, my only child, away from me; and I hardly ever saw him from the age of 4 till the age of 11! Why this was done I'll never comprehend; for I was a single parent who gave her child a good upbringing from being a baby, and I never harmed him and was never a danger to him. Yet I suffered so acutely as a mother from the loss of my son, during those 7 years when I was sectioned, that I kept going "insane with pain." The father, who abused me whilst I lived with him, and threw me out into the snow when I was pregnant, demanded to see "his son" after he was born; then he applied to the courts and continued to harass me until I fell ill; then when I was ill in the hospital he took custody off me, claiming that I was an "unfit mother" because "mentally ill." Why did this happen? If I were a mother in hospital with a broken leg, would I not have had Access rights to my son? Would I have been denied seeing my young son for 6 months at a time? But because it was a "mental illness,"-a broken mind,- and a "mental hospital," I wasn't allowed to see him, no-one arranged that I could see him! I fought like hell for him, and I suffered abominably, and hardly anyone can comprehend what it is like to suffer as a mother in such a way! But this is my story; the story of what it is like to be driven mad by suffering!"

Having now finished the book, having expressed the pain and suffering of my own life and told my story, having "let it go," letting it fall into the endlessness which is God, I can see it is about more than that. It is because it is about more than my own suffering that I have been inspired on Iona to commit myself to being there for others who are suffering similarly, and to work as far as I can to help others.

What is the book really about?

It is about the stigma against mental illness, which made me suffer so much as a mother deprived of her young son. It is about the fact that the only way I could get well and transcend my illness was by escaping from the System, breaking the power that the mental health law held over me. It is a protest of my own, on behalf of everyone who is accounted "mentally ill," an outcry of "Don't do this to us!" We are not to be treated this way, in the way I myself was treated.

More than this, it is about the fact that in that madness I experienced, I "touched" God. It is a strange fact that throughout the centuries people have been considered "touched" by God when mad; only recently are people locked away and discarded as suffering a form of "sickness" or "abnormality." We need to rethink this, so that we respect, we honour those who are mad rather than rubbishing them. My story is about an understanding of God, about the energy I touched, - the energy at the core of the universe which is Love.

This book is indeed "my story," of my own solitary suffering; but all the universal dimensions are what the book is really about.

I have entitled it as I have because the notion of "dancing" with God comes from the Book of the Beloved, Page 20; *for in that mystical story, when God invites "Come and embrace me," I hang back because fearful that to embrace God would entail cold and death-like suffering. I didn't have the courage or strength to embrace him, until he touched the pulse-point of the love within me; then when I did, I found Him "warm and living," and He whispered "Come dance with me."*

This story, which shows my willingness to suffer, forms the connection between the mystical perfect ideal of "saying Yes to God," and my own physical, miserable, abused condition in the conceiving of my son. *For in giving birth, the dance of suffering God led me into, was really the dance of life!*

I recently told someone whose opinion I trust, "no-one will want to read this story because it is so tragic, and so, so sad," and she replied "but what comes across is your courage." And so I hope at the end of the day that my story comes over as life-affirming.

Chapter 2
My Mysticism.

This story about my struggle with the Psychiatric System is shot through by my own spirituality. For spirituality is our "saying Yes to God whenever we experience Him"; and I experienced God in my madness. When I was young, "joyous and eager, capable of ecstasy," I had a revelation about the love of God, which I subsequently called the"Book of the Beloved." And I have come to understand the meaning of this book, contemplating on it every day during my years of intense mental suffering, when the emotions of rage and pain dragged through me like a sea. *Now, years later, I can say I wouldn't want to be without that suffering as it gave me a unique insight into that love. And I offer the book in the hope that others can espy the Love too, without having to go through the madness as I did.*

It is the Love that moves the stars (which I called "the Star-Love," though you can call Him God or whatever you choose); *the Light-Energy which was in the beginning, "in every blade of grass, flowing in every stream, and moving the stars, ubiquitous," "the cornucopia of creativity from whom the worlds tumbled forth."*

And this universal Love, according to my Book, becomes the Lover of the human soul, ie. the Beloved, when she says Yes to him. She is a "maiden" like Our Lady, but precisely because of her innocence and purity she believes what is "beyond the credibility of men's bound minds," and has an inkling of what God can do. *So in the crucial Time-span which was come upon her she did not doubt, but rose beyond herself and transcended herself. She gathered her soul in cupped hands as she vowed; "May everything happen to me as Love wants."* According to my book this is the mighty "Fiat" which brings about the birth of the divine into the human soul, and in Christian terms, the redeeming birth of the Christ-child into the world of time. *"Her words became a pulsation, passing through all the worlds; radiant light-energy pulsed and streamed through her, gathered, centered, streaming in the one direction, with will."*

However, as the first page of the Book of the Beloved makes clear, the implications of this, for the Beloved, is that she must share, partake in God's own suffering; just as Our Lady had to share Christ's suffering under His cross. Hence Page One opens with *the* words; *"the Beloved has received the Star-Love; she has known the Star-Love's Agony."* It is like the imprinting of nails!

The Book keeps returning to the theme of being lost in a cold dark Void, which I identify personally with the Void of madness; (Madness is the void which is left when you annihilate the self). *She keeps clamouring into the Void; "Isn't there somewhere a great enough Love to overcome this cold dark Void of Agony? I cannot reconcile the Star-Love with this Agony; Love is Absent."It is an absence of Love; she feels her soul is not loved and God is nowhere!*

But her Lover tries to compel her to silence, to complete stillness and receptivity, by infinitely repeating truths about love. One of these truths is "Because He loves me He hurts me; the suffering is the Love." And He keeps whispering a new name; "Beloved; Beloved be still." *"Until ultimately she was still; and she heard the whispering which the Star-Love utters in the secret silence to His chosen in all the worlds;" she receives His Love.*

And then the Beloved really rejoices saying; "The Star-Love's Agony became bearable to me, and so shall all suffering be bearable, now that I know I am desired by the Star-Love, and have received Him. And my knowing of Agony and Love together shall be true forever. And the more I am myself, the more I become the Beloved He has chosen, the better I shall understand Love's whispering to me, Love's meaning."

And that was true for me; all of my madness, all of my experience was a leading into the meaning of the love and suffering I was trying to comprehend which I saw burning together in fire at the core of the universe. And I can truly say I have comprehended that Love through my suffering. Hence I will say as I wrote on my original book-cover;-

It is about the "perfect Yes" we can say to God at our soul's centre, and that "perfect Yes" worked out in real human life, amid the reality of suffering and the ravages of human emotion. It is about this endless Energy of Love at the core of the universe, which the author found, experienced, and touched, in her madness. About the dance of her psyche with God!

8

Chapter 3
Beginning.

Journal of 1st September '85: -

"I had a strange, remarkable experience in the early morning; a larger-than-life dream in which all the characters were archetypal, and then when wide awake at the end of it, I heard "the pipes of Pan". Things were a bit strange before this dream, in that I'd got up for a drink, noticing it was dark, and a moment later I realised there was bright light coming through the curtains, and I could hear horses along the street. This dream was full of archetypal figures, such as a true mother-figure, a little child who needed my protection, a bully -figure, and a female soul-friend. I myself was not myself, but someone greater, more good, as if I'd come back in another incarnation, older and wiser in the school of life. At the end of this dream I was listening, trying to find out what mystery was going on among a group of people on horses, and I pierced into a deeper realm, where an artist was telling me how all these images came from "the realm of Los", more real and archetypal; and then when I was listening most intensely, I heard "the pipes of Pan". This didn't seem like a dream; I was convinced I was awake and really heard this music. It was a haunting tune of pipes, Nature's tune, but all created things were making up this music; the noises outside the window were all real notes within this tune. I listened to it intently for a while, knowing that if I moved it would cease. - - "Fled is that music; do I wake or sleep?" - - - I now feel strange and disorientated; my strange dream has made me open, sensitive and receptive to what is strange, to what is "other.""

I was truly astonished, on looking back, to discover what I had written of the night of my son's conception. It was a strange, surreal experience. This is when my story truly began,- when I conceived my son.

This is not to say I hadn't suffered before then. I had long suffered from the ravages of mental illness, which was at first diagnosed as "Schizophrenia". Everything I had done or attempted had been ruined by my falling ill with this terrible "disease". It had first manifested itself when I was a 17-year-old teenager, and spoilt my school life. Then I was brave enough to go to Austria on my own, seeking monasteries and mountains, and I'd fallen ill there and been hospitalized. Then I'd tried university and various jobs, and entered an enclosed Benedictine convent; but whatever I did I kept falling prey to my tendency to become "manic". Doctors kept stuffing me full of tablets to prevent this, but I hated their effect on me, and always stopped taking them. Then I finally came to KirkMichaels university, and despite everything, managed to end up with an Honours degree in English. Then I had stayed in KirkMichaels, largely because of my impossible difficulties with my father. But that's a long story.

It is a long story too to explain how I ended up in Walter's bed. The previous year, 1984, had not been a good one for me. I would not have ended up in anyone's bed, were it not for the fact that I'd had my first genuinely sexual relationship that year. I'd lost my self-esteem at the same time as I'd lost my virginity, because of the fact that the man used me and then, I felt, threw me aside "like a dirty old rag." I had a low self-esteem after that, which left me an easy prey. That summer I went down to Walsingham, and was incarcerated once again in a hospital in Norwich, though on this occasion I wasn't really ill, just religiously excited. But they had got me established on an injection called Depixol, and they made it clear that I had to take this injection ever after; I was going to be forced to take it, despite the dire side-effects. But I couldn't tolerate it, so when I managed to get free, and came back to KirkMichaels, I stopped taking it, suddenly and unsupervised. And I went "psychotic" fairly quickly, - the most psychotic I have been in my life! And at this point I met Walter McKay!

I met him in the job-centre; I was desperately looking for a job and a place to live; he invited me back to his council house. I was slowly but surely going "mad" whilst the Depixol was passing out of my system. He took me to bed with him, and there followed a week of intense and frequent love-making. I didn't know what I was doing. I thought he was "God", and that I had to obey him. He didn't seem to have the wits to realise that I was going completely "bonkers". I became obsessed with different things, and at the end became quite catatonic; I was living in a world of complete delusion. It was an old friend of mine, Vivien, who seeing me obviously ill along the street, detained me at her house and called the doctor. The doctor was called Dr.James, and it was his first encounter with me. Then I was sent to the dreaded Craigdene. This was once in my life that I was genuinely ill, not just "manic."

They locked me up in a "Time Out room", where I lay on the bare floor, unable to speak or move, or to communicate or eat, for 3 weeks. At the end of that time, thanks to the drugs, no doubt, I was a little better and said I wanted to go "home", for I was living a nightmare in there. A strange female doctor came in to see me, and said I could go "home" provided I had somewhere to go to. I cited Walter's as a home where I would be welcomed. This idiot of a doctor said I could go that very day. I was still delusional, and could hardly move or speak. And they let me go, right there and then; I hitch-hiked back to KirkMichaels, being under the delusion that the car's exhaust fumes was benign snow!

And of course Walter took me in at the end of '84. But I was still very psychiatrically ill and under heavy doses of drugs until May of the following year; it is hard to describe, but I was all "stiff" and I couldn't talk or move. And I was "looked after" by Walter in that state, as there was no-one else to look after me. My parents in Yorkshire wouldn't take me in, though I begged them, and I was far too "ill" to find a place of my own to live. I needed someone's support, someone to lean on in a psychiatric sense, and that job fell to Walter. I think he partly took me in out of kindness, but it was largely to fulfil his emotional need of having someone dependant on him; and, as was pointed out to me, it was to have "a woman in his bed." Once there, I was stuck; I didn't have the ability to find somewhere else to live; and it seemed far better to me to live there than in the ghastly hospital. And then time passed; it took time for my brain to get better.

Chapter 4
Trapped.

Time passed, and meanwhile I became emotionally attached to Walter. I didn't have the ability to get away from him, even though he tormented me with his saying of nasty, unkind and bad-tempered things. He kept saying I was selfish and deceitful, for not having sex with him. I bravely resisted for most of the winter, but the result was he kept threatening to "end the relationship"; he kept saying "I want you out of the house", but on the other hand was kind and emotional with me the next day. I couldn't cope; he had me on an emotional string. I intensely hated the sexuality we went through in bed, and wanted to be set free from him.

I felt so unfree, so bound, so claustrophobic, but I couldn't get away from him. I too much feared his anger if he knew that I was trying got find somewhere to live. On one occasion I went into town to see an old university friend, to seek some assistance, but Walter followed, saw where I went, and rounded on me all the way home, calling me a "whore". I felt trapped; I wanted to move out and get away from him but I couldn't; I didn't have the wherewithal, the ability to stand on my own two feet and look after myself, and I knew I didn't. For months I wanted to move out and get away from him. And I spent all my time mourning the past; fearing I had permanent brain-damage, and that I could never be myself again. But with the help of a kind Dr. Abernethy, I stopped taking the injection in March, and gradually it began to wear off. I went to Iona in March, trying to leave the "long dead winter" behind me. I tried to transcend myself, and I felt very "humbled"; I felt God had humbled me by this illness.

But the sickness in my eyes never really left me, and I didn't come back transformed as I hoped. I wanted to leave Walter behind but I found I was physically and emotionally attached to him. He was always being cross with me, and kept threatening "we are finished"; and I was trying to make sense of it and "die to myself". I hated the house; I just wanted to be free from my sense of sickness. I felt that I'd never get better; Dr.Abernethy had said I may always have "residual effects"; I feared I'd always suffer this deadness and dearth of thought. I felt in darkness, hating the way I lived.

Then in April I went back to Iona with Walter. There I plucked up the courage to tell him "I'm leaving you". I told him I was going to go home to my Mum and Dad; he was furious. He wouldn't take any photos of me with the lambs, because he said he'd "finished with me." I was grabbing hold of some hope and faith that I'd get better; I found a metaphor for why I wasn't myself; I decided it was like having a "broken leg" which hadn't mended, and had left me "limping painfully." I tried to see it as "suffering with Christ; I was trying to "patiently endure".

At the beginning of May I finally got better. I was so happy; I felt like an opening daffodil. I was full of laughter, excitement, self-expression; at last I felt I could communicate. My relationship with Walter improved; he was thrilled at my liveliness, and I felt more affectionate towards him. We watched the baby ducklings and the cherry blossom, and I had a wonderful sense of wellness and quickness. Everything was finally going so well, and I felt I was under God's "healing hand."

Then I went down to Yorkshire to visit my Mum and Dad. I had phoned from Iona, and my Dad said I could stay for ten days. I felt well and I was giving thanks. I had been trying not to "strain myself", but just to do little gentle exercises to nurse my "leg", and with my parents this was ideal, because I could join in this "little and humble way of life." I realised I must live humbly this "little way", and not seek ecstasies any more; I must guard against such pride. I blossomed and came to life; but then the stresses and strains of living with my parents meant that I preferred the fresh air and freedom of KirkMichaels. I preferred the way I had felt there, amongst the ducklings and cherry blossom, the week before I'd left. However I contrasted the dirtiness of Walter's house, but my Dad said I should return and clean it. I used to go for long walks, arm in arm with my Dad, looking at all the gardens and the flowers. Then it became "time to go back", and I made the free decision to go back. I felt a pull of affection for Walter; I felt I might now get on better with him, when I was well. I felt I'd "give the relationship a chance," because he'd cared for me when I was ill. He gave me a good welcome, when I got back, and I made the decision that I would try to get closer to God, and become more patient, humble and gentle, by learning to love this one man.

Chapter 5
Trying to Please.

For a month or so I was genuinely happy. I was so glad to be well that I lived in a kind of bliss. I tried to be happy together with Walter, tried to serve him in little ways, tried to reward him for his patience during my long illness. I genuinely wanted to "share my life" with him; I thought I could comprehend God's love through my love of him.
Sex began to work, because I had returning feelings. I was getting to like pleasing Walter, and he began to say lovely things to me and to appreciate me. I started to clean the house, and saw it as a potential "home" for the two of us. I began to delight in doing things to please Walter, giving myself to "human love."

We were planning marriage; we went to marriage lessons with a Catholic priest. I was learning to live a "little life" as a housewife, trying to serve and please. I was full of gratitude to Walter; I saw my difficulties with him in the past as "my own illness reflecting back at me". I tried to get closer to God by being close to him; he delighted in me. There were just occasional small incidents when he became bad-tempered and the air "froze" between us, but I passed over these; I felt that we loved each other, and so could transcend the difficulties. I was always trying to be self-transcending.

At the end of June he went down to London and left me alone at home. I meantime reflected that I wanted to be married and I wanted a man to love; I thought a solitary life was selfish and self-centred. On the 30th June the home-coming turned sour on me. I felt his sexual approaches weren't appropriate, and I was reluctant, and he turned nasty. He said he'd end the relationship; "I'll get another girl; I tell you I'll go my own way, if I feel things aren't right between us." I was very hurt, dismayed, saddened; "after our plans to be soon married, can he say something so callous? After I have committed myself to him, and to loving him, can he so brush me off?" I tried to take the hurt lovingly, but it augured badly.

For the next month we had such difficulties with sex, that I dreaded going to bed. He always used to say I was "reluctant" and "I can't live with a woman like that". I began to feel he wanted me to live with him just for his own sexual gratification. He used to be nasty to me in bed both night and morning, then make up again with me afterwards. I hated the feeling that I had to "submit to sex" all the time; I felt coerced, misused, disgusted and nauseated. "I hate being subjected to sex against my will."

Even my "wifely service", of making his breakfast, etc, became onerous; I began to feel like a slave. He became angry over the slightest thing, like the washing of my hair, and he was always threatening to end the relationship. He kept saying I was "cold" and he "didn't want to know me." Then however he kept making up afterwards, saying "forgive me darling" and "I'm sorry." The feeling that he was oppressing me was building up. In the awful silences when he was angry with me, I used to think "I can't marry him". I felt a sense of bondage; I felt that if I married him, I'd be more bound than ever. But I tried to muddle through; I tried to dwell on the affectionate closeness; I kept telling myself that I had to "accept the pain with the joy"; I started to put his bad-temper down to my own "sinful nature"; I did all the things I could to serve him and please him, and cajole him out of his moods; but I felt really oppressed.

In the month of August things improved. This was because I succeeded in my self-transcending efforts to please him. I kept feeling "Oh leave me alone" under his constant bad-temper, but I controlled my reactions, and always submitted to him. I began to do my best to please him sexually. As a result, our sex-life improved and we began to feel a lot of affection for each other. I had got the idea that he was veritably "my husband", and my duty was to "please my husband". I had also got the idea, from my spiritual books, that my human nature was very sinful and that I should try to purify myself through the love of a husband, and that yielding to him was yielding to God.

Hence life began to improve and settle down. We began to lead an affectionate life which was an interesting life. I was trying to "bear fruit" spiritually by yielding my will to another. *Thus my own spirituality was against me; it was partly my fault, that I became so tragically and deeply involved with Walter, and pregnant on the 1st of September.*

Chapter 6
Dread of Pregnancy.

The 1st of September was the celebration of our being exactly one year together; so we made a tasty meal and got a bottle of strong wine, and became inebriated. And after that we had a veritable sex-orgy. I quickly felt satiated and nauseated, and then something strange happened: -

"I was listening to Walter saying strange things and suddenly I opened my eyes to find that almost two hours had passed. And Walter told me I had been asleep all that time with my mouth pressed against his, our lips sealed together and breathing together. It was at this point that the sourness came. I showed myself reluctant to be sexual again, which was natural, feeling satiated the way I did. But he suddenly and crossly said "Don't bother then!" And then he started to say nasty things, which were all the more hurtful in the light of the fact that this was the anniversary of our being together. The most hurtful thing was "I don't like women who have inhibitions." And as I lay there this just sank into me with hurt. Then all the other things he said kept hurting me until it became a bitter hurt. For he said things that implied that he didn't want to stay with me any longer. He said "I am going to stop trying," and "you have no imagination." The bitterness of the hurt in me nearly made me say; "Alright we won't get married then, and I'll leave you." It was so very hurtful.- -

And then I had the other strange experience that night, when I had a weird archetypal dream and heard "the pipes of Pan." It made me feel strange and disorientated. *And because of my strange dream, I was open, sensitive, receptive to what is other. I felt I had to have an open ear to the mysteries God whispers to us; He is the mystery who is "wholly other."*
- That was the night I became pregnant.

It was a night which contained the germination of what really was wrong between us. I was trying to find and value the "communion" between us. There was a lot of "play" together; I used to pretend to confiscate his sweets for example if he didn't "behave", we played "tig" on the beach, we invented our own play-language. I tried to understand his moods and I took delight in making his meals. I tried to find my happiness in this "communion".

On the other hand I began to develop the most negative feelings when he wanted me to sexually arouse him. I used to lie there, dreading him coming to bed; then if I didn't comply with his demands he used to say the most nasty and hurtful things. He used to say; "I'm going to stop trying," "you don't please me," "you could never make me happy in a thousand years," "you show no interest in sex," "you are not capable of a deep relationship."

On the 13th September, after an incident when he demanded that I get up to butter him an oatcake, after I'd just sat down, I said to myself "I'm leaving you, because you treat me like a slave". That night for the first time I tried to explain to him my feeling, my female feeling about his sexual demands, but I ended up feeling "wounded and bleeding": -

"It was then, when I had done my best at explanation, and had lapsed into angry silence because of his refusal to accept it, that he said the worst things he has ever said to me. What did he say that wounded me so deeply? He said "you have no heart in you; no life, no spirit." On hearing this my anger burst its banks and I said "Oh shut up" and turned away from him. But he continued and everything he said percolated through and wounded me, until I felt I was lying in my own blood. He said "This is the beginning of a relationship breaking up." He said "it raises the question of whether you love me, or whether you are just holding on to a friendly face out of your own need." My anger was giving way to hurt so immense that I could have cried myself to sleep. However I remembered my prayer "I appeal to your grace to shine light into me." And feeling a bit melted by this I made the effort to turn round to give him a kiss; I was hoping that a "goodnight kiss" would bring reconciliation. But his response was negative; he said coldly that he "didn't want to express his emotion." It was again a moment of infinite hurt. I was shattered, wounded; I really could have cried myself to sleep!"

The next day I transcended myself by a sort of catharsis. I realised *Love is inevitably involved with suffering, for it is only when we have a heart open to love someone that we can get hurt. Being willing to be wounded and to bleed is the same as being willing to bear Christ's cross; the wounding and the bleeding are subsumed by the love.* So I asked God to banish all darkness from the sanctuary of my heart, all intense negative feelings, for I didn't want them to darken and poison my heart which I wanted to keep as a sanctuary to love; "Love's sanctuary is the human heart or nowhere." *I just felt that I needed in my darkness to touch God's finger, because he was close and indwelling, and then I would be illuminated by light.*

But there still loomed in my face the difficulties of the relationship. I asked God to banish from me the negative feelings, but if truth be told, I began to feel like a slave, just there to provide Walter with food and sex. It became worse and worse: - "I don't see why I should submit to sex when I hate it." I struggled and did my best to explain it to him: "you mustn't pressurise me with sex; both of us have to be willing, it has to be a free gift." I began to realise that a "wife" shouldn't feel this way; "I don't think he treats me right." I felt how I couldn't go on living that way; "I don't want to be married and bound to him for life."

And then on the 26th September I began to be worried about the possibility of being pregnant: -
"It was fear of having a baby which was dominating my mind. On the moment when Walter got into bed, I didn't restrain myself from voicing it; "Does every woman feel so much fear at the thought, or is it just me?" Walter was sympathetic and comforting saying that every woman is fearful over her first baby. I said how it was worse for me because there was the "added complication" that it might make me ill, and also it was unusual to have a first baby over the age of 30. I also said how it was easier for him than it was for me, because for him it was only a worry over "practical considerations", but for me it was also a kind of "physical fear," at the thought of the pain, the surgical instruments and the doctors in white coats. I really am possessed by fear."

Then I realised, the Thing I feared and that filled me with dread was the point where I would find God coming toward me, was God Himself and a sacrament. I well understood that it was God himself I would find in childbirth; "I believe it is God Himself coming toward me in the thing I dread."

Chapter 7
An Emotional Storm.

On the eve of the pregnancy test results, I knew the likelihood of it: -

"But an emotional event was caused by his sister coming, and by my whispering to Walter during her visit, to enquire if it were possible to watch a special TV programme. It was not until she had gone and the programme was finished, that he made the nasty remark; "You are a bad taste in my mouth." When I realised he meant it seriously, I was hurt and upset. He went on to say how it was impolite to whisper such a thing, as it made his sister feel unwelcome, referring to the fact that it was once her home, accusing me of "having no morality." I was so hurt that I was very close to tears. It came into my head "I don't want you as my husband, or the father of my child." And feeling I couldn't prevent myself from crying, I made the excuse of leaving the room to make a cup of tea. Once in the kitchen I started flooding with tears. - - Soon Walter came in, and I sobbed, "you know I'm sensitive because of this, and then you go and say nasty things; you know I need a lot of affection and assurance." And he promised to look after me and told me not to worry."

I prayed that I should be able to accept lovingly and patiently whatever news I might hear the next day, and to accept it with love as from God's hand. I prayed that I should from His hand accept gladly both good and ill, sweet and bitter, joy and sorrow. For it is God's hand behind it all; and He is a loving Creator. "I accept everything lovingly, as from His hand."

From Book of the Beloved, Page23: - When I am frightened of touching God's hand in the darkness, He assures me that it is His loving hand. "Why do you fear Me? This is the hand, My hand, which created you, which is placed in your being, and from the beginning has loved you." The Love behind the hand dawned upon my understanding; and so I reached out, and touched, and on the instant was filled with light. "I am your comfort and companion," He whispered "and I want you to depend on Me alone, for I myself will lead you." And we went on together, into the dark Void.

1st October 85: -
"The truth is that I am pregnant! We have been through a lot of emotion since we found out the truth this morning; we have gone through a storm of shared emotion. - - I suppose I already knew that I was pregnant before the news came across the phone that the test was

positive; I'd made the comment when I'd got up "I'm sure I'm pregnant." But I was sitting with Walter next to me on the chair's arm when I heard the news, and I just felt benumbed, and clung to him for ages. Then tears came into my eyes, and I cried all morning, not being able to stop.- - Walter is as emotional as I am. He castigates himself for it, saying he'll never be interested in sex again. He bemoans the fact that it will so much change his life; he said "my life is ruined" and called himself "doomed." When he reacted like this I said "Don't be like that; it is a wonderful thing to bring new life into the world." He says he's worried about me, about it making me ill. I said I understand now how girls want abortion out of fear; but I could never do that, - I see it as murder. Walter is aware of how I need to be comforted, saying that I'll feel fulfilled as a mother, that I'll light up with joy when the baby is born."

I felt I should be joyful over the mystery of the life within me, over the fact that I was bringing a new life into the world; I knew we should always say "Yes" to God whenever we experience Him. *Whether it was true in conception or not, I wanted this experience of bearing a child to be a "saying Yes" to God. - "May everything happen to me as Love wants." Though I was crying as I said it, I knew I had to say Yes to this child within me. I prayed that God would enable me to do so.*

From Book of the Beloved, Page4: - When graciously God asks me to share in His great Agony, I am afraid of all the suffering it will entail; and because I am afraid I answer a "Yes but." But He understands me omnisciently and promises, "I will be supporting you, always with you, always sufficient for you; so let your love trust Me." So in the crucial Time-span I spoke my Yes, and He adored and thanked me for it.

After this Walter and I kept clasping each other. Walter said positively that a child would be the bond between the two of us and would bind us together. My reaction was "caring for something you have created requires a lot of love, a lot of giving." But then I began to think how this pregnancy wasn't the way it should be and would ruin my life. And Walter started complaining "I can't go through all that again." I felt nauseated and unable to face reality. Something inside of me cried out "I don't want to be pregnant, I don't want a baby."

I realised that instead of being heartless and negative, I needed to be positive in facing this thing, and cheerful and strong and brave. I knew that when I was sinking down in dejection and heartlessness, feeling "I cannot," God was standing over me with understanding in his eyes saying "Don't you trust me? Do you love me?"

I found I had terrible negative feelings at a concert we went to, of "the Corries": - "Things are not as they should be; it should have been consecrated by marriage, and it wasn't; it should have been a saying Yes to God, and it wasn't; I should love the child in my womb, but I don't; I shouldn't even think of killing my baby, but its in my mind." I kept crying. Walter made it worse by starting to talk about looking after me and the baby in terms of "wasting his life." I felt guilty of my negative feelings. I tried to think what my "soul-friend" would advise; he would say that my feeling, of not wanting the baby, is not so important as my "will" which refuses abortion; moral awareness lies in the will.

I knew "the one thing that matters is that we always say Yes to God whenever we experience him, and I experience him in my baby. "Yes but" is never an answer that God likes; and this is what I have been saying in my non-acceptance of this baby inside of me. To say Yes to God is to say Yes to my baby; and to love my baby is to love God. Instead of wanting rid of this baby, I must really grow to love it. Love is in the will; I will love my baby."

From Book of the Beloved, Page104: - When God addresses me "Will you be my Bride?" I am amazed and confused and plead "I beg of you to leave me; I cannot comprehend what you ask of me." But He says "I am waiting for you to give me the right answer," and I become suddenly sensible that He wants something from me. He lays a commanding finger on my lips; "Beloved I want only one word from you." Suddenly I completely understand what it is; and gathering my soul in cupped hands I answer; "Yes is my one word; let everything happen to me as Love wants."

I found pregnancy ghastly as a physical experience; I felt faint and sick. Walter started saying that he felt "trapped" and that I had "ruined his life". He started pressurizing me into sex again, but I felt set against it: -
"Here I am, on the threshold of so much unwellness and pain, and willing to give a lifetime's commitment and love to the baby inside of me, and Walter has given me this baby by his perpetual oppression of me and demand that I should please him and keep him happy, and all he cares about is his own sexual satisfaction! We've got a baby to consider, and all he cares about is whether he will be kept sexually happy! Well I call that selfish! He has put me into an impossible situation. He is going to oppress me and coerce me on this same point which has resulted in my pregnancy, and I can't

leave him now because I need someone to look after me. That is a cruel blow of fate. I would leave him and not marry him, if I weren't so aware that I need looking after."

There was a hurtful explosion of feeling from Walter, in which he made it clear that he didn't want to marry me. I was feeling "Right I'll leave you, and look after the baby on my own." He was impossible to live with! On my way to church I had been thinking on these lines; "Can I look after my baby without living with Walter? Can I have somewhere to live, and enough income? Can I deny Walter any rights over the baby?" It was becoming such a miserable, impossible situation!

I appealed to God to help me; I had just got over trying to accept this baby, and now I was faced with all this negativity which upsets my security for the future. I felt I had to be brave and take it entirely upon myself. *I felt I had God's assurance that any cross or burden I bore "out of love", was something He would bear with me.*
From Book of the Beloved, Page118: - He keeps demanding "If you love me, carry this cross." I refuse at first, but when I shoulder it the burden is light; and He says "It is I who carry it with you."

I started to feel that I couldn't possibly get married to Walter, as I would feel so oppressed if I did. However I was aware of the social stigma otherwise, and I realised that no-one would look after me and the baby if he didn't. The doctors didn't press abortion on me, as they knew my feelings; I said "I could never stand before God my Maker if I had murdered a baby." It loomed in my mind, from what Dr.Abernethy told me, that if I was not married to Walter, he would have no rights over the child. I was impressed by this because the thing I dreaded was Walter oppressing me over the baby as I could imagine he would do.

My prime sensation was how oppressed I would be if married to Walter; I could imagine what lay before me,- all the squalid arguments, the oppression, the slavery, the misery, the slave-like making of his breakfasts, the entrapment in a small mean miserable life. Even then he was oppressing me by forbidding me to talk to anyone about it! Then I had a powerful dream about a ball of light entering my tummy. And I newly grasped at the idea that I could better assimilate it if I could see the child as God's!

On the 13th October I decided that I must leave Walter: -

"For I see absolutely clearly that I cannot possibly marry him; as a marriage it would never work. I have never really loved him; I've only been bullied, coerced, oppressed by him. I think I have decided, no matter what the risks or the courage required, I am going to leave him. - - As for the baby, I shall accept my responsibility for it, and see God as the father. Perhaps indeed He is, for miracles are always possible. I must accept this baby as coming from God; this means that in a special way that it is *my* baby."

I started to feel that I was accepting my destiny. I saw clearly that the reason I was with child was my fear. It wasn't at all love that led me to sexually engage with Walter, it was dread of his oppression and anger, fuelled by my fear of illness; I would do anything to make possible a life with him because I felt I needed him to look after me. "It was all fear."

Walter was getting angry because I refused love-making: -
"I explained that I didn't want any love-making with the sense of a baby inside of me. This really made him fly into anger. Then he said something which made me turn on my side away from him, - "we're not sexually compatible." I felt how cruel this was to say, after giving me a child. His reaction was to turn his back to me with real violence; and he said something which sounded like the death-blow to our relationship. He said he couldn't marry me because "It'll never work, it will never work in a thousand years!" I smiled to myself, thinking how I could tell him I was leaving him, thinking "out of your own mouth." His final words were "I'm not going into something that will never work!"

On the15th October something awful happened; I phoned my parents and my Dad insisted that I had an abortion, saying "you won't be able to look after it." He kept repeating "It's not alive, it's not alive!" and he offered to pay for an abortion. I was very upset: -

"I don't think I have ever yet been so upset when I put the phone down and hastened into the bedroom. I just sobbed my heart out, convulsing all my body with the sobs, till I felt the baby also convulsed with the pain. Walter rushed through and threw his arms around me as I cried out "I am not going to murder my baby." And he assured me that we weren't going to murder it; then in the end he broke into sobs too. And all three of us were sobbing in a heart-rending fashion on the bed. I say three of us because I felt that the baby was sobbing too; and I had such terrible tummy-pains.- - - I used the opportunity to begin talking with Walter. He had said "I love you both" in his sobbing. So I replied "If you love us, will you help us then?" I explained that if he loved us, he would help get me re-housed, and help with the furnishing and decorating. His reaction was typical and made me see how very selfish he is. For he made it clear that if I moved out, he would have nothing more to do with me. He said "I'll have to forget you then"; "if we're finished we're finished"; "I'll wash my hands of it." Then he said "I'll have to get another girl, someone else to live with me, that I can have a full relationship with." He made it clear that he wouldn't have anything to do with me if I left this house; he even said that he didn't want to see the child, and it would be a good idea not to see it."

I then began to realise that no-one would help us at all; without Walter to look after us, we would be in a bad way! As my Dad had said "the problems were insurmountable." Dr. Abernethy had said that I could go to Craigdene until I would be re-housed by the council. But I realised I couldn't think of throwing us on the mercy of "the cold machinery" of officialdom. I felt whichever choice I made would be the sacrifice of my life in suffering: -

"I have become aware of the insurmountable difficulties of looking after a baby on my own. It would be a life of misery and physical suffering; at least staying here I have the comforts of life,- warmth, safety, enough food, a home, all of which I might deprive myself and the baby of, if I leave. I mean just the practical, physical situation I might get myself into comes vividly to mind, - a bare, uncarpeted, unfurnished room, cold and damp, no cooker, no hot food, no hot water, no-one to help, in a strange and alien place with nothing familiar around me. And I am very aware that if I get ill the baby would probably be taken away from me, and I would fight in vain to get it back. All of these terrible real sufferings Walter can buffer me against, protect me from. - - And hence I have come to see that my only option is to "sacrifice" my own life; I mean sacrifice any happiness I might have had, and give myself up to the misery and oppression. I mean the choice is to sacrifice my own life in that way or to "murder" the baby. And no matter how much my parents urge it, I'm not going to murder it."

Then the woman from the adoption agency came; she was a real "battleaxe," telling me how naïve and foolish I was, telling me I was "selfish like all schizophrenics are." It was she who told me I was naïve to think Walter was "kind" in taking me in; "he just wanted a woman in his bed." She painted a miserable picture of struggling for my rights with a cold legal bureaucracy if I left Walter, begging for housing and having a new-born baby with nowhere to live. And the bureaucracy would take the baby away from me if I wasn't a good mother; she told me I was "not psychologically or emotionally equipped to be a good mother." I was overwhelmed, and realised it just wasn't possible on my own.

I thought, "all I can see is that, unless I murder the baby, I am going to have to sacrifice my life, my happiness for the rest of my life. If I stay with Walter it is the sacrifice of laying down my life, all my own happiness, and everything I wanted from life. And can I murder the baby? Whatever my feelings are, my heart and mind are resilient to that. I ask God to help me choose the path of self-sacrifice."
From Book of the Beloved, Page85: - God once said to me "It is you yourself I want; lay yourself on the altar."

Having thus made the choice of "self-sacrifice" I felt better for a while; I had decided I couldn't possibly leave Walter and set up house on my own. And the social worker Derek Jeffreys came like a breath of fresh air, making me feel more free. It was he who told me I might get occupancy rights to live in the house. He assured me too that as long as I didn't marry Walter I would be legally the child's sole parent and he would have no parental rights. This is so ironic, considering what was to happen in the future. Meanwhile I began to feel I hated Walter and would refuse to have sex with him ever again; "you've coerced me into sex against my natural feelings, and I won't allow it to happen ever again," I said to myself.

The emotional pressure on me continued, until on the 21st October I decided that it was beginning to make me ill. I thought of going to Craigdene to take the pressure off myself, but I couldn't bring myself to do it, as I was too afraid of strange doctors and tranquillizing injections. So I went to a friend's house. Walter was furious, shouting "If we're finished, we're finished; I'm washing my hands of you." It was that day that I realised clearly that he must have contributed to making his ex-wife Rosa ill (she suffered from Schizophrenia too). I was momentarily glad to get away from him; however in the next few days I realised I couldn't do without him, because I was so emotionally attached to him. I couldn't manage on my own emotionally.

It was then that he accompanied me to see Dr.Abernethy. Dr. Abernethy was saying my relationship with Walter was damaging and "You don't need to tell me that your relationship with him stinks to high heaven!" And Walter burst in, aggressively shaking his umbrella, demanding "Will Mairi and the baby be alright? I want to know!" He replied that his concern was with me and my mental health, and he referred to the "present problem in our relationship." And Walter shouted "There is no relationship!" I felt how impossible he was!

On the 24th October a storm descended round my head. I talked to his ex-wife Rosa. And my eyes were opened! In the morning we saw the marriage guidance counsellor, Deborah Gillespie, and there Walter was using my illness against me, saying that because I'm schizophrenic, I am "basically selfish" and "basically childish". And whilst he went on about his ex-wife Rosa, I saw with clarity her side of it,- how Walter had made her psychiatrically ill by so oppressing her. Then when I went to the Cosmos centre to see Derek Jeffreys, I found Rosa there. And I told her what great sympathy for her side of the story I suddenly had, and she opened my eyes!

When I told her I was pregnant, she said how he was doing the same thing all over again; that was the situation in which she herself had been forced to marry him. I had had sympathy for her and some vague idea of what it was like for her, because of the way I see he was treating me. But what she said just devastated me, for I saw it clearly as true, that he would do all those things; I saw it in his nature. For example I'd had an inkling of an idea that if I married him and gave him rights over the child he would use this to oppress me; how right I was! Rosa told me how he used to take her son Andy away from her saying that her illness meant she "wasn't a fit mother." And the irony of it was, it was he who was so oppressing her that he drove her to breakdown. I saw the infallible marks and symptoms of his character, of all the things he was doing to me. Rosa urged "Leave it now, break it off whilst you can, or you'll have 15 years of a most miserable, oppressive, sick life, with a child torn between you."
- - -

I saw it all so clearly then; I saw the truth about Walter; I saw the black and impossible truth of my situation! And I couldn't face it. "How can I go through such a storm and battle with Walter? It will make me ill. How can I go through so much, and be homeless and distressed, all at the time when I am pregnant? There is no-one to help. I have nowhere to go. I don't have the capability to face all this. God help me!"

From Book of the Beloved, Page 142: - In the midst of all the storm God says "Hold to the earth, be still and it will pass over." I tried to commit myslf into His care; "It is I who sustains you and encompasses you; be still."

Chapter 8
November Misery.

After that I wasn't mentally well; I had a minor breakdown and suffered depression. At the end of October I was using the metaphor of a dam, saying I could clearly see cracks appearing in the dam-wall; I could see the symptoms of my becoming ill. I realised that I had to channel off some of the pressure of the water; so for a weekend, I went to stay at my friend Helen's house.

There I spent half the nights being awake moaning: "What am I to do? The picture painted of trying to be re-housed is so bleak, I couldn't face it if I were fit, healthy and emotionally strong, and not close to being ill and pregnant." Basically I was trying to leave Walter. But I had no support from anyone; even my long-term friend Henry said "you've got to be rational and sensible; you've got to go back to Walter." I valued Rosa's sympathetic understanding and she had said, "Get as far away from Walter as possible, as anything is better than going through battles with him." My heart failed me at the thought of battling with him, because I was frightened of him, of his violent eruptions of anger.

I went to Kirkcraig to fill in application forms to try and get re-housed, but everything was so bleak, that I said "Where do I go? I'm done for, I've had it," and I had a great urge to drown myself! I felt I was going to be driven back to Walter as the only place I could find a shred of comfort. And I felt I was becoming ill, and I thought that all were fools in not realising it and helping me. So I put myself in the hospital, Craigdene; it was really in order to get re-housed.

Once in Craigdene I quickly found that I couldn't stand it there. I felt like a prisoner; I wasn't allowed to go out the door, or eat what I liked, or do my writing and prayers when I liked; I was forced to attend "therapy", such as knitting, for long hours, and everybody treated me as "ill" when I wasn't. But for a while I adamantly said to myself "I've left Walter and I'm not going to change my mind." However then the dam seemed to burst, and I couldn't write any more; I had a minor "breakdown".

And my stand against Walter collapsed. He came to visit me and I asked him to take me home on weekend pass; I was back to dependency on him again. I realised that either I stay with Walter with the comfort which that involves, or I'd have to stick it out in Craigdene, that ghastly place, until I should get re-housed. I wasn't brave and strong enough, now that I was "ill"; I arranged for Walter to get me discharged. By the 7th November I was back with Walter!

At first I thought Walter was being nice to me, helping me with the groceries and meals, and I felt a bit better after stopping the tablets I'd been given. But the housing department rescinded my application, saying I'd deceived them. And soon Walter started railing once again for not being "sexual" with him. I reached the pits of absolute misery. Walter started saying to me; "you do all the taking and no giving; you are not capable of giving; you're not capable of love, you're inhuman." I felt how impossible it was to tear myself away, but unless I did, I'd live the rest of my life in misery. I seemed to give in and go completely childish. The only way I could cope with the relationship was to see him as a "daddy" and act like a child.

On the 18th November we first had a "marriage guidance session" with my friends Vivien and Nicholas. We expressed ourselves more clearly to each other than ever before. And I said and realised that I'd always felt coerced into sex with him; and one of the suggestions made was that I should live "like a lodger" with Walter. It sounded all very rational that night but the following morning I quickly realised how "nasty" Walter was going to turn if I attempted the idea. He started saying things like; "if we're finished we're finished; I'll get another woman in"; "you've been using people all your life." It was in vain my pointing out that he had said on the one hand "I'll never throw you out", and was on the other hand saying he'd "wash his hands of me" if we didn't have a full sexual relationship. I felt he was impossible, and I felt how I hated him!

That day I made a crucial decision: -
I saw how Walter had destroyed my integrity, by the way he had coerced me into sex; I saw that it was never a commitment of myself, or free giving of myself. I saw that my conceiving of the child was immoral. And I saw the only solution was to stop being immoral, to cease this way of life, and to leave Walter. And I saw that I had to leave him for the good of myself and the child; I had to get away from him before the child came along.

I began to feel so very apathetic and miserable. My doctor, Dr James, told me I was suffering an "exogenous depression", that is, a depression caused by external circumstances. He also told me that I was so dependant on Walter because, being pregnant, I was driven by the emotional need for a mate. I was also craving for various foods and feeling very sick. There were also money worries. I got no more DSS money, because I was told I'd been defrauding the DSS by not saying we were "living as man and wife." The housing officer also came to see me, and said I must take my place in the queue and wait 7 years, and that you get "no extra points" for having a new-born baby on your hands.

On the 28th November we had another "marriage guidance session" with Deborah Gillespie, and I got really angry because Walter refused to see that I have done any "self-giving": -
"He says this when I have done my self-giving to the core! I pointed out that I had gone into sex with him almost every night all summer, when I felt intensely negative about it, and was only doing it to please him. He replied bitterly that this was "deception", that he had been deceived by me; he started complaining that this wasn't "self-giving" at all. I erupted; it took enormous self-giving to have sex against my inclination! "What about all those hours spent washing, shopping, cleaning the house, cooking meals, washing up?!" It cost me to the hilt; it meant I had to sacrifice all my ideals and everything I'd lived for, to be "domesticated" in that way, to be a "housewife" for him! And he says I did no self-giving! I came down into the mud and the mire, to serve him, to please him! - - Not only have I "come down into the mud" for his sake, being a kind of slave to him, but also my pleasing of him has ended in the result of my "having a baby in my tummy." - - I have also sacrificed my moral awareness and integrity and ended up in this way. It has "borne fruit" in that sense!"

My pain lay in the fact that I had wasted, mistaken, sacrificed in vain, blasted my life by loving a man again. I was aware of the mistake and the sin of human love! I had been brought down into the mud! All this resulted in my seeing with crystal clarity that living with Walter was not for my "happiness and fulfilment", rather it would blast my life, and blast the baby's life. At all costs I had to get away from Walter.- -" For the sake of my soul, and for any achievement, fulfilment, happiness I can find, I must leave him."

On the 30th November, we had a flaming row in the supermarket; Walter refused to give me the extra £5 which he had promised me to pay for the groceries, and he walked off angrily, refusing to help me. I had said to him in anger "How can I trust you to look after me and the baby?" I felt I couldn't trust him to provide £30 a week for us, as he would need to, when he begrudged giving me £5, the £5 extra which he had promised. And I got very distressed and I had terrible tummy pains. I walked back home on my own with the heavy groceries, feeling that all this emotion would give me a miscarriage one of these days, feeling that it was doing harm to the baby. I said angrily to myself "If he can't support me by paying the small sum of £5, how can I expect him to support me when I need it most? I'm going to leave him and take that house, no matter where it is!" And with such distress the miserable month of November came to an end.

Chapter 9
December Tyranny.

On 1st December something happened. That night, when his sister Janet was present, I discovered a new ability to answer back. Walter happened to say "we've got to make sacrifices for a greater cause", and I challenged him "What is the sacrifice, and what is the greater cause?" I found in this way that I could intellectually challenge him. I found that if I asked him to explain what he meant, I could point out his self-contradictions. For example I tried to get him to explain what he meant by "deceiving him"; he said I led him to believe that I cared about him when I didn't. I erupted, "If I didn't care for you, why would I be having sex with you! If I didn't care for you I wouldn't have a baby would I?" Through what was said, I felt I'd triumphed instead of being oppressed for once. I had discovered the power to answer back!

I now found I had power to answer back freely and strongly, in fact daringly. For example when he refused to peel potatoes, I commented, "For someone who claims that they don't need me to make meals for them and that they can manage perfectly well on their own, you don't show yourself very capable of it!" I said "Have you ever thought why I should make meals for you every day whilst you are watching television? I'm not a slave you know, I don't have to do it!" For example when he said housework was "trivial", I answered back "If you think it's so trivial why don't you do it? What you mean by trivial is that it is beneath you and too unimportant to do. But if the housework were left to you, this place would be a pig-sty!"

Thus I suddenly felt freed from the emotional tyranny that Walter had exercised over me. I thought this a wonderful thing; I realised it must be because I was no longer afraid of him. Walter's reaction was to turn all morose and sorry for himself. I found that I could even refuse to let him cuddle me in bed. And thus with this ability to answer back came, not only a new sense of triumph, power, freedom, but also a new sense of myself, of my integrity, freewill, ability to love or not love.

I began a new journal with a severe indictment of "the father of my baby". I realised I did not in fact "love" him because "there is not a single thing I admire or appreciate in him": -
"He has not a single virtue or admirable soul-quality; in fact everything I see in him I deplore and hate; he is arrogant, pompous, selfish, inconsiderate, self-conceited, proud, self-centred, foolish,

unintelligent, lazy, ungenerous. - -The list could go on; he is not a "good" man. He has really revealed his true colours. He is basically stupid, unintelligent, and insensitive, in that he doesn't even realise or notice his own motives and self-contradictions. He is incredibly vain and self-conceited, in the way he claims to be an intellectual and a "philosopher". And yet all his words and talking is an ego-trip; he says nothing, is incapable of addressing himself to the point, but just comes out with a waffling that he repeats on every occasion in front of other people in order to inflate his own ego. As for his laziness, he never does a stroke of work, though saying he must "get on " all the time, and claiming in front of others that he has to devote attention to me, making this out to be an act of great "self-sacrifice." As for his meanness and tight-fistedness with money, I witnessed this when his teenage son came to ask £2 off him, to get the bus to visit someone in hospital, and he gave him a real "dressing down", shouting "do you think I'm made of money!" He is always going on about "not earning", though this is his own fault and laziness. "Does he think I'm going to trust him to support and financially provide for me and a child when he is so mean as well as so stupid?"

The idea of adoption suddenly really appealed to me; this was because I had with my soul decided- "that I wasn't going to distress the baby beyond what it has suffered already by bringing it into the distressing situation that exists between me and Walter; I am adamant about that." Walter accused me of seeking "the easy way out", saying adoption was "cruel" and meant bringing a child into the world to "let it suffer." But I saw it as "the most loving choice." For - "I'm not going to be with Walter; it would be cruel to the child to bring it into the midst of such a distressing relationship. This child has suffered already so much distress in the womb, it is going to need a wonderfully warm, affectionate, loving atmosphere to grow up in, if it is not to be permanently harmed. As for the alternative of my bringing up the child on my own, it would be a cold, friendless, poverty-stricken situation, removed from everyone I know, and I'm not sure of my capabilities of bringing up a child on my own in those conditions. Thus if I were considering most the baby's welfare I would choose adoption. For then it would be in a warm, caring , stable, loving atmosphere from the beginning of its life."

"Walter made a song and dance about the idea of fatherly "rights" and that he too would suffer because of giving the child up. He actually said "I'm going through this pregnancy too; why should I go through all this and then have the baby taken away from me!" I pointed out that it is me alone who is going through the physical misery of pregnancy. And I'm going to make sure, for all Walter's protesting about the way he'll contest it, that he doesn't get the chance of looking after it and caring for it. The fact that I dislike all the traits I see in Walter doesn't help me to feel positively towards the child. If the child were the baby of a husband I loved, I feel that I could love the child and lovingly bring it up. But when I don't love the father, I can't love the part of him that is in the child. And what's more, I see it as "a child of sin" rather than a child of love. So as my unkind father suggested, I have a very good reason for not "wanting" the child, for devoting my life to bringing it up."

Thus after all my black sea of suffering, I found myself emerged "with a sense of myself, strong and free, able to make loving choices." How it came about was a mystery to me; "perhaps it is one of those mysteries that can only be ascribed to God." From then on I felt I could coolly wield intellectual power when there was a problem.

One night he complained when I wouldn't give him cuddles, saying "Do you want to make me suffer?" I replied that I was only trying to lessen my own suffering; "by realising that I have freedom, that I have choice." He complained, and then started threatening me, "If you're not going to give me any warmth, then I'll make my own decision, I'll do something." I replied coolly "What are you threatening me with? What do you intend to do?" He said back "I'll go with another woman." At the end of this altercation , I was smiling to myself "with the sense of triumph, freedom, power." And he went all morose and unhappy. I said to myself afterwards, "Serves him right if the tables are turned. I don't care; I have no sympathy. He oppressed and tormented me, and he's not going to do it any longer; so now he is suffering and feeling sorry for himself because I'm answering back and am no longer under his thumb. Well I'm free from that strangle-hold, and if he suffers because I'm free, I don't care!"

However this new-found liberation didn't last long before it became difficult to maintain. I struggled with it, and soon felt under his tyranny again. I found I couldn't always answer back when I got really hurt by the "nasty things." For example one night he accused me of "not being normal"; "there's something wrong with you sexually;" "you're useless as a woman," "you don't know what love is." I realised I was allowing him to oppress me again. I wondered if we could ever establish a free and adult relationship; I felt it would never work, because he wasn't capable of changing. He claimed he wanted a "free and liberated woman" to live with, yet he bent all his will-power to keep me oppressed.

On 9th December I found myself feeling "used", "abused" in bed again, whilst trying to avoid his temper, but he still said nasty things to me: -
"What is the point of letting myself be subject to that, to avoid his temper, when I am subject to his temper anyway? It is the most pernicious form of oppression, to allow oneself to be sexually abused; I lay in bed feeling that I was powerless to assert my freedom or integrity. - - This is really terrible, that I should feel so oppressed again, with all my sense of "myself as a person", my freedom and integrity, gone! When Walter was saying "you are destroying my life," I felt like saying back "you have already destroyed mine." I feel that by robbing me of my freedom and integrity, he is actively destroying my soul."

On the eve of 11th December, which was my 32nd birthday, I was moved by a letter from my soul-friend. He urged me to continue "saying Yes" to the child. He sent me a photo of a little child which said "Whoever accepts/ takes up such a child accepts/ takes up Me." For the first time I felt that my child was loved; I felt Pater Leo's total loving acceptance of me and the child inside of me. And then I made a soul-deep decision; that I was going to accept/ take up the child as I would take up Christ. I decided I was not going to have it adopted, but I'd take up the child to nurture and educate. *I asked God to teach me fully this deep, spiritual, loving acceptance of my child, and all that in the future it would bring me.*

The next day we attended the "marriage guidance counsel" with Deborah Gillespie. And we talked about sex. I said I didn't intend returning to those days when I felt sexually coerced and oppressed; I saw it as wrong if it didn't have my whole self consenting to it, with all of my freedom and integrity. I said I wouldn't engage in sex when it was soul-destroying, instead of being positive and whole and expressive of love. It came out that Walter thought that sex was wonderful and beautiful when he himself got sexually satisfied; and he went on about the importance of sex to him. I said; "If you just want a woman to have sex with I don't feel that you are loving me at all; you don't like me with my freedom and integrity, you don't accept me as I am, so I don't feel that you love me at all." I had already thought the day before, that I had never truly been loved by him.

Afterwards we went to "McGregors" coffee-shop, and Walter went all sullen; "I've got better things to do; my life is going to be different from now on; I'm not going to waste my life; I intend to make a decision; I can go with another woman; there is Betty waiting for me down the street." And then he started threatening that he would go away for Christmas. I felt oppressed and sat in silence, feeling that life was nothing but misery and pain. I thought it was a hopeless relationship; it was impossible for Walter to learn and change.

I decided that the thing to do was to be more concerned for the child in my womb than for this hopeless relationship; I needed a deep and loving acceptance of the baby. I began to experience it as a spiritual force going out from me, to make my baby feel "loved in the womb."

We had a terrible conversation one night, when he found a new threat. He started talking down to me again, saying "no-one has ever loved you before I did; you've never been capable of a real relationship", and when I answered back to this, he started saying that he would "make other arrangements"; I said it was a waste of electricity if we separately cooked our own meals. He replied "no it wouldn't, because you would be paying for it." I was mortified by this new threat. When I had mentioned being a lodger earlier, I meant not sleeping with him; what he now meant was that I should pay for rent and bills! I had always given the whole of my DSS money for the food for the two of us; I didn't have money for rent and bills. He started saying I didn't do any self-giving, so I pointed out all those hours of slaving away that I did for him. He said back "That doesn't count; that's nothing at all, that's not giving; I could pay someone to do that." I was mortified. I felt really bullied and coerced into silence, as he kept talking down to me and threatening me. I was thinking to myself, "Don't think that I'm going to stay with you when I'm vulnerable with a new-born baby, because you can threaten me even more then."

Meanwhile I had written to my parents. I had sent a card to them saying "Christmas is about a baby being born." My Dad had suggested an abortion again, saying "we are adamant that you are not coming home in that condition." My Mum said "it is a terrible thing to bring a child into the world without having loving parents and a loving home to come to"; and I replied "this baby seemingly isn't going to have two loving parents and a home; it is only going to have me."

On the 14th December Walter made me very emotional when we had an altercation about the extra £4 he had promised to give me. He refused to give me the money, when I was going shopping, saying "he didn't trust me", "wanted proof of what money I spent", was going to "do his shopping on his own." I was quaking with anger as he laid into me, knowing that this emotion wasn't good for the baby. He finally gave me the money, but he blocked my entrance out of the door, shouting that if we were finished he wanted the £4 back! I went shopping, highly distressed, hating the way he was threatening me. But then, before returning home, I decided on a strategy; I'd say "I'm not going to do all the cooking and shopping for you any more; if you are going to threaten that I should live as a lodger, - right then we'll do that; then you can't threaten me with it any longer." I tried annulling the threat in this way, and it worked; I suggested he made his own meal and he backed down. I felt that I'd won for myself a little more of a foothold.

I felt I hated my state of existence, in which I was treated like a slave, and had to endure repugnant kisses in order to avoid anger and distress, in order to make life tolerable. "When I think of the alternative, my stomach turns with dread of the future; it seems a better choice to take the circumstances of my present existence and try and make them tolerable; though I know this is not the brave thing to do." *And I asked God to help me to be brave in facing the future, and brave in being "true to myself," rather than trying to "make life tolerable" in this way.*

One evening, returning from a "marriage guidance session" with Vivien and Nicholas. I had a glorious sense of triumph when Walter insisted that I tell him what was in my letter from Pater Leo. I considered this a "nugget of gold", which was held secretly and silently in the depths of my soul. Walter demanded to know what it was, saying it must be to do with him; I coolly remarked "he didn't even mention you." He again demanded that I tell him, but I was adamant that I wasn't going to "share my soul-life" with him; I felt there was great power in my silence. I nearly said to him "you can't demand to share my soul-life like you demand your dinner or demand sex!" I did say something to the effect that he had possessed me bodily but that he couldn't expect that I share with him my soul-life as well. This experience gave me the sense that my soul-life was valuable; a sense of my soul's worth.

The days were hastening towards Christmas. There was a calm sea for a while; I was just glad when I wasn't distressed. I told the Social worker that I had to find a home for the baby, and I was playing a waiting game. I started to keep whispering to the baby "one day we'll get away from him."

An unhappy Christmas day came; there was trouble over the turkey, and I felt I was being treated like a slave. I thought "I am tired of living like this, in all this bad-temperedness and painfulness, with no love there at all." However I was cheered at Midnight Mass by seeing my friend Henry and feeling that he had "a bright warm place in my heart". I thought how Christmas is about that "bright warm place", and so I felt a touch of God's love, even though I felt there was no love in my life.

The next day Walter was abusing me again, and I was gazing at the crucifix whilst he was doing it, praying and saying to myself: "you have my body but you can't have my soul. You have no control over my soul; my soul is my own." And as I lay there gazing upwards I got a triumphant sense of my soul's freedom. *"I felt gloriously, triumphantly, that though I am imprisoned in this situation, and though my body is abused, yet my soul is a thing winged and free, which can't be imprisoned or controlled or touched."* And I whispered *"one day we'll get away from him,"* which had become for me an expression of hope.

Chapter 10
Breakdown.

Friday 27th December '85: -
"What has happened this night is the final catastrophe - the cutting of the thread. I am crying now after the most violent anger. "Don't worry, baby, we're on our way" are the words that made me start to cry. It is done, and it is said. The decision has been made, and told. The threads have been cut.- - It has been made clear to me that I am "a stranger" in this house and have less right to be here than his brothers and sisters; as I told Walter shaking with rage "if I am counted as a stranger in this house then it is no longer my home"; "you are cutting off me and the baby." Their family can keep the house and I will find a home elsewhere. - - It took a last straw like this to make it "decided", irrevocable, told in the open. And I am not going to be softened by Walter into changing my position. When I was still trembling with anger on the bed he came and stared down at me using words like "selfish" and I screamed in emotion "Go away". But now whenever he keeps coming in the bedroom I just say coldly, calmly the words "Go away". I realise I'm going to have to be hard, shell-like; but I shall remain cold, icy, unmoved, for it is "decided"!

What had happened was this: -
Walter had told his brother it was alright to come, and his sister on the phone said he had a right to invite his brother to stay in his own house, especially as it was their "home" in the past; I defended myself, "What I object to is that Walter invited him without considering or asking me, and it's my home too you know." "But he is our brother" she said crossly, and I replied calmly "But he's a stranger to me." She shouted angrily "it is you who are a stranger in that house!" How deeply that offended me and distressed me! It was I who had made this horrible house into a "home", cleaning, caring for it; the man who lived in it had so abused my body as to give me a baby; it was to be "a home for me and my baby." Now I found it belonged more to spectres of the past. "Alright then, let them have it; I will find another home for me and my baby!" And I said back to his sister in trembling anger "You say that when I am bearing his baby!" And I slammed the phone down; it was like a tearing in my emotions; my affection and attachment to this one-time "home" was broken! It was done, torn like a curtain! My attachment to this house was gone, and with it my attachment to Walter, for they always went together, intertwined and inseparable,- my need for this "home" and the man to support me whose house it

was. Now it was gone; and what was left was "a cold, dead, icy, hard feeling, and the fact of finally facing the frightening future awaiting me."

There followed a long night of distress and sleeplessness, and a long marathon of an altercation in the morning. At the end of it I felt leagues had been travelled and nothing was the same.

It made me angry and bitter when Walter said "Now I know we're finished, I can live my own life again, I can make a fresh start in the New Year." I said back "That's fine, you do that, after leaving me burdened for life and facing a frightening future!" It was not fair that he should so easily leave this relationship behind, when I was left with a baby. This was something I keep reminding him of; there was a baby between us which is a "fruit of this relationship", which in a sense bound us together for all time, which he couldn't so easily leave behind. It upset me when he said in bed about 2am, "Once I've finished with a woman I never look back."

Things had been said which couldn't be unsaid. I had tried to assert that I was a "lodger" in that house, until I could leave; I had tried to make that bedroom "mine"; I had left a note on the door to say I was in pain and felt ill and was going to sleep, but he burst in at midnight, and made me emotional and angry till 2am. Instead of leaving me alone, he distressed me further and deprived me of sleep. I went to lay wrapped in a blanket on the settee, with horrible tummy pains, but this marathon argument carried on; Walter ranted and raved at me till 2pm the following day. It ran through every emotion in the book; from over-the-top laughter, to wailings and floodings of tears, to iciness, bitterness, to trembling rage. And Walter played shamefully with my emotions; at one moment he was bitter and hurtful, at the next he begged for kisses and threw himself in tears on my breast. The doctor when I phoned at 8am had told me to stay in for a "restful" weekend; when Walter said he had to look after "an invalid", it finally stung me into getting up, and washed and dressed. I decided it was now "already over" and it was best to remain "cold".

After this I tried to maintain my position a "lodger," refusing to do the "slave-like" chores, and continually retreating to my bedroom; but Walter couldn't and wouldn't accept this. He kept bursting in to my "sanctuary," with no respect for me or my space, saying "I will start treating you as a lodger, then you'll be sorry," and yelling at me "I want money." I was trying to transcend the "cold, hard, bitter feeling" I was left with. On the Monday morning I went to see a solicitor, about my legal rights; I came away saying "Isn't it wonderful to know that in the vulnerable position that I am in, the law allows no protection whatsoever!"

It was later that day, the 30th December, that the complete cataclysm happened: -

"It has been the longest agony of a day, in which I've burst into hysterical sobbing three times, for my emotions are stretched to such a pitch, and I feel so ill, so tired, in so much pain; because I was deprived of a night's sleep by Walter and his brother. Once was with the health visitor this morning, once in a shop, and the third time when hard bitter things were being said between me and Walter. He said "you are hating me," and I sobbed "I don't hate you Walter, but it's because I feel so ill, that my emotions seem all hard and cold and bitter." And I made clear to him what made me so "bitter"; the fact that he could "walk away," "leave this behind," "live his own life," in the way he kept boasting, whilst I am left looking after a baby for 16 years, facing a miserable future. And the last thing I said to him also makes me bitter; "you must realise that in distressing me you are distressing and harming the baby."

"It is precisely because he is so distressing and harming the baby that I am determined to leave him. But he is too stupidly insensitive to see this; he accuses me of being "too easily upset". "The selfish bastard!" was what I said to myself, bitter and sleepless at 5 o'clock in the morning, whilst all the noise was going on. He is a nasty, wicked, unkind, selfish, insensitive, inconsiderate man! It is his brutish insensitivity that causes me so much distress; it is this which makes him come storming into the bedroom when I need to be alone, without respect for my person, my space, my aloneness. I told him in front of his brother, "You show no respect for the freedom, the worth, the inalienable rights of the human soul." Then I used the tactic of putting a chair behind the door.

"God help me! I've taken more than I can take, but it goes on, distress upon distress! It is too late an hour now for me to go anywhere, but go I must if I want rest or sleep. And I must have that precious sleep; sleep that "knits up the ravelled sleeve of care", "balm of nature".- -

"I practically begged his brother on my knees, to have the decency and kindness to allow me to sleep tonight, making clear to him how in need of sleep I am. He flashed with temper and claimed his right to go to bed at what time he chose, being "nocturnal". I am being driven out, pregnant, from what was my only home by an insensitive man who doesn't respect my right to sleep! He said "I know what you feel like, I like to be on my own too, I like peace and quiet too", and I turned emotional and said bitterly "It's not a matter of that at all." "What is it a matter of then?" he called after me. Something in me snapped, and I shook with emotion, screamed "Ask the doctor if you want to know" and slammed the door. - - - A minute later Walter came in, intruding on my sanctuary, standing over me, saying "you are too easily upset." Aware only of his "stupid insensitivity", and hating the thought of my baby inheriting it, the next thing I said in a bitter voice was "Get out!" "That is no way to talk to me" he replied, and I said back "What, no way to talk to the father of my baby!"

"And then I thought something and said something which is the most wicked bitter thing I've ever felt in my life. It wasn't good and loving like I've been trying to be, but I was at the end of my tether, made ill by all this. I am cracking up; this is destroying me; such bitterness issues from a crack in the texture of my being.- - *This wicked bitter thing sprung from the feeling "I hate your stupid insensitivity, I want no part of you, I will give you back what you gave me." What I said in words, what sprung out of me in bitterness and hate, was: - "Now I know the feeling that makes mothers murder their babies; if I could, I would tear this baby out of my womb, and leave the dead thing on your doorstep!"*- - A moment later when he'd gone, I disintegrated, flooded with tears in piteous emotion; it can't be counted as crying; I wailed, screamed and howled."

Chapter 11
Leaving.

The following morning, at 7am on 31st December, I had left that house and left Walter. I never went back. I realised I had to go somewhere to get some sleep, because Walter and his brother had now deprived me of sleep for several nights, and my tummy pains were dire. It was deep snow outside. I always said, for years afterwards, that Walter "threw me out, pregnant and homeless in the snow"; this is what it felt like, though perhaps in reality I had to "escape".

I went to the only place I could think of going; - to the Health Centre to see my kind GP, Dr.James. I had to wait an hour, miserably, and then at first he showed an unsympathetic attitude, saying there was nothing he could do unless I went to Craigdene; I said I'd rather die than go there. He went out of the room to make a phone-call; and when he came back he seemed transformed; he was all pity and kindness and gave me the glad news that I could rest and sleep in the local hospital here. I felt God must have "touched his human heart". *I felt astonished that I should find "mercy, pity , peace and love" dwelling in his heart, when I couldn't even find it in my Dad! ; "I mean how could he in a trice come back as if his heart had been stirred and touched by some angel of God?"*

He showed me out the back door of the Health centre, as Walter had come after me, shaking his umbrella, and was in the waiting room. And I plodded through the thick snow to the hospital along all the back-routes, so that he shouldn't find me. At first I was grateful to be in the hospital, where it was warm; Walter pursued me there, but the nurses turned him away; I felt anguished.

I wrote a letter to Walter, saying that I was "driven out" of what was my only home; what was done to me was beyond my human capacity to forgive; "together you seem to have succeeded in destroying my soul; I have turned bitter inside". To drive out a pregnant woman into the cold of January, with no recourse, like this, was "an abomination". When I was trying to escape and rush out in those few minutes, he was ranting and raving - "You haven't paid me yet; I want money!" - - " Isn't it wonderful! He drives me out, pregnant, with nowhere to go on New Year's Eve, and then demands money for such a privilege!"

"Today in some ways I have "won," in finding a place away from Walter to get rest and sleep. And yet ultimately "I have lost". For now he knows the "trick" which makes it impossible for me to stand against him

- he deprives me of sleep! Why does this mean I've lost the battle? I found out from a solicitor that the law allows no legal rights to someone in my vulnerable position; but even if I succeeded in getting rights of "occupancy" in that house, he could continue depriving me of sleep! As I said to Dr.James "without sleep you cannot defend yourself; it's what they do to break down prisoners when they torture them." I've lost what was never a fair battle anyway; in fighting with Walter I have absolutely lost!"

The way Pater Leo prayed I should know "the peace and joy of Mari," with my baby loved in the womb, when I had said such a bitter wicked thing, made me keep sobbing. It was due to the contrast of the tenderness, love and acceptance there should have been in my heart, to the hardness, coldness, bitterness that was dwelling there.

And then I couldn't sleep the next night. Sleeplessness has always been a sign and symptom of my becoming "ill". It was now 1st January 1986, and at 7am, I phoned my Dad, and I begged him, absolutely begged him, to let me come home for a while seeing I was "pregnant and homeless in the snow", but he refused. The hospital wouldn't provide food and drink when I needed and wanted it; when you are pregnant you become physically distressed by your body's need of nourishment. I begged all my friends on the phone to help by bringing in food, but they refused. I was determined to be "strong and brave," and not go back to Walter.

"Though I'm distressed by hunger, I've said with adamant steel "I will not beg of Walter if my life depended upon it." I will not be driven back to him by physical distress and need; if I can't make a stand against him now, how can I ever hope to in the bleak future that faces me? - - It is everything on earth, all the gold and silver in the world to me, I will pay anything, though it costs my lifetime to repay, but I will find the warmth and nourishment to alleviate my distress, and make me well, and enable me to stand against Walter and face a future! But I will not beg! I have begged again of my father this morning; there is nothing worse than being refused when you have begged. What a harsh cruel bitter world, when even my own father turns against me in my most need, even after my begging!"

Things became worse, for I was anguished: -
"I weep because I am so desperate that I have in me the wicked bitter thought, - driven to it as my only choice, rather than destroying my soul, - "Then kill it! Give me an overdose of the sleeping tablets, and kill it! At least then my father will allow me a roof over my head!" Yes, after

all my "protection of the baby," and desire to know "love and acceptance," I would kill it as my only remedy!

An unkind Doctor came in and threatened me in the place where I have come for rest and peace and relief from distress. When I asked him "If I take too many sleeping tablets, will it kill the baby?" he replied "All that question tells me is that you are threatening to commit suicide." When I said something else, he replied "All that tells me is that you are trying to convince me of how desperate you are, to make me feel sorry for you." "You have a choice" he said, never making clear to me what the choices were.

"Here I am on the verge of making the choice to kill my baby at the risk of my own life, as the "best" thing in a desperate situation, and he so insults and belittles me. - - And I have to swallow every vestige of respect in taking it, otherwise I am out on a park-bench in the cold tonight, or I collapse my stand against Walter. I must, I must maintain this stand, because If I don't, if I can't do it now, it will never be possible again! That is why I say, why I think it is preferable to kill the baby, even though it is an abomination and a mortal sin, than to ruin, destroy my soul for the rest of my life! Either way it is a choice of death. My only freedom is choice which way to die!"

I hardly slept again that night, though I was impressed by the kindness of a nurse. I thought in the night how I was going to leave the hospital. I had sent for a priest, because I felt so badly over that "wicked bitter thing" I'd said, and the next day Paul Thompson, the Anglican chaplain came to see me. I confessed to him the whole of my experience with Walter, and how I'd finally said, "If I could, I would tear this baby out of my womb and leave it as a dead thing on your doorstep." I communed deeply with him, and through that, I felt once again a love and acceptance toward the baby. He told me that God stood in the same position of love and protection toward me as I did to the baby. He told me "the preservation of your soul depends upon your love of the baby." When he left I felt such sweet thankfulness, and that the distress had been lifted off my shoulders.

I decided I would make my stand upon " the freedom, worth, inalienable rights of my human soul" and be strong and brave to face the future. For there was always choice; and I would make my choices in the spirit of divinely-given love and acceptance! - - I would protect my baby, show love and acceptance toward my baby. From that moment, that point, I felt I was free "to go out into the world loving and protecting my baby."

45

I made my plans to leave the hospital. I tried to get my act together and get dressed and packed; I tricked the nurses into giving me the tablets I needed. My soul-friend Pater Leo had written that he prayed I should know "the joy of Maria, the peace of Maria, when she carried her Lord in her womb and full of peace went over the mountains in intimate communion with her child." It made me feel I wanted to go where I could be alone, in communion with God and the baby; to some deep dark hidden place. And so I left the hospital in secret, pretending to the nurses that I was going to collect something from Walter's house.

I had a most beautiful walk through the dark, star-lit park. I can remember hastening along feeling that I was close to God and loving and protecting my baby in the womb. In reality I was manic, but I thought it was mysticism. I bought food from a local shop and went to a bed and breakfast establishment.

The next morning, after another sleepless night, I woke with a horrid eye infection. One eye I could hardly open at all. I was struggling to find somewhere to stay that I could afford; I met Paul Thompson along the street; he said he would let me stay in his university apartment for a few nights. I was struggling along there with my bags, barely able to see when I came across a police sergeant who was looking for me because he said I had "absconded" from the hospital. I was trying to trust in God to protect me; I felt that God would provide "angels." I was praying to God "give me the ability to touch the pity in human hearts."

At the end of my journal I wrote: - "the deep wonderful communion with God. He is the father of the baby. Trust .Angels. KirkMichaels is full of angels. Be guided. I am Maria. God's child in my womb. Deep and wonderful knowledge. I bear Christ in my womb. Christ."

And I was "mad"! I had deepened the valid idea of knowing the "peace and joy of Maria" into the mad idea that somehow I was a second version of Our Lady with the Christ-child in my womb! After that, I can't remember exactly how it happened, - I think it was the friendly police sergeant who took me to the police station and called a doctor, - but they sectioned me, gave me an injection, and took me to Craigdene.

46

Chapter 12
The Craigdene Pregnancy.

Waking up in Craigdene after being pumped full of Largactil is a horrible thing. Your mind lurches around and twists around and feels thoroughly sick and disorientated. And the nurses seemed to be there to torture me. They kept grabbing hold of me and giving me injections. I fought back at one stage; Dr.Abernethy told me to stop "beating up" his nurses. But Dr. Abernethy was relatively kind to me; I was there on a month's section; I was in the normal ward, Ward 19; I wasn't psychotic at this stage, just manic. I bore it bravely, making plans to escape when the month was up. Dr.Abernethy was a doctor who treated his patients with respect, unlike the Dr. McNeill who succeeded him; he made a "bargain" with me that I should continue to stay in the hospital voluntarily if he allowed the section to lapse. However I didn't keep my side of it; when I became voluntary, I used the pretext of visiting Walter on a home-pass, to escape from the area. I got a taxi and ran out of the house before I could be stopped, and got the taxi to Langport railway station. I then made my way to a monastery I know at Abbotsford; it was the only place I could think of going. I remember it was deep snow at the time, and the taxi from Haddington to Abbotsford nearly couldn't make it through the snow.

When I reached the monastery guest-house I felt I could rest there for a while; I didn't have any money left. I remember I phoned my Dad from there to ask if he'd send me a small amount, say £50, but he refused. Somehow the police were alerted to where I was; I was astonished and felt threatened when the father guestmaster told me that the police had phoned to ask if I was there. He said they were looking for me, because I wasn't officially discharged from the hospital, but they would leave me alone there because I was no longer on a section. But I felt my liberty was under threat. So when I met someone who was from "SPUC"(Society for the Protection of the Unborn Child) and based in Glasgow, who said they could find me somewhere to stay without it costing money, I readily leapt at the chance; I went with them to Glasgow in their car. I remember the long journey under all the motorway bridges.

The charity had a house in Glasgow for unmarried pregnant mothers, but there wasn't room there for me beyond the one night. I remember feeling safe at last in that the police wouldn't be able to trace me; I thought I might be as a "missing person" on the TV. The next day they moved me on , accompanied on a train, down the west coast to a town called Girvan; they ran a "mother and baby home"

47

there. I hoped that here at last I could wait out my pregnancy. However I reckoned without one thing - I hadn't been taking the psychiatric drugs that I'd been taking in Craigdene, and without them I rapidly became psychotic.

The warden of the house must have begun to notice my strange behaviour. I gave all my gold and silver ear-rings away to the teenagers there. I started going around in a taxi all the time, with a "personal chauffeur", saying that I had plenty of money to pay him. I bought expensive clothes, saying I was going to have plenty of money once my books were published. I went to see the local priest, saying I was an important person, and that I knew the devil by sight. I remember how the "devil" was to me my image of Walter McKay, and I thought he was "coming after me". I remember how the priest's housekeeper was alarmed when I assumed the right to go in and use the telephone. All these incidents of "weird behaviour" must have built up in people's minds. The next thing I knew there was an ambulance at the door for me.

Now I had put blessed "Walsingham water" at the threshold of the house, assuming that no evil could therefore cross it. So when these ambulance people came in, I thought that their coming was "ordained by God", so I packed my stuff and quietly went with them. I kept asking where they were going, but they wouldn't tell me. I somehow thought it was No10 Downing street; I never dreamed it was a mental hospital called "Rannock" in Ayr.

During my few days stay in that hospital my delusions continued. All I was aware of was this bare white room with a bed with bed-linen on it. And the room was locked. And very rarely someone came in to give me food or tablets. My perception of this room fluctuated between an inner room I was trying to get out of, and a room or house I was trying to get into. Whichever way it was I kept banging at this door shouting "let me out", "let me in". For some strange reason I kept stripping the bed of the bed-linen, and throwing it as a pile against the door. I thought it would then be a "sea" that people couldn't get over if they were intending to do anything nasty to me. I felt I had to have the "bare pillow" and the "bare mattress", as these I felt were "clean." I remember seeing "Cleosan" written on a pillow and thinking it was Anglo-saxon for "clean". But nobody ever took me out to the toilet. So I kept weeing on this bed-linen that was up against the door. And the more I exhibited this behaviour, the more people kept coming in, clearing away the dirty linen and putting fresh linen on the bed. I felt it was some kind of never-ending game. I was as placid as a child whilst they did these things, and just ate and drank whatever they offered me. It was like another world, which I felt I could never escape from. And then finally someone strapped me to a mattress, which must have been a stretcher, and carried me out of the room. And that was the beginning of another ambulance journey.

Back in Craigdene I was not treated well. I was put in the time-out room, of the lock-up ward, Ward 6. And I was left there for what seemed weeks. They didn't treat me as humanely as in the hospital I'd come from. They left me on a bare mattress on the floor, with no light or window, except the artificial light they put on before rushing in. And they kept rushing in, sitting on top of me, giving me a injection and rushing out again! I was totally swamped by these injections; no sooner was I struggling to the surface from one but they would give me another one. They later told me that the drug they were giving me was "Pyraldihyde", "which they give to sharks"; it was something which wasn't supposed to do damage to the foetus. But they never fed me! I sat at the door for hours in the dark, shouting "if this is a hospital you are obliged to feed me!" And of course, being pregnant, I was going wild with need of nourishment. And also it was time-deprivation; there was no way I could know whether it was day or night, unless someone opened the little hatch in the door. When that was opened, to look in at me, I could see the outside window in the corridor, but otherwise I could have no notion of daylight or darkness. Sometimes I heard the other patients traipsing down the steps in the morning, and I used to knock on the door, for someone to open the hatch, for some relief from my solitary confinement; just to see a face! And it seemed to go on for centuries!

And then I was let out to see the Mental Welfare Commission. All these people do really is back up the doctors and back up the regime. They took me out of my "time -out room" to see them. As I went through the dining-room, they were serving bread and butter pudding. This has always been a favourite of mine, but now my body's need of the eggs, drove me crazy to get some! They made me wait in the queue. Before it got to my turn I was led away to see the doctors from the Mental Welfare Commission, up the stairs. They asked me all manner of questions, partly designed to test my orientation in space and time; I could quote my dates with accuracy, but this wasn't enough to convince them of anything; I must have exhibited very poor responses as I was snowed under with drugs. When I was released from the room, I immediately went back to the dining-room, for the much-desired bread and butter pudding. The big burly nurse in front of me said "You're too late," and emptied the remainder of the tin into the pig-swill bucket! I remember going physically crazy watching this lovely food thrown away in front of my eyes! It was an act of wanton cruelty!

They kept letting me out of the time-out room after that. I was taken to the toilet, and bathed, and allowed out for meals; I always felt that the Mental Welfare doctors had complained of my treatment, though I don't know whether that is true. But I was always marched around between two nurses, in different colours of ward pyjamas. I wouldn't walk on the corridor floor, and a poster in the surgery had impressed me which said "Beware sharps!" So when asked why I wouldn't walk on the floor, I replied that there were "sharps in the water." I used to think I could turn over the TV by sticking my forefinger in the radiator pipe and the pointing at the television. I still thought I was Maggie Thatcher with power to give posts in my government. I remember when my GP Dr. James came to visit me I told him that I'd put him in charge of the Ministry of Health!

When Dr.James did finally come and visit me, I remember running along the corridor to embrace him with great glee. He told me he had come "for the baby's sake", not for me. He must have been called in by the nurses because of my abnormal blood-pressure, etc. He examined me and pronounced that I was suffering from "Pre-eclampsia." Apparently this is a dangerous illness during pregnancy which means the mother or baby can die. I was pleased though because it meant that at last I escaped the ghastly place, as I was rushed by ambulance to the nearest hospital for antenatal care - Strathwells in Invertay.

Having this Pre-Eclampsia I subsequently found, permanently damaged my eyesight; and I have always felt that I had a deep-down soul-choice between my eyes and protecting the baby within me. But in effect, as I have since realised, Dr.James played his part in God's gifting me with a son; by taking this caring and swift action he saved my baby's life!

It was now March, and I remember seeing hosts of daffodils in the roundabouts in Invertay. They looked after me in Strathwells; they were very kind to me. I was now 7 months pregnant, and I remember the joke of the doctor saying that lying on my back I "looked like a stranded whale". I also remember how they did a scan on me and found out it was going to be a boy. It was then that I decided I wanted him called "Gabriel", as that was the name of the

50

first archangel; I wanted him to be "like an angel of light to me." The trouble came when they wanted me to leave; after a week they suddenly tried to whisk me away in a wheel-chair, and I dug my heels into the floor, shouting "Craigdene is a torture-chamber; don't take me back there; I tell you it's a torture-chamber!" But they didn't take any heed of me and I was delivered back to the place.

Chapter 13
Birth.

By the beginning of May I wasn't considered psychotic any more, and I was just left depressed; so I was transferred back to the normal ward, Ward19. I was terribly conscious of the fact that I had been "crazy", and tried to come to terms with it. I remembered how I thought I was different people; how for example I thought I was Princess Diana, about to come out of hospital with her second baby; whoever I saw on the television I thought I was them, contrasting this "real world" of real people with what I called ordinary "black and white people". And now, one month before my baby was due, I came down to reality with a thump, and felt as the nurses said, "flat as a pancake." A nice doctor called Dr.Pickwick called it "post recovery depression." At least I was living in reality! Before I had left Ward6 the minister Paul Thompson had been to see me, and he said; "At least now you are living in reality, where God is; God is in reality, and you must live in reality where God is."

But reality was hard! They were gradually reducing the medication I was on, but I didn't come round as I expected. I was dreadfully depressed. I so reluctantly got out of bed in the morning, only to lie inert on the settee in the sitting-room; consciousness was pain! The nurses, who were quite kind here, kept urging me to motivate myself, but I couldn't. I kept asking "Will I feel better when the baby is born?" And the nurses kept assuring me that I would, since my hormones would change. But life was so miserable for me that, after Walter started to visit me again, I started going out on "passes" with him, because I so desperately needed his support.

Walter kept trying to persuade me to go back to live with him, and he was endearing and kind to me, and it was very tempting. But I realised in my heart of hearts that living with Walter just wouldn't work, and it was an easy way out. The harder way, but the way I should take, was to wait for a house which the council would offer me, and so live on my own to bring up the baby. It seemed an almost impossible thing to do; I felt I just wasn't mature enough or clever enough to bring up a baby on my own; and there was my illness which was such a danger; I felt I just didn't have the guts! But I was back in Dr.Abernethys care now, and he and the social worker, Derek Jeffreys, assured me that a council house would be offered to me in the month after the baby was born.

And so the month of May passed miserably, and I kept moaning to the nurses. The baby was overdue by a week; it was the 5th June when my waters broke. I remember it well; I was in the dining room eating sago pudding and prunes at the time! An ambulance was fetched and I was taken to Strathwells. I remember still feeling so depressed and forlorn that I said to the nurses in the ambulance; "I'm psychiatrically ill aren't I?" I was frightened; frightened of child-birth and frightened that I'd never get well.

The birth wasn't easy; I was in labour from 12 noon till 10.20 at night. I hadn't properly been taught breathing exercises, and I was dead set against having an epidural, so they gave me "gas and air". But this made me what the doctor called "away with the fairies." I was listening to the music of "Jesus Christ Superstar" at the time, in the labour suite; and it seemed to me that all the archetypal ideas I'd had when I first got ill about my being a second Virgin Mary, were true and valid; and I shouted out "it's all true, it's all true!" I'd had too much "gas and air" and they took it away from me! The next thing I knew they were saying the baby's head was too big to get out, and they had to give me an episiotomy. *Finally the ordeal was over, and I was given a little baby boy to hold.*

That night I was left in the recovery room, as there wasn't room on the ward, with this little baby in a plastic cot beside me. I put the baby onto my bed to cuddle; a nurse came and told me not to do this, as I might suffocate it, but I did it again when she had gone. *I talked to the little mite; I said "your name is Gabriel" and I said, with all the power of my soul, "And I'm going to live with you and not Walter." I held true to that decision.*

Various people came to visit me, to see the new-born infant; they kept me in Strathwells for a week. Among the visitors were Walter; and I told him straight about my decision; "I'm not coming back to live with you; I'm going to live with the baby on my own." He was so angry that he took away again the bunch of flowers he'd brought for me and marched out! All I needed now was the soul-strength to keep to my decision.

I realised I had to say "Yes" to God in looking after this baby. I knew I should want what God wanted, and I felt God wanted me to keep my baby and look after him, because He had given him to me. I remembered how Pater Leo said I must "take up" this child, as I would take up the Christ-child, in love and acceptance.

I had to take the baby back to Craigdene; I had to wait there till a council-house was offered. There I was given the "Mother and baby room", in which to keep the baby in a cot which was provided. A layette had been provided for me by friends and by some kind nuns that I knew. I struggled, in my depressed condition, to feed the baby, change its nappies and respond to its crying. I had the perpetual chore of making up bottles and sterilising them; I had begun in Strathwells to breast-feed, but my breasts had become so incredibly sore, that I had changed to bottle-feeding after a week. The bottles and the nappies seemed to go on ad infinitum! With such reluctance I got out of bed in the morning, to see to the baby before breakfast. The nurses needed to positively bully me into the task of being a mother. I remember one of them bullying me into the job of cleaning and vacuuming the baby's room; I was so reluctant to do anything at all. And I had to take the baby for walks in the pram, endlessly going round the grounds.

But I was convinced, despite the difficulty of the task, that looking after the baby was what God wanted me to do. And so I was trying to be strong about it. The idea of adoption had been banded around by my friends. I remember one of my friends accompanying me on a walk with the pram trying to tell me I should give this baby to people who could adequately care for it, insinuating that I couldn't. And I felt that I couldn't too! But I saw the idea of "giving away" my baby as a wicked temptation that I had to resist.

I was sure that trying to be as Pater Leo said "a good strong wise mother" would transform me into a better person. I had to believe that there was a purpose in it, had to trust God to give me the strength and the grace to be just that, - a good mother. I had to trust he would give me the nitty-gritty strength to look after my baby when that was what He wanted me to do.

Soon I was given a house; it was in KirkMichaels, just down the road from where Walter lived, but I had no choice but to accept it. I remember going to look at it with the social worker Derek Jeffreys. The grass at the back was waist deep, with big chunks of corrugated iron around it; we looked through the kitchen window and saw a bare red brick floor, an old gas fire and various bags of rubbish; when we looked through the living room window, we saw all the old wallpaper hanging off, where the workmen had torn away the curtain rail and put in a fire-place. I looked at it all in dismay; I was disheartened; it looked a horrible house, and I had no-one to help me to make the place liveable in.

But I rallied my spirits and tried to tackle it. Dr.Abernethy now gave me a new type of drug, called "Sulpiride", to help tackle my depression; it worked well; I remember Dr.Nightingale reporting back that I thought it "the best thing since sliced bread." For the next month, whilst based in Craigdene, and my baby looked after there, I bussed into KirkMichaels on a daily basis, to try and make the house a "nest" for us. My Dad offered to come up for 5 days to do basic decorating for me. I remember well him arranging to meet me on the corner by the golf-course, and complaining to me when I ran to greet him that I was wearing too many layers of clothing "for the middle of summer." I helped him to do woodchip in the living room and one bedroom, and to emulsion it; I found it hard to put up with his bad-temper; I remember him remonstrating with an electrician about a faulty socket. It wasn't finished within the 5 days as he had difficulties with the "whitening", but he insisted on leaving. I had no money of course to furnish the place, but the council gave me a bed and a cooker, and I got a carpet, and furniture second-hand; and a friend of mine provided a cot and a pram, and various other baby things from an NCT second-hand sale. A man from the council emulsioned the kitchen and bathroom walls; I bought second-hand curtains from the newspapers-ads, and a nurse gave me an old fridge. Meantime I went on shopping trips to Inverlang and Kirkcraig, to buy all the household items I needed; and I visited the local "Nappypin" to buy things like socks and vests for the baby.

It was really incredibly difficult, and took a lot of courage, to look after my baby adequately well in the hospital on the one hand, and to create a "home" in KirkMichaels on the other hand, going every day back and forth on buses. I had to manage everything adequately well, so that the doctors and nurses would be convinced that I would be well enough to survive on my own,- so that I could one day cut free of the hospital and look after my baby alone. It seemed to take a superhuman feat to convince them of this! But finally the day arrived; it was 31st July 86.

As a mother I struggled to say Yes to God, if not in his conception, then in accepting and loving my child in my womb, "in the crucial time when the depths of my thought touched infinity." For that reason he was not born out of a man's lust, but out of a greater Love in my own soul!

Chapter 14
Early Days.

From Book of the Beloved, Page 20; God invited me "Come and embrace me," but I feared it would mean sharing in His Agony, that His touch would be cold and death-like, and that I wouldn't be able to bear so much; and a great struggle went on between my love and my fear. But He graciously bent over me, saying "You must trust to my love." And because He touched that pulse-point of love within me, love cast out my fear. And when I voluptuously embraced Him, "the music of the stars was present to me, and I found His closeness warm and living, and He whispered "Come dance with Me."

The birth of my son left me feeling very scared. And it was in fact only the beginning of the trauma of my deeper suffering. It was indeed a dance of Love and Agony God was leading me into. But I can see looking back, that the dance of suffering He led me into was really the dance of life!

So I was left with a new-born baby to look after on my own. It wasn't really "on my own", because quite a lot of support was put in. Every morning and again late afternoon a home-help came; three days of the week I was taken to Eastvale day hospital, taking the baby in his Moses basket in the ambulance; and the two other days each week I got visits from the community nurse and the health visitor. But life in those early days was hard; I was very bored with the routine of baby-care, and I was still depressed; I spent half of my time falling asleep.

On the 31st August it was the baby's baptism; Paul Thompson baptised him in St.Stephen's chapel, and I gave him two Godmothers and two Godfathers, and we had a reception afterwards which my Mum and Dad attended. I remember how my Dad badly cut his hand with a two-edged knife when cutting the cake. I called the baby "Gabriel". That same day I started writing again. And I said to Gabriel, "you are a little human soul that I am caring for and loving."

In September Walter started calling round, to see the baby, and I let him in. However I was realising it was a mistake, as I didn't really want to get involved in a relationship with him again. But he took me out on occasion, and I appreciated it when I was so bored. I kept trying to make resolutions not to let him in; I wanted to keep to the resolution I made the night Gabriel was born.

I still felt "dead" mentally , and wanted to be more active and alert, so I made the decision to go out and visit someone every afternoon, instead of going to sleep. This worked wonders; gradually during October my mental life revived; I started reading baby-care books and taking delight in the small things Gabriel did and learnt every day. My writing and my prayer-life revived. I started going out in the evenings, to evening classes and talks at the chaplaincy, and to "Gingerbread" and the Baptists meetings. Then I started going to "Mothers and Toddlers"; by going to various of these, I ended up going out every morning. I developed friends to visit, and I took the baby round to visit students. I got a pushchair for Gabriel at about this time.

I also began to take more interest and delight in Gabriel; at first he had been a thing whose nappies I changed. But I began to be interested in his "little life", noticing all the little things he learnt each day, like shaking his rattle or putting his fist in his mouth or holding his toes. I began to work out how I could make him laugh or cry, and the reasons why he cried. I was trying to be a "good mother", talking to him and playing with him and being patient all the time. It dawned on me that I must take full responsibility for his growing up; his "goodness" depended on how I trained him and cared for him; he was "my own son" to train and teach.

It was at this time, in October, that I was introduced to my new psychiatrist and my new social worker. The new psychiatrist was Dr. McNeill, who has done so much damage in my life. The new social worker was Philip Davidson, who I instantly took to, and who was a great help in those first 5 years. I liked him enormously, because he was wonderful with the baby, and spent long hours with us. He immediately applied himself to improving our life, like increasing our DSS payments; he later got me electric central heating and a phone put in. The first thing he talked about was how he wanted me to build safeguards in my life. What he meant was safeguarding my baby against my illness. I remember him well talking to me in a café, with Gabriel in his push-chair beside us, pointing out that when I was "psychotic" I had poured hot tea on people's heads in order to "baptise" them; he pointed out that I must make sure never to do such a thing to the baby. So he set up a meeting with all my friends, to get them to keep an eye on me, and report if I should show signs of becoming "ill". He made me feel that I was in charge of my own life, and he was full of praise for me.

On the 26th October I finally made the resolution not to let Walter in the door again. He had continued to visit, and I felt I didn't want to accustom the baby to his "Daddy". And then on that night Walter turned nasty, accusing me of being "cold" because I wouldn't kiss him; he shouted "I'm the father of that baby, and nothing will alter the fact that he's my son." I had to tell him to go because he was upsetting the baby. And it made me think thus: -

"He is going to interfere with the baby's life; he's going to tear my child away from me. He will come offering to take him out, tempting him with sweets and toys; there will be arguments in front of the baby. It will always be like that; bullying and blackmailing from Walter. - - I agree with Vivien, I mustn't let Walter exercise a hold over me; nor must I let him harm, "blast" the life of my baby, because that is the very thing I made a stand on in the first place, which caused me 7 months of suffering. It will be very difficult to refuse to let Walter in, because he has wormed his way back into my life; but I am going to be strong; my prayer is "make me strong." *Yes, I have made a resolution; Walter comes not a step further into the life of my child. I have got to put a stop to it now. I make a resolution and a promise; God help me to maintain it.*"

A few days later Walter called again, and I felt I was an idiot to let him in. But I told him of my decision: "What would you say if I said I don't want you coming round any more?" I said, "I don't want you popping in and out of the life of my baby." He became quite violent and shouted "Nothing on earth will ever stop me from seeing my son; I'll go to prison, I'll commit suicide, but nothing will stop me!" I pointed out that I could stop him. He turned to threats; he said he'd get professional help to get his name as father put on the birth-certificate. (I had only put the mother's name down.) I had a hard time getting him out of the door: - *"I refused to take back what I'd said; Let him ramp and rage, let him threaten; I have the power to stop him from seeing his so-called "son". I don't want Gabriel growing up with the awareness of such a man as his father; and that is my final decision, which I will not go back on!"*

It was 3 weeks before he came back. I had become quite determined to stop him from seeing his son and exercising an influence over him. I tried to stop him coming in the door; "you're not coming in" I said, as he pushed his way in. "I want to see my son; he's my son." He threatened that I'd suffer for it if I didn't let him in. "I'm the father; he's going to want to know who his father is." I shouted "Get out of my house!" After that incident I got a chain put on the door. I was determined to keep to my vow of "not letting him a step further into the life of my child"; I saw it as part of being "a good strong wise mother."

Meanwhile I was blooming in my motherhood, as I became ever more aware of how to "nurture" my child. I came to believe that if I was a good mother it would make him a good-natured child. Sometimes he was screaming and squirming and wouldn't eat; but I tried to show an infinite patience. I tried to treat him as a "you", rather than an "it" who gets fed and gets his nappies changed. I tried to see him as a "little intelligent soul" who I was caring for. I thought "I can be like Maria, saying Yes to God through the constant loving care of my child."

It was about this time that I obtained a high-chair and a playpen. Meal-times became more interesting as he was gradually weaned off the milk and baby-food. I made him milled food, and spent long ages trying to feed him; I tried to be patient with him at mealtimes, to make it enjoyable for him. I started to play lots of games with him, singing nursery rhymes. I started to build a good little relationship with him, and began to feel he was my "companion". I remember looking at his little form in the playpen one day, and thinking how sweet and adorable he was. I thanked God for the tender moments each day when I felt close to him and bound up in his own little life.

Meantime my relationship with the support services was changing. The home-helps gradually stopped coming, though I painfully missed them at first, and I gradually stopped attending the day-hospital. There was a case -conference, at which everybody expressed themselves as wonderfully pleased with me; they thought I made a good mother.

Christmas-time came, and I didn't enjoy the day itself, because I was unexpectedly disappointed that we couldn't go to my friend Helen's house to have Xmas dinner with her and her family. But we had a good Christmas season with lots of friends around us, and I provided lots of toys for the baby, to try and make it special for him. Going into the New Year I said to my friend Vivien "what a lot of horrible things has happened in '86"; and she said back "Look at the good, hopeful, happy things that have come out of it!" For I was now set up with a home and a baby, and with medication which would hopefully keep me well, and I myself had changed for the better. And so I felt I was in a new, positive, hopeful situation, as we went into 1987.

Chapter 15
A Promising Year.

I was very happy in 1987. I took delight in baby-care. Everything looked promising, as I began to feel and look well. I became a radiant mother. I had lots of friends. I found life stimulating and interesting.

Everybody agreed what a superb mother I made, and I was happy in my baby-care. I tried to care so much for Gabriel as to make him a happy and contented child. I played games with him; I tried to train him. I was patient and kind when he was fretful at mealtimes. One of my concerns was that he should put on weight; he was always getting weighed at the time. We spent all our time going to "mothers and toddlers", and visiting other mothers and children. I thought I had a future happily watching my child grow up.

I wrote to my soul-friend Pater Leo saying how a "beautiful new little life" had come out of all that horror and suffering; a little child who can look forward to the future with hope and joy. I wrote, "This little child has come out of all the messiness, suffering, darkness of my own illness; something living and light-filled has come out of what was darkness and death."

Soon I realised that Gabriel was growing out of his babyhood, when he suddenly learned the trick of flipping over onto his tummy when I'd left him on his back; for it meant he had become fully mobile. He crawled everywhere and got in my way with his baby-walker. I began to see him as "a proper little person". I tried to be kind to him and reward him with affection and make him happy; I tried to make him feel loved. He became my little companion, and I took pleasure in looking after him.

Meantime the social worker Philip Davidson was coming a lot and spending time with us, and being wonderfully kind. He did a great deal for us in that year, getting grants for me for central heating and for decorating and for baby things. A mark of his care lay in the fact that he read my journals regularly, as a means of checking that I was alright. He also went ahead with his plans of having meetings with all of my friends, to build a support system round me, telling them to keep an eye on me and report any signs of my illness; his idea was to safeguard the baby against the illness in this way. Dr.James was also a great support, and we saw him a lot for minor ailments. Dr McNeill seemed alright to me at the time; he wasn't then the ogre he later became. I believed that the Sulpiride would keep me well.

Right at this early stage, Walter's threats became real. He had visited once in January, but I hadn't let him in; I told him "you haven't any legal or moral rights." I said to him "it isn't fair when I spend so much time, money and effort looking after the baby, and have him 99.9% of the time, to have you coming along and just visiting when you please, saying "I'm your Daddy", when you make no contribution to his life whatsoever." It was in my mind how he used to say "a baby would ruin my life." He himself wasn't willing to look after the baby! Anyway he threatened me saying "If you don't let me in, I'll do something about it."

He made another visit on the 9th March, which left me frightened and shaking. He tried to push his way into the house, when I had made the mistake of taking the chain off the door. I explained that I wasn't going to let him in, as I didn't want the baby to have "a daddy floating around." He then threatened me; "There's a new law out this year and I'm going to get my rights" and "I'll wait for you along the streets." He became irate; "I'm going to see my son; nothing will stop me from seeing my son; you can call the police if you like but I'm coming in to see my son." I was alarmed. Adrenalin rushed into me and I launched myself at him, pushing him out of the door and down the steps. And I locked the door saying "Get out of my house." It left me frightened and shaking.

It was thus on the 10th April that I first went to see a solicitor, Mr.Sutton. It was Philip's idea. That day Walter had pursued me along the street, and it frightened me. I'd had a word with Walter's ex-wife Rosa, and she said she would do anything she could to support me, even saying in court that he was an unfit father, but warning me that, if made an enemy of, he was "cunning and persistent." Dr.James had also said he would do his utmost to support me, saying he remembered the days when I suffered under Walter's vile temper. Philip encouraged me to go see this Mr.Sutton; it was his idea of a "pre-emptive strike." He said it was best to get the battle over and done with, rather than having a threat hanging over my head for the next 16 years. This is ironic, looking back, as the court-case lasted 13 years.

On the 15th April I first got a letter from Walter's solicitor; it made me very worried. I was worried that it might make me ill, as it made my mind race, but Philip rushed round to help. I asked Dr. James if he would support me, saying to him "if he was so vile-tempered and unkind as to drive me out pregnant and homeless in the snow, it's his own fault that he can't see his baby." And I wrote a letter to

Dr.Abernethy, saying "it would be terrible if my little child should be harmed by that vile-tempered man getting access; I would do anything to prevent it."

Thus alarmed, I went to see my solicitor, Mr. Sutton, but he soothed away my worry. He said the letter was a good thing, as it meant it could be conducted in a "reasonable fashion" between solicitors. He said we had a good case; Walter shouldn't pursue it if the worry of it could make me ill; "his solicitor is presumably reasonable and kind." And so I left, feeling it was all in the hands of "reasonable and kind" people.

I went to see the solicitor again a week later with Philip. And it was suggested there that Walter could see the baby without me; "over my dead body" I reacted. I explained how Walter distressed me when I was pregnant. Mr.Sutton said it was clear from Walter's character that he was pursuing this just to get at me. And I thought this was true.

Meanwhile Gabriel started to walk; it was like "breaking the sound barrier." I was realising how much easier life would be if we had a phone and a "playroom" for Gabriel; I petitioned Philip for these things, as they would improve the quality of our life. On the 5th June we held a great celebration for Gabriel's birthday .

There was an odd occasion of my seeing Walter in his house, when I went in because he said he had birthday presents for Gabriel. When he pleaded "I want to see my son", I was adamant "my decision is No." I said to him "I don't want the two of us to continue a relationship with you; I want it to be finished, over with, in the past, done with and finished." He threatened that he would tell his solicitor to go ahead with the court case; then he made pleas with tears in his eyes that he "loved" the baby. I felt that I shouldn't have gone in, feeling it was like "a spider's lair"; I managed to get out by saying "I'll think about it." The next day I swore to Vivien, "I will not set foot in Walter's house ever again"; I vowed to have nothing more to do with him.

On the 16th June I got a legal letter by recorded delivery at 7.30 in the morning. It said Walter was taking me to court for "declarator of paternity access." In it he claimed that we were "living together for a period of years as man and wife." It upset me; I thought how untrue this was; it was just over a year I was with him, and only a short part of that did we have sexual relations, and he didn't financially support me. When I saw Vivien, I moaned "Oh dear" as she hugged me. I agreed as she said that "it is best to get it over with"; she said it was better happening now than when Gabriel was 5. Little did I know at the time how many years the fight would drag on!

About a month later I happened to encounter Walter as I was walking past his house. "You never came back to tell me of your decision," he said. "Well you went ahead with the court action," I replied. I said "I don't think you'll win a court-case," and he threatened "you'll find out." I hurried past feeling scared and upset. I said to the baby in the pushchair, "Don't worry, I won't let that nasty man near you." *And I said to myself, worried, "I bet he's going to claim that I'm an unfit mother." It was a prophetic thing to say!*

Meantime in mid-July, I went for a holiday down with my parents. It was a really good enjoyable experience, because they loved the baby, and enjoyed playing with him. It was fun, though their restrictive language of "you can't , you mustn't, you'll have to" started to bother me. Coming back home, I felt it hard afterwards looking after Gabriel again completely on my own.

And then in August I took a psychiatric tumble. I phoned Philip saying I might be getting ill, because my brain was getting "overactive". I felt it was urgent, saying "within a couple of hours I shall be on the other side of the great divide, insane instead of sane, with no more insight." Philip rushed me to Craigdene in his car. I trusted him utterly, as though he were a Sir Galahad; I consented to go to the dreadful Ward 19, because I trusted him. We had deposited Gabriel with Vivien, and she agreed to look after him at my house, where all his baby things were. I was later annoyed with Vivien for her lack of sense in baby-care, but she did manage to look after him. I hoped it would be a positive feather in my cap, in that I myself had "pressed the alarm buttons"; I said it should make people trust me more rather than less.

This was the occasion when Dr.McNeill put me on Lithium. My first reaction to it was dreadful nausea, diarrhoea, and an itchy face. And Dr.McNeill forced me to keep on that drug, and those symptoms continued for seven whole years!! He forced me to keep on it by keeping taking blood-samples, which showed if I was taking it regularly; blood-samples are necessary, because if not "in the therapeutic waveband" it can become toxic. *Lithium became the bane of my life, as it had the dreadful side-effects, but never worked on me.*

However at the time I felt the Lithium a small price to pay, because after just three and a half days I was discharged from Craigdene. For I seemed OK. Whether it was the Lithium which rescued me from a psychotic episode I'll never know; but Dr.McNeill took a blood-sample and to my astonishment and delight, said I could go home. When I got back home I found a topsy -turvy house and Gabriel running about like a wild thing, but I buckled down to child-care again. When Dr.James came to visit me I told him I thought my illness just recurred at regular intervals. As for Philip, he was pleased that our plans for "the care and protection of Gabriel" had been a success. I was just thankful.

Chapter 16
A Second Year of Happiness.

In the second year of living with my baby at 109 Drumchapel Drive, I made lots of home-improvements. I got a play-room decorated for the baby, with a safety-gate at the door; this meant I had somewhere to put him. I got central heating put in, so we had warmth and were no longer dependant on the coal-fire. I got a second-hand automatic washing machine, so I needn't struggle with the old twin-tub. I obtained better wardrobes and better armchairs. I got a phone put in, which saved me the torment of trying to phone from the public phone-box. All these things improved our quality of life and made it more of a "home".

I led a busy life. I made lots of good friends at the "Mothers and Toddlers", so life was a perpetual round of visiting and being visited. I took delight in my baby, and watched with glee all the new tricks he learnt, like clapping his hands, stacking bricks and dancing. I spent hours reading him books, and playing games and rhymes with him; I watched with interest how he began to connect the word with the thing, and began to talk. Everybody said what a good mother I was, and everybody said how "easy to relate to" I had become; I was relaxed with people.

I was in my prime, and the health visitor Mrs.Bloomfield remarked on how very attractive I was looking. But I wasn't in the least bit interested in "finding a man", because I had my child as my companion, and wasn't in the least lonely. I still had a "support team" round me; my GP Dr James, Mrs.Bloomfield, the community nurse Ted , the social worker Philip, and my home-help Jan. I was told by Dr.James that Walter wouldn't win the court case: "It's not just me, you have the whole team behind you" he said. I didn't want Walter disturbing us, because we were getting on so well on our own.

On the 12th October I got a citation from the court. I felt upset because it said things which were downright untrue. The most painful thing it said was: "the mother is emotionally and psychologically unstable, and therefore the child needs a father." I talked to Vivien and Helen about this, and they both said that all it needs is the medical profession to point out that Walter would distress me and make me ill. The court-case began, from this point on, to dominate my thinking and my conversation. A few days later I saw my solicitor Mr. Sutton, and he said the case hinged on whether he could get the medical evidence to say that Walter's access would cause a deterioration in my condition. I said I had lots of witnesses, and signed legal aid papers, and left feeling the matter was in good hands.

It was at this stage that I approached Dr.James about him helping; I saw him as my chief witness, and knew a lot depended on him. When I explained to him that there was a thin line between being "stable enough" to make a good mother, but "unstable" enough to risk becoming ill by Walter distressing me, he had the idea of what he could aver: the trauma of the time when I was living with Walter had left such scars in my psyche as would be re-opened by contact with the man. He took some of my evidence down on his tape recorder, but he said he needed to know exactly what Walter said and did; he told me to look it up in my journals. He said "we must be thorough", or I might have Walter "hanging round my neck for years." I was reluctant to do it, because I didn't want to relive the trauma, but I did do my homework for him.

And then, on the 4th December, I related the whole saga for him, from my journals, and I felt it like a catharsis; it was like a total "confession". Then I felt how this one man held my destiny in his hands; the story had been told to him alone, and it was up to him to exercise his power to keep Walter out of our lives. *I said "it would be a terrible thing if we are burdened with Walter after all I've suffered to get away from him"; "it's all up to you; nobody else knows the story."* He said he would make a report of it to my solicitor. I trusted him completely; and as it was, in the event when he gave his evidence, he didn't fail me.

At this time my parents came up for a couple of days; it was all "feasting and fun", and they brought Xmas presents. I was proud of my house and proud of my baby. My mother said "you can tell how well you look after him." Philip met my parents and we had a profound conversation together; my mother told him what an exceptionally good child I was, and how bright I'd been at school. Philip confessed that the support team had thought I wouldn't be able to cope when Gabriel got more active; "but she has risen to the challenge marvelously."

About this time Gabriel started having tantrums; I found it hard to have the patience as he threw his bricks around and screamed. I was dismayed at my child's will-power. I wrote a letter to Pater Leo, saying I believed that as a mother I could influence my child's will-power, my child's soul. I kept looking for advice from other people.

As we were moving toward Xmas, my solicitor worried me by the idea of Walter raising "an interim action"; he was asking for Access to give Gabriel Xmas presents. Dr.James said he would "scotch that" by producing his report. Dr.McNeill was less than helpful, suggesting that Walter could well visit the child without my being present. I was talking about the issue to all the friends I visited. Henry Maple played "devil's advocate", saying "What was there to hinder Walter taking care of his child whilst you are ill?" *I reacted "Make me ill and then look after the child?- that's evil!" In the event that is what he did!*

When Walter's other son Andy visited on Xmas Eve, I expressed my emotion to him: "He hasn't paid a single penny toward the maintenance of that child's life; - why should he have the pleasure of seeing him? Why should he have the father's rights without the father's duties?" I went on, "we are getting on very well the two of us together; we don't want Walter interfering and giving us emotional hassles." Andy admitted that he was torn apart by his mother and father for years; "such emotion could make me unwell," I said "which would do harm to Gabriel, because our welfare and well-being are inextricably bound up together." All I wanted was for Walter to leave us alone!

On Xmas day itself, something happened to be said which touched on a sore spot in me. We were having Xmas dinner in Ernest and Helen's house. Ernest said I was bringing Gabriel up very well, as it showed by his intelligence and individuality. I replied that I was finding him difficult to handle; right then I found him difficult to feed. And Ernest said back "Well of course he has the wiry frame of his father." *It was like a wound! It touched on that same sore spot, that feeling of there being a part of the father in the child, which made me say that terrible thing in December '85 ("If I could I would tear this child from my womb and leave it as a dead thing on your doorstep.") It made me want to purge and murder and kill.* I thought it a terrible thing for Ernest to choose Xmas day to make such a remark.

On Boxing day I made a profound realisation, which radically helped in my handling of Gabriel ever after. What it was, watching him screaming in a tantrum, was this: *"you behave like this because you were distressed, you suffered emotion before you were born, when you were in your mummy's tummy; so really, you are hurt." This realisation that my child was "born hurt" helped my patience with him enormously.* Instead of losing patience with his tantrums, I saw that it was for me to heal that hurt and love him better. From then on I became more relaxed with Gabriel, and more patient and kind.

In January Philip put it into my head that I could have a "boyfriend", but I dismissed this as I was devoting myself entirely to being a mother. Philip also informed me that I had, according to Dr.McNeill, a "Schizo-affective disorder", basically a form of manic depression, rather than Schizophrenia. I was pleased at this, because I knew that manic depressives could be very creative people. It was about this time that I became concerned about the low Thyroxine levels in my blood, caused by the medication; a vivid picture was painted to me of the bad effects of low Thyroxine levels.

At this time I felt more emotionally mature than I ever had been before. I had become more relaxed, with more flexibility and elasticity. I also felt more "spiritual" than I had for a long time; though I didn't spend long hours "contemplating" like I used to, because I felt Philip wouldn't approve. I was loving the task of being a mother; I was delighted at my child's increasing understanding, watching all the endearing things he did, with floods of affection for him. I had students coming in to play with him, and a constant round of mothers and babies to stimulate him. Some of the mothers, like Rachel, had become good friends of mine. There was a "rosy glow" about life, and I really loved my child enormously.

But my happiness became slowly spoiled by the impending court case. I was devastated by a visit to Mr. Sutton, when he let me know what a big event it would be. I thought it would be little thing gathered round a table, but he let me know it would mean a cross-examination in a witness-box, and it would last all day. It reminded me of "Kramer versus Kramer" when she is reduced to tears; I felt petrified at the thought. Mr Sutton said "it would all have to be gone into," though it would take several more months for "adjusting the evidence." It was so much of a bigger thing than I had anticipated. I was so upset going home on the bus; at the thought of Walter seeing my child, I declared "I won't let it happen, even if it means leaving our lovely home; I'll go away, I'll go away somewhere."

When I talked to Philip about my feelings, he said that I mustn't "go away" when I had built "a support system" round me. I said I'd have to be "brave-hearted" about it. We mentioned "proof of paternity", and I explained how, in order to accept the baby when I was pregnant, I had to say to myself that God was the father, saying Walter and I were never "married" or united in our minds and souls. The thing is I couldn't emotionally accept Walter's paternity. There was an occasion when Walter's mother and sister came round to see

Gabriel, and I hit the roof with pain when they remarked that he had "the look of a McKay" about him. I thought to myself how, if Walter lost the court-case, I would reject him and all his family out of my life entirely. I accidentally met him along the street on one occasion and felt a real hatred of him; I thought with dismay how I would be churned up like that every week if he succeeded in getting access.

On the 16th May when I saw Mr.Sutton again, he said he was going to ask for a "Social Circumstance report". He really churned up my emotion by telling me what Walter claimed about September '84; that I "had sexual intercourse with him, then moved in to live with him." He made it sound as though I were willing and culpable in going to live with him! "But" I replied, - and it was a big but,- "I was extremely psychiatrically ill at the time." I said the point was I wasn't in my right mind, I was ill. Mr. Sutton didn't seem to take this in; it struck me later that he probably thought I was "just a wee bit depressed" at the time; when in actual fact I was "floridly psychotic"; I thought I was Our Lady and Walter was St.Joseph, or even God at the time! I came home very upset, as these memories were stirred up in me. My blood boiled at the thought of how Walter had abused me. I shouted at Philip down the phone that "he exploited the fact that I was floridly mentally ill in having a sexual relationship with me."

On the 1st June the Court Reporter, Elizabeth Waters, visited me, to make a Social Circumstance report. She was impressed by my immaculate house and by the interesting life I had created for Gabriel. I painted Walter black: "I will not let that nasty, vile-tempered, violent man near my child!" My emotions were strong; "Why should I let this nasty man pour his violent emotions over this little, vulnerable, happy child, blighting his life?" I said how Walter had abused me when I was ill and vulnerable; "How could you trust the care of a vulnerable child to a man like that!" Elizabeth Waters asked me "Why is it you don't want Walter to see your child? Is it because he will directly harm the child, or because he might make you ill?" I claimed that it was the harm he'd do to the child. She said I should tell Mr.Sutton that Walter would do harm to the child, regardless of the mother's mental health; (for of course our court-case had been built up around the deterioration it would cause to my mental health.). I got very emotional.

The 5th of June, which was Gabriel's birthday, came and went. I regarded that day as the "best day of my life so far," and I learnt a new easy-going, relaxed attitude, which was like a real enlightenment. Walter's sister had come with presents, and I said I might "work something out" with Walter; but the next day I was adamant against him again; "if he never sees his son again, he simply has what is coming to him; it's a kind of natural justice."

A few days later I saw Mr. Sutton again and persuaded him to hand over to me the medical documents, to let me read them. Up till that point he had refused to let me see them, so as not to upset me. I told him how I had become much more well, and more capable of handling it, and I wanted to be involved. I was really chuffed when I saw that this eminently rational man had altered his attitude toward me, and saw me as more "grown up"; I felt like an airforce pilot "getting my wings". I then read the reports and thought they were very true; they were brilliant medical reports, saying the interference of Walter in our lives would be very dangerous. I thought to myself "how can Walter's flimsy word stand up against the opinion of 3 eminent doctors and psychiatrists?" I evaluated it as "we have a very good case."

On the 17th June I had a session with Mr.Sutton, sorting through the documents and making replies. Walter had said he was "a stable person who can give the child a stable and caring upbringing." This made my blood boil; I complained of Walter's desire to dominate and abuse; "am I going to let this brutish man dominate over my child? - Over my dead body!" We got somewhere with the documents that day, sifting the truth from the untruth, and achieving a "true statement". It was a joint effort, as we thrashed it out together, and then we sat back and smiled at each other. I saw the exercise as a matter of "fighting for our life of shared happiness."

Soon after, when I came back from visiting my parents in Yorkshire, where I felt oppressed and claustrophobic and not free to be myself, Philip told me something. He said he had been asked if he would be the supervisor to take Gabriel away and round to Walter's house. It made me hit the roof; "such a thing I will not tolerate!" I then went for a walk along the beach, where I became worried that Elizabeth Waters was going to recommend it in her report. I thought of the "nasty man" having influence over my child, and I felt how "I would spill my last drop of blood to prevent it." It was then the desperate thought came into my mind, along the beach: "I'll go away, I'll take Gabriel away with me!" And I seriously pondered on taking him away to Austria. I made the decision that that I'd run away to Austria if the court should grant Walter access: "I will, I really will; I have sworn't!" I said, echoing Hamlet. And I hugged Gabriel; "I will protect you, my child!"

Then I talked to my friends about the idea. Agnes, who was herself a solicitor, pointed out to me that it was not a violation of the law to go and set up house somewhere else in the country. I realised that my idea of an escape to Austria was a mere wild dream, but I could feasibly make a fresh start somewhere in England. I realised that at the moment I couldn't do without Philip, who was my chief support in the system; but I thought that if ever Philip left his job, then I'd go. This idea of being able to move house filled me with a sense of choice and of hope. I realised what I couldn't stand about the court case was, that after all I'd suffered to get away from the man, some faceless persons should impose upon us this dark and miserable fate of having him influencing our lives. Rather than that I decided, I would have to leave behind my house and my support-system; I decided I would have to. *In effect, after 24 months of baby-care, the years of my happiness were over!*

As an unmarried mother, things were stacked against me; my life has been blighted by Walter, and his burdening me with a child! When I said "no matter what suffering I go through I won't kill a baby," I didn't know what suffering it would entail.

Chapter 17
Days of Torment.

And then on the 3ʳᵈ August '88 something cataclysmic happened, which left me sobbing and howling. What happened was, I found out by going to see my solicitor Mr.Sutton that the court reporter Elizabeth Waters had recommended that Walter get Access. The news knocked the bottom out of my world; I came home sobbing and howling with the pain; it sounded like a primal scream.

It seemed that Walter would be granted Access; evil and harm were coming on my child's head. I felt like committing murder to remove Walter from existence. My initial howl of pain was followed by a great ache. "I've no alternative; we will have to leave all this behind." I had lost, and it sat like ice or stone at my heart. I thought what a stupid woman Elizabeth Waters was, in that she had ignored all the weighty medical opinion, and just accepted the word of Walter and his sister that he made a "wonderful father." My net feeling was one of stony cold incomprehension that such an unjust evil thing could happen.

That night I couldn't sleep. I looked out at the world at 6am. through dull and despairing eyes; the world seemed to have gone grey, the heart seemed to have gone out of everything. I felt I was made of stone. I made phone-calls in the morning; one of my friends suggested I thank God for the evil come upon me, and "offer it up to God"! Mr.Sutton was cross and impatient with me, and I felt he'd recommend we dropped the case, and I felt dissatisfied with him. I found out by phoning around that I could do a council-house exchange, but I wouldn't be able to afford the furniture removal, so I'd have to sell everything. I had come to a decision in the middle of the sleepless night, and that day told Philip of it.

I had said to myself in the middle of the night; "there are more important things than houses; like what? -like the health of my child's soul." Philip said it wasn't as simple as that; it had a "two-o-clockish distortion to it." I told Philip of all the thoughts and feelings that had gone into it; how heavily we would "lose" if I lost my house, but how Gabriel would grow up free with his soul in a healthy atmosphere; "my child's soul is at stake." I said that as well as the damage from Walter, there was also the wound in me which would warp my child's soul. I said that for example if Gabriel reported "my Daddy says," I would erupt. "The wound in me, if prodded and poked and made raw in this way, would serve to warp my child's soul." I said basically it was a choice between "home" and "soul". Philip pointed out that to take Gabriel way from his "home" would also do harm to his soul's health, and "home" doesn't just mean "house" but everything I have put into it, like the support system and the structure of a rich life. He said the "stability" of this home is a precious thing, plus my friends in this home would act as a balm to my wound. But I told him I still believed it was a dichotomy and choice of "house" against "soul."

The next morning I got a letter from my soul-friend Pater Leo, and read it in bed; I dissolved into tears when he said that he "wished Gabriel would grow up healthy/whole in body and soul." I wrote straight back, saying *"the only way to avoid Walter's evil influence over my child's soul, the harm and the warping of my child's soul, is to leave behind, not only my home which I've laboured so hard to create, but all the attachments I have to this place, to my friends, to all the wide circle of this happy life we are living."* I asked if we could come and live in Austria. I said I couldn't understand how God could allow harm to my child's soul.

That morning I had the thought that I would murder Walter, but watching Gabriel eat, I had a much more terrible dire thought; "I will kill *him*." The feeling behind this was the desire to speed him quickly on his way to heaven, whilst he was still pure and innocent, before his soul can be warped and harmed. Then, knowing I couldn't do this, my lesser thought was- "adoption". *And suddenly a light came into my eyes, as I saw this as a real solution. "If he was taken away from this place into the care of loving parents, then I would experience less of a loss and Gabriel himself would have a better life. I would rather lose my child that way than wittingly to damage his soul."* And then I saw it as the most loving thing to do, and the best solution.

I was in contact with my best friends, Rachel and Kate, and they understood; they said they felt rather "helpless" when I asked for solutions. And the Baptist minister Arthur Wilkinson listened like an open channel to God. I was seeking for a God-given answer, some guidance on my dark way, and all three of them suggested the same; that Walter might not exercise his legal right of Access, once it was granted. I thought there was hope in that. Meantime I noticed how my dire thoughts were affecting my feeling for Gabriel. It was a terrible thing to think- "I keep Gabriel and lose everything, or I lose Gabriel and keep everything." It served to twist and thwart my natural mother's feelings. And so I pushed him away, saying "I have no feelings for you; I don't care for you when I might lose you."

On the 6th August I went through long realms of suffering, until I caught hold of an answer, though not a nice, good or loving answer. I felt I shouldn't have been left so acutely alone at the weekend "to stew in my own anguish." My feelings for Gabriel turned callous; I told a Craigdene doctor on the phone "I don't care if he has a dirty nappy, I don't care if he eats." I realised that if I became psychotic, the first thing I'd do is harm him! I tried to get another doctor to remove him from my care. The terrible answer came to me whilst watching Gabriel eat.

I'd already had a couple of intense thoughts: "the worst thing is if I ceased to love Gabriel because he is sandwiched between me and the man I hate." And I was thinking how my feelings could only be understood by someone who had gone through the impossible thing I had done, "of learning to love and accept the child in one's womb, whilst hating and rejecting the father." And I was aware of how there is "my own salvation at stake here as well as the child's." Then as I say I was watching him eat, and I had this thought that I could thrust him onto Walter and say "he's all yours, I want nothing more to do with him."

And then a mad wild gleam came into my eyes as I espied the answer! Yes I could threaten; I could triumph in this way. I could say "if you insist on having access, then I relinquish care and responsibility for him. Here you are, you can have him, but you can't have his toys or clothes, he comes to you naked. Damage him all you like; I don't care because I don't love him any more. It's all or nothing; it's me or you as the only parent." And I reasoned it this way; he wouldn't be able to look after a 2-year-old by himself, and if he tried it he'd fail. Then I would triumph rather than Walter, and also it would protect the health and capabilities of loving in my own soul. *And I thought how easy it would be to effect; "all I have to do is pretend to be mad; all I have to do is threaten to relinquish care and love of Gabriel."* I thought and plotted about it.

I thought further about it as I gave Gabriel his bath; "I can simply feign psychosis and the social workers will remove him from my care; if they have him adopted, that's what I wanted, as it removes him from Walter altogether, and if they give him into Walter's custody, it won't be for long that Walter could endure that, and he would still go into care." And I had no affection for Gabriel at all whilst giving him that bath; I felt my anguish had permanently injured my feeling for him. I was reconciled to losing him. "Well I had him for two years; I'll

74

just pretend that he died." And thinking how it was similar to my first week of breast-feeding him before I went onto the bottle-feeding, I said gaily "Well at least I gave you a good start!" And thinking how it was similar to sending him out into the world as a teenager, I said gaily "you're out in the big wide world now; I hope you'll come back to see me when you are 16!"

What I felt toward Gabriel had radically altered in the space of 24 hours; I had reconciled myself to losing him, and had removed my affection from him. He seemed to mean nothing to me any more. I thought how he was Walter's child, and therefore I could never really love him; I would get rid of him I thought and start again; "perhaps I can find someone I really love and have another child; this is Walter's child, and he can have him; I am not going to look after him or love him. In a sense, really, I have already lost my child!"

On Sunday the 7th August, full of this "terrible answer" I had found, I travelled down to see Paul Thompson in Edinburgh, seeing him as an open window, from which light could be shed upon my dark way. He made me see more clearly, and he made me relinquish the intention of doing something drastic to get Gabriel taken into care. *I had quite frankly had the idea of abandoning Gabriel somewhere and going off by myself, putting a note round his neck- "my mummy doesn't want to care for me any longer." I felt something tragic had happened to my soul, which had damaged my capabilities of loving.* But I decided to wait and "give Philip a chance", who would come on the Monday.

Paul Thompson talked with me for 4 hours, and he approved of the broad road of my decision to choose adoption as my only salvation. I told him of my thought which dominated the train journey,- "If he's half Walter's I'm certainly not going to look after him." And I explained how impossible it was for me to realise Walter was the father and continue to love and care for Gabriel. I told him all my thoughts and feelings of the last days, without crying. *Paul's final words were as regards Gabriel being "half Walter's"; - "he is wholly God's, more God's than he is yours."* I wrote this down and made a summary of what he said. *He approved of the solution of adoption, "but it must be a loving one"; it must be done out of love, rather than as a means of triumphing over Walter. And if I choose the path of adoption, I must go on loving Gabriel. He said "your salvation and Gabriel's salvation are inexorably linked"; this is what he had originally said when the wound was made in December'85.* Then Paul explained how the solution of my wound, as it was patched up when Gabriel was born, was temporary because untrue. It isn't true that Walter has nothing to do with him; this solution had fooled me for years, it being a blind refusal to see Walter as Gabriel's father, although it had enabled me to love the child. So now what shall I do, asked Paul, when this solution had come to an end? I moaned "How could God let harm come upon my child's soul?" Paul replied "Who can tell what God is going to do?" He gave me a few additional clues; that I shouldn't pretend I'm an unfit mother; "don't pretend anything." And he said "don't decide anything until you see what thoughts and feelings last."

I left Paul and we returned on the train. I noticed on the train how my attitude toward Gabriel was changed; I let him run about without any care for his welfare. I thought how he must feel that his mother's affection had been removed from him, without understanding why. When we got home I spurned him away, and acted as though I didn't care about him. Then it occurred to me how it wasn't that I didn't love him, but that I didn't care for him, because I couldn't care for him if I was going to lose him; "I will continue to love him, that's why I'll suffer the pain of losing him." And it was brought home to me what Paul had said about "the judgement of Solomon"; *what I am doing out of a greater love is "letting go"; I will relinquish him rather than halving him." And I thought it out; "I am relinquishing the care and responsibility of my child, because the most loving thing is to let go; but I would still love him in a higher sense." I realised that my motherly feelings of "care" had only been destroyed because of the fact that I saw myself as losing him.*

Philip came the next day, saying "I've just come to listen." And I told him everything that had happened, and all the dire thoughts and feelings I'd passed through. I concluded "now that I realise Walter is the father I don't want to look after him anymore; because of the way I feel, it makes me an unfit mother." His deep response was "I share the loss with you" and "I share your tears."

God was put back into the picture for me that day; he had been missing in my anguish. I came to believe "this is what God wants me to do"; God had brought my path to a dead end, and he would free me and liberate me, as I could see he had other plans for me. I looked at this "knot" of Gabriel's conception, which included Walter, me, the child, God, my soul and Gabriel's soul. I saw that because of it I must forever be bound to the destiny of my child's soul: -

"But it is false, it is insoluble, because he was not conceived in love. I now say "he is not mine" because there wasn't love at his conception; ie. the conception was sin. All this really that I suffer is payment for my sin. I think that because Gabriel wasn't conceived in love, therefore he was never really mine; therefore it has had to be a reparation for my sin that I have loved him and lost him. The words are in my head "the wages of sin is death." So the solution has had to be, ultimately, that which originally came out of the wound; ie. "I would tear this child from my womb and leave him as a dead thing on your doorstep." (I know the key lies in solving this somehow.) This ultimately, you see, is what I'm going to do, though not in hatred but in the spirit of oblation, for I have indeed imbued him with life."

Being at the Lammas Fair with my friend Kate that day significantly improved my feelings for Gabriel. I had the terrible thought, comparing Gabriel's slowness to talk with Kate's infant, "that Walter is the father is probably the reason he lacks intelligence." But I was solaced by talking with Kate, who had been in a similar situation, about how we would conduct a campaign to enforce fathers to totally leave the mother and child alone. I realised how I could still love and care for other children, and so felt that I still loved and cared for Gabriel as much as any other child. I realised how I must be careful "how to obtain what I most want." I didn't want Gabriel to be messed around and left in the custody of Walter; "I want him to be quickly and quietly spirited away into adoption." I realised "I will weep tears for the rest of my life for the loss of my child; I will also die of loneliness." I realised "it is best to lose this child who was not conceived in love; perhaps then I will find the man I love and have another child. I feel I know why God instituted marriage."

The next day I wrestled with the theological point I had discovered; ie. *"Because Gabriel wasn't conceived in love he was never really mine; it is therefore a reparation for my sin that I have loved him and lost him."* That "knot" was exceeding my comprehension and I wanted to ask everybody about it. I thought it out this way: - "He came out of my womb, but that doesn't mean I'm his mother. Because he wasn't conceived in love he is not completely my child. I love him in the highest sense, in that I am thoughtful for the good of his soul, whilst having no motherly attachment to him. I have surrendered him up into God's hands. I am going to relinquish Gabriel into the hands of the man who will damage his soul, saying "I leave it in God's hands, I am not going to make myself responsible for preventing it." In a sense what I am doing is a great surrender to God's will." My friend Rachel certainly saw it this way; *she said it was like the sacrifice of Isaac; it was the same "oblation" because in the same way Abraham believed it was what God demanded of him.*

And so I had decided that I was no longer dedicating my life to the upbringing of my child. I found I no longer cared "a fig" for the support-system or for the law; I was willing to go to prison to effect my intention of getting Gabriel adopted. All fear of my illness had gone; I thought "the beauty of it" was that I had power in my hands by the fact that I could refuse to take my tablets. When I met my "community nurse" Ted, I made this clear to him, and he said "you mean you are going to use that as a tool!"

The next day I approached both the visiting catholic priest and the Baptist minister Arthur Wilkinson. The priest talked a load of nonsense to me; "rejoice and be glad," he said, "because in this mother's pain of losing a child you are actually sharing by this sacrifice in the suffering of Christ." I thought it was a sick religion which could tell me to "rejoice" over it! But Arthur Wilkinson had a deep understanding and left me peaceful. I told him I was willing to make this oblation of "surrendering my child to God", and felt it was what God demanded of me. He said back "it may not come to that"; God might "provide a ram." He told me that Gabriel had been "given to me to love."

I wrote a letter to Pater Leo, saying what I felt about this "knot" of Gabriel's conception. I had always believed that conception should be a saying Yes to God, and in this case it wasn't. So I wrote, *"His coming into being was not a wrapping round in the womb of the love of God. It is true that the necessity of surrendering my child up and knowing the mother's tears of pain for the rest of my life is the direct consequence of the fact that he is not wholly mine. And the reason he is not wholly mine is that I didn't conceive him within the womb of the love of God."* I thought afterwards, "because my child isn't wholly mine I can only love him as wholly God's; he is lent to me to love." I realised "I was wrong in thinking God wants me to dedicate myself to his upbringing; even if I keep custody of him, I still won't be dedicated to him anymore."

The next day I talked with my friend Rachel about this "knot", about Gabriel not being "wholly mine." She said she wondered how women feel when they have been raped. I said I thought how conceiving a child "in the womb of the love of God" means the child isn't "half and half", but wholly the mothers and wholly the fathers. I said I'm saying I'm not Gabriel's mother because he is not "flesh of my flesh and soul of my soul", because my soul didn't take part in making him. *"Because the consent of my soul didn't go into his making, I am not his mother."*

Dr.James came. I said to him "I want you to facilitate Gabriel's whisking away with the least possible pain to him; facilitate Gabriel's passage through his pain." He pointed out to me "the meaning" of the Abraham and Isaac story; the point where the angel says "Stay your hand; I was only testing you to see how far you would go."

And Philip came. He said "Mairi don't be so belligerent." He knew I'd told Ted that I'd use my illness as a tool. I said I intended to contemplate again; he said "Do be careful". I told him I had been prevented from abandoning Gabriel "because of my feeling for you." I was speaking with a trembling soul; I felt how I really loved him. I thought how I wanted to say to him "I promise that in this matter I will not do anything you don't want me to do."

The next day when he came back, I said about Gabriel "the consent of my soul didn't go into his making"; he said back "people learn to accept the mistakes that are woven into the fabric of their lives." I said I could accept the motherly care of Gabriel, but "I refuse to allow this child to be influenced by such a depraved character whilst he is in my care." He asked about my "practical intention"; I said I wanted to start contemplating again. Then I said what I wanted to say, with head bent and trembling: "I promise that in this matter I will not do anything you don't want me to do." He replied "you give me great power and responsibility which I will try and shoulder gently." Then I said trembling, after a pause, "I am enabled to say this because I really deeply and utterly love you." - - You could have cut the air with a knife! I said I'd go and get Gabriel, but he said "sit down there and listen to me." And he gave me a long professional talk, which ended "the bottom line is that I can't love you back!" I explained, embarrassed and at some length, that it wasn't "human love" which needed reciprocating, but had the quality of the love of God, in that it was utter and pure. Philip finally went, saying "Oh good, I don't feel so worried now!"

That evening, being terribly hurt as I was, I tried to rationalize things by arguing to myself that really I was "loving love", and meaning that I loved God. However I realised that when I said "I will not do anything you don't want me to do", I was ensuring that my love of Philip would guide me. I was ensuring that I'd be guided by the love of God, by submitting my will to Philip.

79

I had a most brilliant idea in the early light of the morning when the next day dawned! I was incredibly clear-sighted, and lucid, as this idea fell into my mind. - - I would take Dr.James to court with me on Wednesday, to say to the judge "How can you be so blind?" He could point out that Access would dismember the mother-child relationship. And meanwhile I would get everyone to pray that the judge's eyes be enlightened. - - *(This idea worked! It must indeed have been God-inspired!)*

I later that day wrote to Pater Leo again, with my final conclusions: - "It is not true that I am to dedicate my life to Gabriel's care and upbringing. Gabriel is my mistake; a child who is the result of the mistake of my soul. You must know, Pater Leo, that I feel quite frightened at the prospect of what may lie ahead of me in the future. *We do not know what lies ahead of us in the mists of time, and I cannot tell at all how long this child will be with me, whom I love with such a deep human love, or whether I may have to lose him altogether.* The very likely conclusion will be that this child will be given over to the depraved man who is his supposed father, where he will suffer so much, whilst I myself will go to prison."

I now felt suddenly drained and exhausted, after a week of intensity. Giving Gabriel a bath, I thought "I am reconciled to losing him; it is only a question of the different degrees and manners, both for me and for him. If I yield him into Walter's custody it would be like handing him over to the torturers; I couldn't tolerate that. If only I could put him in to Pater Leo's safe and loving, prayerful hands!" And I thought how Gabriel would be safe in Austria, and it gave me a gleam of hope, though knowing "I dream of happiness which can never be."

Chapter 18
Day of Triumph.

It was now Sunday 14th August, four days before the court-case hearing on the Wednesday, and we knew that the court reporter had recommended Access. Yet that Sunday I had a genuine ecstasy; I was in the Baptist church, singing a song, when it happened. I had felt in the morning that a fog surrounded me; I feared that the result of the court-case would be that I'd go to prison; I was heavy-headed after all the torment I'd been through. But I was ravished by the love of God when they sang a particular song; the song was "Shine Jesus shine, fill this land with the Father's glory, blaze spirit blaze, flow river flow, flood the nations with grace and mercy, and let there be light." It flooded over me like a wave; I thought of how I could put Gabriel into Pater Leo's hands, and I thought of my love of Philip, and I was in a veritable ecstasy. Light and hope shone into my soul; it was like embracing Christ.

But that afternoon I had a corresponding bad experience when the new Catholic priest came to visit me. I felt he was an unenlightened priest, as he merely asked questions in order to judge and condemn. He actually suggested that I marry Walter as "reparation for my sin"! And then he said it was "sinful" going to visit Paul Richardson, when he had been a veritable soul-friend for me, as he was a non-Catholic minister, concluding "it was of course utterly wrong and sinful to allow Paul Thompson to baptise your child." I was so horrified, that I practically threw him out of the house!

Dr.James came that night. I had had this idea, with clear-sighted eyes, early on the Saturday; my plan was to ask Dr.James to speak in the court, and then to get everybody, everybody I knew, to pray for me on Wednesday morning. So when Dr.James came, I said "Just the man I was wanting to see!" He said he would indeed speak in the court.

On Monday morning I first went to see an independent solicitor, before I saw my own; and he painted a really black picture, saying I would go to prison, if I couldn't and wouldn't comply with any court-order made. I felt the blackness in front of me like a wall. Then I saw Mr.Sutton, and impressed upon him how "keeping Walter out of my life was essential to my sanity", and how granting access was "risking the child's life." Then I said "We have a plan!" I told him of my idea of getting Dr.James to speak in court.

That evening Philip acted like a theologian. He told me how there was a sense of guilt, sin, mistake in me, and how I must forgive myself. "There is forgiveness that can take on that level of guilt, of sin; it is there, it is full and it is free." He was talking of Christ offering himself in complete sacrifice on the cross. He said how acceptance of the forgiveness is difficult, but it would allow me to live with the mistake. I realised it was true that Gabriel was a consequence of my "mistake", and I needed to accept God's forgiveness.

On the Tuesday Dr.James visited again, and this time he pointed out the danger of saying what he was going to say; that "if I become psychotic the first thing I'll do is kill Gabriel." The result might be that the judge takes Gabriel out of my care. He pointed out that I myself might be called upon to speak; as regards this, Philip told me not to read the psalms whilst waiting as I'd intended, as it would put me in the wrong frame of mind. That day I told everybody how much was riding on the morrow.

Wednesday 17th August dawned. I knew it was going to be one of the greatest days of my life. I prayed fervently before setting off; "I abandon myself to Your will; Your will be done." Dr. James took me to Kirkcraig in his car; he, Philip and myself waited all morning in the court; when I got frustrated Philip whispered to me "Accept the things you cannot change"; it was recessed for lunch. I thought this meant Philip and Dr.James would have to go off to their afternoon engagements, but they both made phone-calls to cancel their plans. We had lunch together in Philip's room which was in the nearby hospital; I felt so cared for and loved by these two professional men. We waited in court again; I was aware that many people were praying for us; we didn't know whether Dr.James was going to be allowed to speak. Suddenly Philip said "Off you go," as I had promised I would go out whilst he spoke. I prayed outside in the corridor. Then I was called back in, and I couldn't believe what I heard the judge saying! *His final words were "Interim Access would not be granted!" I couldn't believe what I was hearing!*

And so incredibly, unbelievably, we won! The judge didn't listen to the recommendation of the report! I felt that he did have his eyes and heart opened by God's grace and light! The threat of Walter over our lives was gone! I did ask the solicitor, Ms.Humfrey, "What happens next?" but I was too jubilant to hear her answer. Philip said coming back in the car that it was "totally resolved, all over bar the shouting!" The jubilation of the three of us, as we came out, was so great that we danced along the street in the pouring rain! Philip brought me back in his car, and we were talking and laughing, over the moon! Once home, I phoned everyone to tell them of the good news.

The next day I felt my soul was singing a Magnificat; there was an endless hymn of thanksgiving in my heart. I was happy and relaxed, and celebrated with friends. I felt that Walter's power over us was broken and shattered; I felt there was a future in front of us. Everyone, especially Pater Leo, said it was a "miracle." I felt a hymn of praise and thanksgiving was rising from the whole of KirkMichaels!

I felt that all ways of thanking Dr.James were inadequate, when I bought him a thankyou card. I was aware that the vision I pursued of getting him to talk in court was not a human plan. I wrote to him, about the Isaac story; "When the attitude of Abraham's heart was right, desiring what God wanted, God brought a miracle about."

Then I saw my solicitor, Mr.Sutton, jubilant. I asked "What happens next?" He said that if Walter pressed it to a full court hearing or to an appeal, he was so unlikely to win that he wouldn't be funded; "he would need a new convincing argument, and he hasn't got one." So it was indeed "all over bar the shouting."

Then I talked with Philip. We talked deeply and sensitively about the "I love you" business; I said how my love for him would guide me, rather than "tend toward union." I said how Paul Thompson had said that I should continue to be guided by him, because he was close and contactable, because he was wise, and because he "cared for my well-being." He said he was willing to continue to guide. I then asked him whether I could "contemplate" again, and he said it was OK if I were careful. I then told him that it was no coincidence that after I submitted my will, it was then that early Saturday morning, that I had the "vision" of what I should do; ie. to ask Dr.James to speak in court. *I said it was like "a vision", saying "do this and you shall be saved." We agreed it was in the order of a "miracle." Philip then told me this: - the judge pronouncing judgement, saying "therefore interim access will not be granted", speaking from on high, was like God saying to me -"you are forgiven!"*

I thought about this, and how it was a resolution of that strange sentence of mine - "it is therefore a reparation of my sin, that I have loved him and lost him." The next morning I got letters from both Pater Leo and Paul Thompson, and they both spoke about "forgiveness"; about how the answer to sin is to accept God's freely offered forgiveness, because we can't redeem ourselves from our sin. I realised "I do feel forgiven and saved." I wrote back that the event for me was "something like the children of Israel crossing the Red Sea"; it was an initiation and a miracle, an event from which they could date their lives, for "they were liberated from the power that evil and sin had over them."

And on Sunday I got Arthur Wilkinson to read out in the Baptist church, after thanking everyone for their prayer, - *"Mairi feels liberated from the power that evil and sin had over her; she feels forgiven and saved."*

Chapter 19
Increasing Intensity.

After that fortnight of dark intensity in August, normal life closed around me. But in the coming months I gradually became more intense in my suffering again, *until I had an "enlightenment experience" which solved the suffering, but also made me lose touch with reality and go into "madness."* There were certain elements which, on looking back, clearly caused it.

Dr.McNeill stopping my Sulpiride didn't help. Sulpiride was the medication I had been on for over 2 years since Gabriel's birth; Dr Abernethy had given it to me. Dr.McNeill had introduced me to Lithium in August of 87, and that is supposedly the medication for manic depressives. In mid-October Dr McNeill, after reading through my early hospital notes, pronounced that I wasn't "schizophrenic" but "manic depressive".   He said that I never showed the classic symptoms of schizophrenia, like hearing voices; I had a "mood disorder" rather than a "thought disorder". He diagnosed me as "purely manic depressive" and therefore said I wouldn't need the Sulpiride. I was thrilled to bits! This was because I always thought of schizophrenics as failures whilst manic depressives were usually very creative people. And it all began to make sense to me; when I was suffering intensely "like Christ on the cross" that was the "depressive" side of the illness; Dr.McNeill said that I probably said it "due to its intensity." When I asked him why I had recently been "psychotic," Dr.McNeill said that was "just a more pronounced swing."   Things about my illness became clear to me. And I was proud to be a manic depressive!

Philip didn't help; by struggling with his new-found role as my "soul-friend", by whom I would be "guided", he did me a great disservice. He actually led me on, into dangerous mystical territory! I had not "contemplated" for years, knowing it was dangerous to my mental health, but when, at the beginning of September I showed him my "Book of the Beloved"(the mystical text about God's love that I'd written in my youth) he was so enchanted by it too that he gave me permission to contemplate upon it every night!   That was a big mistake!

I had a deep, intense, golden time with Philip for the most part in these few months. Having decided he had a "theological hat" to put on, as well as his "social worker hat", he delighted in delving deep into religion with me. I felt he was my "soul-friend" as much as Pater

Leo was, and for a while that relationship held good. The fact that I had confessed I loved him in August, didn't spoil our relationship.

We talked deeply about why I felt "guilt". We talked deeply about my knowledge of the love of God; I said how my "mistake was unforgivable because I had "a blueprint" for the love of God; it was then that I showed him my "Book of t he Beloved", and he remarked "rarely does a thing of such beauty come out of madness." We talked about how I'd written this book; how I was in Austria, knowing Christ's suffering, and the next year I was there in ecstasy, when I understood God's love. And so the book was an expression of a "bipolar mood disorder", and yet it is strangely beautiful and intense; this was a fact I now "took to myself with shining joy." I explained to Philip how, because of this book, I felt "a sense of sin" in giving myself to human love, because I felt I must "give myself to God alone". He replied that it was like a "young girl's first love"; he said it gave added purity to my youth but perhaps now I could go beyond it; he hoped I would find someone who would give me "warmth and affection and cuddles."

We had soul-deep talks like this on a regular basis. He wanted me to give a talk to his students in Invermount about my experience with the Mental health services; I was in complete command of my audience for an hour's lecture on the subject, and I concluded: "All people like me can hope for, is to be gifted with a social worker as caring and dedicated as mine."

However then the "soul-friend" thing started to fall apart, and my reaction, - my dangerous reaction, - was to decide I'd do without "the support system" and "go off on my own." Philip occasionally hurt my feelings, by intimating "everything you say is hyperbole, with you everything is so excessive", and putting it down to my illness, my "handicap". I was mortified on these occasions. But on a visit in mid-November, he hurt me very much. He said I was too full of myself and always thought my suffering was greater than anybody else's. I thought how he was talking like "a well-trained social worker" rather than a soul-friend. I was trying to explain how I felt "guilt" because I had "betrayed my own powers of loving" when with Walter, although it wasn't my fault. I said it was rather like the sufferer from child abuse bearing guilt for the rest of their lives. Philip on leaving me commented "we've solved it; in my head I knew I wasn't guilty, it's just that I had these feelings of guilt in my heart." This hurt me as he drove off, saying to myself "knowledge of good and evil comes from the heart." I felt he had really failed me; he hadn't thoroughly understood me, he hadn't given me an adequate answer. Then, feeling really hurt, my extreme reaction was; "Philip is no longer my soul-friend; from this moment on, I relieve him from that role." And my dangerous reaction as a consequence was; "I'm not going to submit to the support-system any longer; I'll go off on my own."

Another thing which "didn't help" in my progress towards mania was the legal situation. Although my solicitor Mr.Sutton had intimated to me that it was "all over bar the shouting", in mid-September he changed his tune. He told me the matter would be carried to a full court hearing in January; he said Walter's legal aid certificate covered it till the conclusion of the action. I was surprised and heavy-hearted; I felt that the threat was hanging over my head again. I was dissatisfied with Ms.Humfrey's attitude; she tried to prevent me from getting involved. When I insisted, she reluctantly gave me the papers for "adjusting the evidence," which churned up my feelings about Walter again.

And then there was this occasion when Walter accosted me along the street. He said "I want to see my son." I said he was an idiot to pursue the court-case because if he'd leave us alone, I'd let him see Gabriel in future years, but now he was putting us through such anguish, I'd be resilient against it. I begged him to "leave us alone." He shouted at me "he's my son too you know; he's half and half!" *I really went beserk inside, screaming with anguish inside of me; "after the way he abused me and left me with the burden of caring for this child all on my own, he then says the child is half and half!" I thought how he said "half and half" as if Gabriel were a possession; he was like Shylock, "and like Shylock his motive is revenge."* I was all churned up inside as I had vivid memories of how he treated me; "I hate him, he is evil."

When I went back to Mr.Sutton I told him how Walter triggers such a deep pool of guilt and anguish that it disables me from caring for my child. I asked if I could get an injunction to prevent him from approaching me, for I realised that if he lost the court-action he would accost me all the more; he wouldn't stop pursuing me. And Mr.Sutton replied that No, an injunction to prevent his approach could only be used if he caused "great fear and distress" by threats against my life; and even then it couldn't prevent encounters along the street, as it was part of his civil liberty to walk where he chose. I realised how Walter was "free", free to pursue us for the rest of his life; no law on earth could prevent him approaching us and saying things to us. I saw that the law cannot legislate about "inner reality". *My only hope was that by analyzing my interior guilt and anguish, Walter may be bereft of his power to trigger it. And so I set off on the dangerous path of trying to analyze all my guilt and anguish.*

This sense of guilt and anguish reared its head in the Baptist church one Sunday. I had been having difficulty with Gabriel, because he was throwing things around and being a naughty 2-year-old; I had been struggling to find a way of coping with him. I realised in the church "the solution lies in my being able to feel that I love him." I thought how he was "born wounded, born hurt," and remembered how distressed he was in my womb when I was pregnant. And then I had a strong sense of "sin" about those days when I was living with Walter. And I saw the entanglement of love and sin. "Is there not great enough love somewhere to cope with my sin, to redeem my sin?" And I sobbed my heart out along the nearby lane.

I realised then that the reason I couldn't cope with Gabriel was because his origin and my love of him are all bound up with a deep burden of guilt. I realised that I would always suffer because of the legacy my illness left me with. I began to feel a kind of rage against God. "Why is it that God puts such a burden of guilt upon me for something that wasn't my fault?" When I asked Philip this on the phone, he sympathetically replied "our mistakes remain with us forevermore and get compounded as we go on."

Then on one occasion the health visitor Mrs.Bloomfield said something which triggered a mass of anguish again. She told me that Walter had approached her superior saying, "Why has no-one told me about my son and how he is getting on? I demand to know!" Emotions gushed up in me; I felt I loathed him; "Why is it he hasn't cared to know for the last 2 years? It was because a baby would be a burden to him, but now at this age he thinks he can have some pleasure from his son." I went on "he forfeited all rights as a father when he maltreated and rejected me; in rejecting me he rejected the child." My thoughts went on like a nuclear chain-reaction: - *"How do I overcome the guilt which is deep down inside of me, as deep as I am?" I realised that terrible sentence of mine when pregnant, - "If I could I'd tear this child from my womb and leave it as a dead thing on your doorstep,"- was uttered from my need to sever my life from Walter's for my soul's salvation; the child would bind me to him forevermore. I felt Walter would pursue us forever, and would never leave us alone, for that connection of the child would always be there; it wouldn't come to an end until he died or the child died or I died. I raged against God, because that "mistake" in my life was the result of my disabling illness; "how can God so blame me as to put a burden of guilt upon me because of my illness?"*

I realised I couldn't tolerate the suffering involved in taking on my guilt. I desperately thought *""I will leave my mistake behind; I'll go and make as new life for myself elsewhere!" And then, during that evening, Gabriel happened to babble "why, why?" and it took on a new meaning. It seemed to mean "Why did God allow this mistake, and why do you have to so suffer for your guilt?" And I clutched him saying "I don't know sweetheart!" And we clutched each other "like two souls sharing a shipwreck."*

Then on 18th November, having determined to leave my soul-friend Philip behind and "go off on my own," I had an experience of "transcending". I felt I embraced my aloneness; it was a positive, liberating freedom. The night before I had cuddled Gabriel in bed, and felt indeed that we were "two souls together in a big wide sea," on the same raft together, and I felt swamped by love of him. And then in the cold sunshine of the morning I felt free to go anywhere or do anything. I took Gabriel to the castle-grounds where we sported among the sunlight and wind and waves and seagulls. We had a day of freedom together. I felt I was "gone beyond", like "Jonathan Livingston Seagull" when he leaves the pack behind and soars into transcendence on his own. I palpably felt my "free-doom," having choice to go anywhere. I felt I had become a mystery to everybody else, and nobody could say anything relevant to me. I was in fact losing my grip on reality, but to me it seemed like "embracing freedom."

It is clear looking back that I was becoming "manic," as one of the signs of this is when all my friends seem to turn into enemies. I was becoming so aggressive, feeling that no-one could understand me, that I fell out with everyone. For example, I fell out with Vivien, because I was angered by some little thing she said. I was deeply offended by the "Homestart" people who came to help me and babysit for me. And my parents came up for a couple of days, and I was angered by them, as they undermined my sense of "freedom." I fell out with the community nurse Ted; I was saying my madness is a capability, a part of me and not something to be afraid of, and he said I needed him to watch me and protect me from my illness; "society pays me to prevent you from being ill." *I replied aggressively, "You make it sound as if it is you and me against my illness; actually it is you against me; my madness is on my side!" He looked at me and I looked at him, and I had a sense of danger.*

I was still suffering this "existential anguish", which I expressed vividly to a few people like Rachel and Paul Thompson and the Baptist minister Arthur Wilkinson. When it was suggested that I "forgive Walter", I said "some things are unforgivable; violating another human soul so as to destroy its capabilities of loving is probably unforgivable by that person in that life-time." I had black thoughts of killing and of suicide. I seriously considered killing Walter, thinking it was like "Tess of the D'Urbervilles", when you get a sense that it was right to kill the man. I thought of suicide because "everyone has a right to limit their own suffering." I thought I would be sent back in another life to work it out again; hence suicide "is not a way out but a way in", a way to get back to God and ask him things. When I saw Dr.James I was honest enough to tell him that thoughts of killing and suicide were in my mind. Philip was trying to help and to "be there for me". We had both agreed that he was to give up his role as "soul-friend", but he was tentatively feeling his way forward, wanting to respond to my need. I told him that though I'd rejected the support system, I saw himself and Dr. James as greater than their roles and would remain open to them.

And then my deep dark mood of mind perceived a solution. I suddenly thought how I would have enough rage to kill Walter, if I could get into that state of mind I was in, in February'86, when I beat up all those nurses. I thought how at one stage I was fleeing in the snow to get away from Walter, and the next moment I was doing all I could to get back to him to kill him. "What did I understand on the 14th February '86 which so turned me round?" *I remembered how it was as if I had come into contact with some "burning divine energy." "If only I could touch that point again!"-* I was getting into dangerous waters here!

And then on 25th November I foolishly went to see a psycho-analyst called Denis Tait. He was very soul-probing; he said "it is not the facts but your perception of the facts that need to change." When I said how I perceive Walter as the devil pursuing me, he pointed out that he was probably just "an insignificant little man." We talked about my "rage against God" and why I couldn't consider what happened as "God's will." He told me to get in touch with my knowledge of the love of God, as this would cure my rage. He said he wanted me to be "free and whole," free of the past and able to face the future; I felt positively hopeful on leaving.

I went straight from there to see Dr.McNeill, and that was a dismal and negative experience. He said he wasn't happy about my seeing a psycho-analyst and that he was "worried about me." "I'm the trained psychiatrist" he said. I got cross that he saw everything in terms of mental illness. He demanded to know everything, saying "I'm worried about what you are keeping back." I got offended and wouldn't tell him my deep thoughts; "I suggest that you discuss it with Philip; he's not worried." I had had a long talk on the phone with Philip that morning; it was a perfect, still, deep talk, in which I got the sense that "he knows where I am."

The next day I became even more intense and aggressive, having an almighty row with Dr.James' receptionist, telling her she was power-mad and using her job to "attain her meglomaniac ambitions." Then I had this intense experience on a bus, after having had a dream about beating Walter up; I realised Walter was indeed a "pathetic little man", not "great" in any way. *My image of the devil and this "little man" had separated out; my perception had indeed altered. Was I becoming "enlightened" or was I becoming "mad"?*

I had said to Philip in that "perfect, still, deep talk" on the phone that always my illnesses is twinned with my enlightenment, because *"whenever I touch the point inside of me I seek, its energy cracks me up."* I said I could see the point; it was the point where *"I died".* I explained "I have spent all my life trying to die," to get back to the origin, the centre, to my knowledge of God's love. I said "When I find out how to die, I'll do it." I said "If I die again, I will then have the capability of killing Walter." Philip said "you mean you will kill him inside of yourself and so break his power over you." I replied, "Yes, exactly," glad that Philip was coming with me on this. I said how I felt my Grandad was very much in my life at present; Philip understood this and I felt our communion was very deep; I said how his archetypal figure "directed me heavenward." Philip said, mystically, "perhaps you want to die in order to follow him and get further instructions." I felt "he truly does know where I am." So I got this clear in my mind; *"If I die, interiorly, I will have the capability of killing Walter inside of myself." But I also had the worrying thought, "I am not sure that I can control what I may unleash."*

The next day I did it; "I died" to myself!

Chapter 20
Death and Rebirth.

On the 27th February '88 I died to myself and a week later on Sunday 4th December I was sectioned and hospitalized, but I am convinced, now as then, with all the written evidence in front of me, that I was not "manic", not "ill"; I merely had an "enlightenment experience" which people misinterpreted. I wrote when I came out of Craigdene two months later:-

"Yea, I really did die inside; and it was followed by a wondrous experience of rebirth and new life, and the sense of God's love flowing through me. It was a magnificent thing! And after that, the week after, I was full of a wonderful enlightenment about what Death is and what it means. - - - The first thing that happens after an enlightenment like mine is that the Universe attacks you. It is unforgettable and unforgivable as it means I have lost two months out of my life. But note: my Enlightenment remains valid."

On the 27th November "something mysteriously happened to me," though I couldn't tell the hour when it happened. After writing the night before, truths leapt out at me with crystal clarity, then I saw things and knew things ever deeper. I saw "it is when you stop striving; you really attain to something when you cease trying." I saw "to die deep down means yielding to God's will and God's love." I saw it was true "it is not Walter I have to fear but the devil; I can be freed from the power of the devil by God's almighty power and love." And I cried out in bliss, "I have experienced salvation at first-hand!" And I was flooded with the sense of being loved. I felt something was happening inside which was God's mystery; "I've touched the centre inside myself where I die." But the truth was more like "God is doing it; it is He who is touching me." I couldn't know when or where or how it happened. It reminded me of what an Austrian monk once said of Christ's resurrection,- "No-one knows the hour."

I wrote to my soul-friends, but couldn't explain "where I am", because it was "a landscape I do not recognize." "Have I found the point inside of myself where I completely yield to God's love? Have I done it? Has it happened?" Then I happened to watch a "Narnia" film, and saw how the land lay in the power of the white witch, in the grip of winter, ice and stone, until Aslan comes. *In the same way I realised "something that was stone inside of me has melted", and it let "a warm gush of peace and joy and love flow over me." I realised in the same way I couldn't break the power of the devil over me, but Christ both can and does." I felt my powers of loving had been "released, let loose."* And then to my utter astonishment I discovered that I had begun a period (after having no periods since Gabriel was born). *And it seemed to me like a miracle; "by God's own touch" my womb was shedding blood again! And I felt I had got in touch with the same point inside myself as when I conceived Gabriel.*

The next day I wanted to tell Philip about this "mystery" that had happened to me; I wanted to say- "If I said God has touched my womb, so that the melting at the heart of me has manifested itself in my body, would you understand what I meant?" But when I tried to explain he asked if I were talking about death "metaphorically", and then he tricked me by leading me into answers and then applying the measure of "mental illness". I wanted to share this great secret, and I felt I couldn't forgive him for turning it into an exercise for judging my closeness to "illness". Then I asked if he'd keep this secret if I told him it, and he turned away in his soul and said "No!" He wasn't daring, warm, loving enough to leap in when invited! I listened to his answer with a kind of infinite sadness and pain.

I then realised that "nobody could come with me"; I'd found a realm of my own aloneness where I walked in touch with God's love, but it "precluded relationships in the world of men." I said to myself, "How far are these cold cerebral men from ever understanding this mystery? They can never know what it's like to feel God's touch upon the womb, releasing the blood, the warm sweet life!" I realised I had to keep the deep dark mystery; the words came flooding into me whilst sitting in pain under Philip's eyes,- "Now that you know, keep silence!"

"I really died, and now know rebirth; physical death is merely when it expresses itself in your body. The suffering which was my sickness was my dying, my trying to die; my dying is my healing. *When I really died, life flowed through me. It is re-birth."*

I had this sudden and complete remembrance of the night I conceived Gabriel (when I heard the "Pipes of Pan"). And I saw that I had been mistaken about it, and about the sin in Gabriel's origin. His conception was all to do with meat and wine. *"My sensuality and my body went into his making. And though I didn't consciously and rightly yield my whole being to God, yet yes, it was God I yielded myself to."* It was *"more like yielding my body to the rhythms of the earth."* "And now God has touched me again in the same way, in the same place, and in doing that he has healed me; God has touched my womb."*

"It is the woman who is in touch with the rhythms of life; it is the man who says Yes to the woman; (the passive and yielding roles are the reverse of what is apparent.) - - And death and life too are the reverse of what is apparent. If life is a holding back from death, that is the death; whilst in embracing death we find rebirth. - - And rebirth is the "living warm gush of life." Who said it was resurrection? Who wants to be raised from the dead? "You must be born again" said Christ; he did not say "you must crucify yourselves and be resurrected." Look, I have come through the same experience as Christ; I died completely, and the fact that I found rebirth and have come alive again, has manifested itself in my body.- - The rest is silence and a finger pointing the Way. - - Yes I know the Way!"

Chapter 21
Enlightened.

I understood all of the Zen koans and I understood all of my "Book of the Beloved." I spoke in koans: -
"Have you arrived?" - "Well it depends what you mean by arrived, because in reality I've never set off. I've simply found out where I am all the time."

To the health professionals trying to judge my state of mental health this was disconcerting. Philip and Dr.James both came round frequently that week, but they didn't see enough in me to call me "manic". *And indeed I wasn't "manic"; I was in a strange state of mind. I felt I had realised something or experienced something which gave me a special "knowledge" like Christ or the Buddha: I also felt I could never communicate it: -*

"I cannot communicate this knowledge to others; I can only lead them by the same Way to the same point. That point is where God's love can touch them."

What exactly that "knowledge" was, is impossible to say. I discovered it through an experience of death and rebirth, but it was really the "touch" of God's love. Philip came round demanding to know what it was, and I spoke mystical things to him: -

"I am always willing to hold doors open for you, but I think that you have permanently shut one."

"I pity you; you missed the best opportunity God ever offered to you. And this was because you wouldn't leap in, you couldn't love, you wanted to remain aloof and safe inside yourself. And that is the way to miss salvation."

"You think you can stand on the edge watching things. That's not the way God works. If you don't jump in and give yourself to it (this warm heart of love) you are forever far removed."

"You may have the earthly power invested in you to force your way into my home, into my "space". But what if the space is empty?"

"How can you demand to know the Truth? Truth is a gift you need to accept."

Philip sent Dr.James round: -

He asked "And what is it that you wouldn't tell Philip ? What is the great secret you have discovered?" The reply came: "Nothing, there's nothing to tell. I simply realised something; but so what? We realise something every day."

He said it sounded like "a lovers' tiff" with Philip . Then he accused me of lying when I wasn't. "The only untruth I told was in pretending there was any truth that I was lying about."

I promised to tell him if I were "going off the rails."- "What rails? There aren't any rails!"

"There's nothing to tell; it was between me and him (Philip), and now he declines to share the secret, it is between me and nobody!"

Philip came back again: -

"I told you not to lay that trip on me again, and you sent someone else to do it. Do your own dirty work! Did you expect to find out what you missed knowing?"

"Why can't I stand on the edge?" he asked. "Ask God that, not me; consult the book that you carry with you."

"Do you mean to say life on earth is for entertainment's sake?" he asked. "No, it is a pursuit of the Godhead. But once the Godhead is found, then life is entertainment."

"You sound like the Buddha" he said. "Do I really? Fancy that! It must be because I have found out what he knew."

"All I've done is realised something about Death. But you can't realise this thing until you really die. And you cannot do that until you can plunge unreservedly into the fiery heart of love."

"Did you really expect to find out what you missed knowing?" "And what have I missed knowing?" he asked. "If I die before you do, I might just hand some knowledge onto you. But don't bank on it."

Then Philip and Dr.James came together, to ask me more questions: -

"What gives you the impression that I know something? I know nothing at all. That's what I know - Nothing."

"What worries me is that whenever we ask a direct question, it comes back to us in an indirect way," said Philip. The reply came, "As is the case of all arrows which are shot into open air."

"It is you who is asking indirect questions. What is it you want to know? What I know is what you want to know."

"What is your state of mind?" they asked. "What state of mind? I haven't got one."

"All I can say is, If you don't want to listen to my silence, don't enter my house."

Because I had touched that point where God touched me, where I found the secret of death and rebirth, I felt I had a special knowledge. But I didn't go around trying to tell others it, rather I knew it was dangerous. I felt it was the same knowledge that the Buddha or the Christ had; *I didn't think I was the Buddha or the Christ, rather I felt I had the same "knowledge" as them.* "We all have to be careful what we say; when you consider that something Jesus said got him crucified. "Now that you know, keep silence" is good advice!"

"The best thing to do is to leave the doors open, but not to let anyone know that anything is there. - - That's what people do with God, - lock him up. So as to protect themselves from him. God isn't "safe" you know! - - When people think they are protecting God, they are really protecting themselves from him.- - What is the point of locking doors? All space is God's; people lock doors to keep God out."

The deep "realisation" I had was about Death: -
"I loathe Death. This is what death is; a struggling to hold onto life. When you really die, in a warm gush of self-giving love, then you really find life. They are sick because they are trying to die. Life is trying to die. *That's what life is; the effort to die; if you cease the effort you do die. For death is a yielding, a giving-up, a head-long rush into the fire of God's love. When you really die you do not "pass on," you are extinguished."*

I couldn't stand my long-beloved crucifix any longer: -

"I loathe that crucifix; it is all cold and dead and bloodless! What a horror of a thing! "God is not dead of the dead, but of the living." I will go and throw it into the sea. Its image has bound me long enough. It is a "graven image."- - So I did throw it into the sea, together with my pen. And on throwing the pen I said "there are no magic pens"; and after throwing the crucifix I remarked, "at least I gave him a watery grave!"

And how was I looking after Gabriel during this "enlightenment" of mine? Well he was never in any danger from me. Rather I treated him like "a little prince." I listened to him, I let him do anything he liked, I tried to teach him, quietly and carefully. He wanted my clock, and I gave it to him, saying "a soft tick at the heart of things is very comforting." He wanted to be in the living-room rather than his bedroom, so I converted the living-room into a bedroom for him, moving round the furniture. I paid meticulous attention to what he said and did, trying to understand him and teach him. I realised a lot of deep things about the things he was trying to express; for example, how he said "bye-bye" when he wanted to be alone, or wanted people out of "his space." I thought my role was ultimately to "teach him" what I knew.

I do not remember how I was hospitalized; I do not think Dr.James or Philip had anything to do with it. It happened on a Sunday. One of my friends came round, and thought I was "strange", and she saw I had turned the house round, and I think she just assumed I was "ill". And I think she alerted the hospital. She took Gabriel away, to look after him, whilst all the nurses dashed round in an ambulance to section me and lock me up.

"I think it is the secret pleasure of the System to catch me, like a sweetie in the teeth."

I remember I was very angry at the time; I was angry because I wasn't ill; you can't be angry when you are truly "manic". Gabriel was looked after first by Elizabeth, and then, when she went away, by Helen. For almost two months I was locked away in hospital without him; I was very angry. Philip, acting as my social worker, tried to arrange it so that Gabriel was brought in every day to see me. But I was so angry at the situation that Elizabeth and Helen didn't want the responsibility of visiting me; I can remember once striking Elizabeth across the face with the flowers she brought me. Other brave souls sometimes brought Gabriel in instead, and they fared better with me, as I wasn't so angry with them.

On one occasion Helen's husband Ernest brought Gabriel in to see me. And I remember quite clearly walking along by his side with Gabriel in the pushchair, feeling angry and wanting to goad him, seeing he seemed so smug. So I said, just to goad him, "I threw my crucifix into the sea (I did this because of my realisation about the nature of death.) -"I threw my crucifix into the sea; it was just as well I didn't throw Gabriel into the sea; it could just have well have been Gabriel!" - - And he believed what I said, and promptly went and reported it to every body else, including Dr.James and Philip, saying "Mairi said she nearly killed Gabriel by throwing him into the sea!" It was a load of nonsense; I was never anywhere near hurting Gabriel!

I was very angry with Philip of course. I felt he had betrayed me. And I felt that, luring me on as he did about my mysticism in the Book of the Beloved, and then refusing to commit himself to the secret I had to tell, refusing to "leap in after me", as it were, that he had somehow "abused me". I told people he had abused me, although I meant it in this mystical sense. I remember when they took me to court to put a six month section on me, in front of the sheriff, I said "Don't take any notice of what Philip says; he abused me." I was asked whether I meant he had "sexually abused me", and I was confused and couldn't answer that.

The thoughts I wrote down in the hospital show a mood of mind which was perceptive and enlightened in a wistful manner, rather than being "manic." And I really couldn't comprehend why I was being locked up, or why I couldn't see my baby son; and as always in Craigdene maltreated.

"It is the gap in the worlds that I have discovered; I know where it is. - - I can say nothing about everything, because I know everything, or Nothing. I know the God who dwells in "black holes". - - As regards light and darkness, darkness was there first. Light can lead into the darkness, but the quicker it is put out the better."

"It is the characteristic of all people who are lost, that they desperately want to know where to find something. - -You don't invite guests into a warm place, if they are going to bring the cold in with them. - -You only need an umbrella if you are trying to keep dry; and if that is the case, it is best not to go out those days. - -Nothing that is true is written down, and nothing that is written down is true; this is by definition, as truth is a living thing."

They eventually let me out, at the end of January, and I felt violated and still very angry with everyone, especially the health-care professionals. That's when I wrote; "the first thing that happens after an enlightenment like mine is that the universe attacks you. It is unforgettable and unforgivable as it means I have lost two months out of my life." I also wrote; *"What hurt me so much was that what I was understanding was so precious, and they tore it away from me. It doesn't make sense, it isn't fair, and I feel bitter about it."* I did feel very bitter.

And in that "bitter" state, partly as a reaction against the health-care professionals, and partly as an acting out of my "enlightenment", in which I no longer feared the "insignificant little man along the street," the first thing I did was something stupid. Dr. James afterwards always said that it was the most stupid thing I did in my entire life! - - What I did was take Gabriel down to Walter's house, to let him see him.
What I wrote was; "Acceptance is recognizing the fact that Walter is the father of my child, and accepting him as well as the fact; and being willing to like him and kiss him on the cheek."

The thing is, feeling bitterly that the professionals were my "enemies", I saw Walter as an ally in my life-struggle. I let Walter see Gabriel frequently in the following weeks. The result was, he never had to fight the matter through the court; the principle was established, by the solicitors, that Walter had Access rights. I didn't realise at the time what battle would ensue; I didn't know what I was doing. If I had "stuck to my guns", Walter would probably never have won Access rights, as he had already practically lost the fight in the court. *It was indeed the most stupid thing I've ever done!*

Chapter 23
Walking on.

Then after all this traumatic experience, I picked myself up, and put the pieces back together, and walked on.

When Christ faced the man who lay on his stretcher in leaden despair, His bright eyes were beaming a challenge; to rise up and grasp life, to discard despair like a garment, and walk into Life as open affirmation. Salvation came to him as in that moment he rose to Life and grasped it; and this saving action in his soul showed itself as a sign in his walking away.

So I picked up the pieces and walked on. "The good thing was that all my pain and guilt and rage over my situation was solved, resolved, dissolved. The irony of it was, something happened at the same time to make me bitter."

Gabriel was returned full-time to me. I was worried about his bad behaviour; he seemed to have regressed in everything, and had learnt to say "No." I once said to him, fed up of his "No", "Are you going to say No to everything I say?" and he replied "No"! I put it down to him having been undisciplined in the last two months. I started spending a lot of time taking Gabriel places, rather than the endless round of visits with mothers and toddlers; I took him to the castle and the cathedral and the botanic gardens. I found him cuddlable and cute.

However I felt bitter. I felt my home had been violated. I felt bitterness toward everyone who had been involved in my hospitalisation. I hated the "support system". My hatred of Philip stretched to the heavens, and I had a hatred of Helen; I felt Gabriel had been divided between two mothers. When Philip insisted I let Gabriel see Helen, I took him back saying "I'm your Mummy, it's me who is your mummy!" I refused to discuss anything with Philip, thinking him arrogant and pompous. Only Mrs. Bloomfield did I find kind; she told me that I wasn't the type of person to remain "bitter" for long.

Feeling like this, I took solace in taking Gabriel to visit Walter, letting him play with him and going to the beach together. I felt it was "right" to have Gabriel relating to the two adults instead of just one. I had accepted, through that "enlightenment," that Walter was the father of my child. I felt I didn't hate him or fear him any more. However I soon found him starting to "bully" me again. He started demanding more visits, more than once a week, and I found out he had applied for custody. We began to talk about what he wanted put into a "legal agreement." It was a case of "give him an inch and he takes a mile!"

I began to feel warmer toward Philip. He tried to talk about my illness, pronouncing "it's like a moth going into a candle." I accepted I had some kind of "breakdown". However I also saw that what I realised during that "enlightenment" about Gabriel's care was all real and true; I had tried to give him access to me at all times, gave him full use of his toy cupboard, abandoned the safety-gate, got him to help with housework, tried to teach him at all times. And I still kept doing these things. I became a much better "mother".

By March I was becoming more whole and more "sane," and the bitterness left me. When I saw Dr.McNeill he said that my "creativity" was bound up with my illness. I told him I didn't feel "safe" with medication any more. He said that Lithium and Sulpiride together should do the trick. He made me feel that I had to sacrifice my intensity and creativity in order to be a good mother to Gabriel.

Meanwhile my solicitor Mr.Sutton, when I told him I was allowing Access, said he would make a "joint minute"; this would be a legal agreement which would obviate the need of a court hearing. He suggested an access visit of two hours on a Wednesday in my presence; this would last for 6 months before reviewing it; then we could see if Walter would stress, worry, or bully me.

But Walter was already beginning to "stress, worry and bully me". I had tried to pin him down to make an arrangement of giving me £15 a month, toward Gabriel's clothes. (He had never contributed anything to Gabriel's care, though he was earning money.) But Walter responded "just leave it to me, depend on me, you can trust me." But I knew I couldn't trust him. I remembered his meanness with money; I remembered how he treated me when I was pregnant. I suddenly realised, one day at Cameron Park, that his aim was to bully and coerce me. When I talked with him about access times and money, I found him "slippery as an eel."

Then on 18th March I had an argument with him, which caused me a great deal of emotion. He made me angry as he tried to wriggle out of the agreement. The stipulation that he should pay £15 a month was part of my agreement to let him have regular Access. He said that day "he doesn't need £400 a year spent on him Mairi." I was angry at this statement as we had agreed that he should spend the same amount as myself, so here he was dictating to me how much I should spend on clothes! I was left raging blindly. I thought "if I can, I will try and prevent his access." I told him "the arrangement is off!"

So I decided to take it back to the court case. I decided, feeling his tyranny over me, "I just can't go on like this! - I think the reason he came into our lives was, not to see Gabriel, but to have in me someone to bully and coerce." I thought to myself "I suffered enough when I lived with him; why should I continue to suffer just because I had a child!"

I went to see Dr.McNeill about it, and he was most unkind. I asked if he would "back me up", saying that the emotion and stress Walter caused me were not good for me. But he wouldn't promise to assist me. He said "but you have been under this stress since Gabriel's birth, and you have remained remarkably well; first you say it happens in cycles then you say it's stress from Walter that causes it; you keep changing your mind." I pointed out that I can hardly be trusted to make a sane decision, letting Walter have access like I did, when I'd only just come out of a mental hospital! He replied "I can't tell that you are any more sane now that you were in January." And then "here's the rub"! - *I didn't like the idea of remaining a sectioned patient (I was still under section 18 of the mental health act, which lasts 6 months); he told me he only needed to sign a piece of paper every 6 months to renew it, and made it clear he intended doing it. He said it would then be easier to get me into hospital!*

(NB. Dr.McNeill had me continually sectioned from then until August '95, and during that 7 years I was taken back and forth to the hospital like a yoyo, my freedom always under threat.)

I then went back to my solicitor, and I had a horrible talk with him. I said "I can't tolerate Walter any longer; can we go back to the court with it?" He was cross with me, saying "will you stop messing me about!" He said "the legality of it is" that the law grants the father's access to the child. He said we could never win the court-case without Dr.McNeill's support, as it was he who was the consultant psychiatrist. "If Dr.McNeill will not say that stress from Walter makes you psychiatrically ill, there is no argument, we have no case." *He said there was a real risk Walter would get custody. I felt absolutely beaten. I looked out of the window at a grey and hopeless world; I felt cold and too benumbed to cry.*

104

After that Walter's visits became a torment. I asked him "Will you accept 1-3pm Tuesdays supervised by Helen?" He replied "well of course I'll be wanting to take him to the sea and the woods and the playpark." I sat benumbed; I decided I'd rather stay with them, then suffer the worry of Walter taking Gabriel places.

Philip's great sympathy helped me to get back some of my old feeling for him; he said "you are rightly feeling very angry and very sore." Dr.James said in alarm "don't sign any legal agreement." His opinion was that Walter only wanted power over me, to bully and coerce me and get back in my life again; he said he was using Gabriel as a pawn to get at me. He suggested that if I allowed Access to Gabriel without him seeing me, Walter would get fed up of it and decline to come. Philip agreed that, without me being there, Walter wouldn't persevere in exercising Access. So I thought my "best bet" was to say it should be "at Helen's house under Helen's supervision."

And so I went into a sad and miserable Easter, aware that some legal agreement which I didn't want, was imminent.

Madness is the state which refuses to face reality. The road out of madness means taking pain to yourself. There is always a way back, for those brave enough to take it.

Chapter 24
A Summer of Conciliation.

An unhappy summer was spent, negotiating Access with Walter. At first we arranged for two hours of Access at Helen's house, then for a time Access was supervised by myself, with lots of extra "unofficial times" together, and then finally, by the end of that summer, it was agreed that I hand Gabriel over for unsupervised Access on a Saturday morning. I struggled with it; it was something I didn't want to do, but I was forced to move forward by the agreements we made with the "Family Conciliation Service."

My initial feeling about allowing Access at all was negative: "he abandoned me with this child through his birth and for 3 years, and now expects to come waltzing along to get a bit of pleasure from him!- Over my dead body!" At first I was convinced he wouldn't persevere with Access if it was at Helen's house, if I wasn't there. But Helen said how well they played together and how it was important for Gabriel to have a relationship with his Dad; "it does him the power of good to have a play with his Daddy."

In mid-April I saw my solicitor Mr Sutton together with Philip, and he said that he had spoken to Dr.McNeill, and he refused to say that the stress would cause me psychiatric illness. *"It is obvious!" I said in a rage; "what's the difference between the case last August and what it is now?"* He replied that I'd spoilt my own case by allowing Access from January to March. I felt in an impotent rage, and Philip sympathised, "I understand your fury."

I started letting Walter see Gabriel at my house. On one occasion I felt a bit sorry for him. But on another occasion he was interfering with the potty-training, and I felt he was "competing" for control of the child. I thought of all the misery this Access was going to entail.

We had the first meeting of the "Family Conciliation Service" with Netta Waterston on the 7th June. I had already seen her early in May, telling her how resentful I felt, and she kept telling me that Walter was "his Dad" who had a "deep emotional bond" with the child. The first proper meeting was as emotionally charged as a volcano. Walter began with 3 demands; he wanted three hours instead of two, he wanted it at his house, and he wanted to be called "daddy." *I was speechless with rage; I said I didn't want Access at all, but had been bullied and coerced into it; "I've looked after this child all alone for 3 years and that makes him mine!"* Walter was shouting too, then I suggested that we "start again." Netta asked how the Access was going, and I said I didn't like the way Walter competed for control. He apologized for that, and we started talking to each other. Netta's conclusion was that we both wanted a definition of limits round the thing. We came out, and due to the release of emotion, we were all and sweetness and smiles. Walter was all lovey-dovey, and we agreed that we had perhaps a "love-hate relationship."

Meantime I became angry with both Philip and Vivien. Vivien had complained to the Social Work department, saying that the way I talked meant I shouldn't be looking after Gabriel, and she wanted him to be adopted. So I was angry with her. As for Philip, he wanted to renew my section. *I was outraged; "you can't do this; surely the law won't allow you to certify me as mentally ill when I'm not!"* He said it was to facilitate my being hospitalized and to force me to take my tablets. I saw it as a threat to my freedom; "I won't allow it, I'll appeal!" But I knew it was as good as done. And these things made me feel much more positive towards Walter. I saw Philip and Vivien as my enemies, and Walter as my friend and ally. I began going for walks with him in the evenings.

I was very angry with Philip, after I got an official letter about the Section; I felt I really hated him for a while. I told him I was going to "cease co-operating"; I told him that he was trying to "force me to do things against my will", but the   professionals needed my co-operation. It didn't do any good; I was re-sectioned.

I found out that having to admit Walter into my life spoilt my attachment to Gabriel; I couldn't love him fully whilst realising that he had half his origin in this "father." I was becoming more "careless" about Gabriel. I thought "I don't want to live out a mistake"; I felt I would only look after him for 16 years in a muddled way "as payment for a mistake."

There was another Conciliation service meeting on the 29th June, in which we talked earnestly for two hours, and it made me feel more positive towards Walter. It was agreed that "bonus time" should remain as my free gift, and he said he wanted to be put as the father on the birth-certificate. Netta drew up an agreement to sign. Again we were all nice to each other on coming out, and Walter took us for lunch in "Littlejohns." I was beginning to see him as "friendly" to me instead of a threat.

On 21st July there was another meeting, which brought about a real catharsis. At first I simmered with rage when Walter complained that I was no longer turning up for evening walks. I said I endured Access visits because I had to, not because I wanted to; "I'm forced by society, forced by the law." Walter threatened and ranted and raved. Then in no time we were all warm and melted toward each other. We came out all lovey-dovey, and he took us for tea in the Pancake Place.

Meantime we were going for Summer outings together, to Cawdor castle and the Deer Centre and the Highland Games and Cameron Park. He had all these "unofficial times" as well as the official Access. I rapidly realised that I wasn't enjoying these trips. Mrs.Bloomfield said Walter was playing "happy families,"- "daddy, mummy and baby bear all going on a jolly picnic together."

I watched Walter with Gabriel and decided he was acting more like a Grandad than a father; he just wanted the pleasure of playing with him, rather than the responsibility of being a father. I remember watching him once from a refreshment tent thinking how he acted like a fool, an imbecile, and wishing that someone else was the father of my child. I felt what an idiot I was to get saddled with a man like this as the father of my child!

I decided I wanted these "unofficial" Access times to stop. I realised Walter was greedy and untrustworthy where Access was concerned. I realised "I don't want him in my life; I don't want him in my life at all!" I thought how hard it would be to give Gabriel up to him for two hours a week, but it would be better than having a life dominated by him. *Again I felt outraged by my situation; "Why should I be dogged by this man for the rest of my life because I have this child!"*

On the 1st August we had a horrid time in Cameron Park. I handed Gabriel over to Walter for a time, whilst I wandered alone in the greenhouses. I was thinking there how I'd have to harden myself to handing Gabriel over, and would have to trust that Gabriel would realise as he grows up that Walter was an "imbecile". But then Walter didn't bring Gabriel back to the rendezvous. I was furious, when I finally found them, saying "how can you be counted as responsible?" Walter replied "if you are going to be unpleasant, I'll apply to have Gabriel on my own." And all the way back he was playing "emotional games" with me.

108

Then I had an earth-shattering talk with my friend Agnes, who could give me advice because she is a solicitor. She said that, if I handed the matter over to the court, they would rapidly give Walter an extension in time and in freedom; he would be given a whole afternoon to take him where he liked, and soon he would get "residential access." It would go on increasing, and there was nothing I could do to stop it. I was benumbed with pain.

For a while I seemed to descend into the depths again. I talked with Philip about how Walter had damaged my very soul and it was essential to separate my life from him. I told him I had to love Gabriel less as a means of protecting myself from too much pain. *I said I couldn't invest so much in him only to have him "served up as a morsel" for Walter. I felt how I was "stuck in a knotty muddy mess."*

In this black mood of mind I started thinking about Adoption again. I thought it might be the "least damaging" for Gabriel; "I'd rather see him go sailing off, happy and whole, rather than seeing him damaged as he grows up." Then I thought "perhaps no matter how much he is damaged, I can heal him by loving him." Then I thought how, if I gave him away, I'd end up a bitter sour old maid, saying "I gave away my child when he was 3." *This thought made me realise that Gabriel and I belonged together, for our soul's salvation. "Motherhood is part of my salvation; I can't deny his conception and birth took pace in my body; I've got to go through to the end with it."*

It was at this stage that I started contemplating again, in a bid to find some solution to my suffering. And I found a solution in my Book of the Beloved; I realised that suffering is without ending until death; the book was all about suffering. I realised that "the existence of my child flagellates me"; *the existence of my child was my torment. But it wouldn't cease. I had to "accept the idea of endless suffering."*

I saw "I will be looking after a damaged child"; I foresaw all the messy heartache with him. I decided "I mustn't do anything which would make things worse for Gabriel." I winced with pain when Helen said that Gabriel had "an anxious look about him, that a 3-year-old shouldn't have."

On 16th August there was another Conciliation Service meeting, at which it was agreed I had to give Walter unescorted Access,- two hours on Saturday morning on his own with him. Philip had given me the advice that I must do this "not because I want to, but because I have to, as a decent, responsible, law-abiding adult." I tried to control my emotions; we argued about the best day to have it, and the Saturday was my own preference, so I could go supermarket-shopping. Then Walter asked what I did the rest of the week, and I shouted "Why should I tell you? I don't want a relationship with you." I was very tired when we finally got an agreement that I liked. Again Walter and I came out as friends; "there's no point in being enemies is there?" I said. We went for coffee and pancakes in the nearby "Pancake Place". I said to Walter "what it is, is that I have a very messy emotional relationship with you." He said back "well look at it this way, - a lovely son has come out of it;" and I found it touching.

The next day I saw my solicitor Mr.Sutton, and he was very negative. He said "the damaging emotion comes from you; it is you who have the mental illness." He said Walter could turn our argument against us, and there'd be nothing to stop him applying for Custody again; if we were obstructive over Access he would attempt to seek Custody; he would be likely to win in the matter of Custody in the long term. He said the more emotional I became, and the more I got ill, the stronger his case became. I left feeling benumbed with pain. I saw a future of never-ending heartache and pain.

(NB. This is what happened; Walter sought for Custody and used my illness against me, claiming it made me an unfit mother. And I suffered years of heartache and pain, because my child was taken away from me.)

My soul-friend Paul Thompson had a talk with me one night, and I told him how I foresaw a future of suffering. He told me "all relationships involve suffering, but relationships that are more worth have more suffering in them." He re-iterated what he had said before, that my salvation was bound up in my love of Gabriel. When I contemplated that night I saw "the absolute identification of love and suffering at the heart of the universe."

When I saw Dr.McNeill a few days later I told him how I'd resurfaced out of the depths of suffering again by realising I had to "accept the idea of endless suffering"; that I had to "say Yes to the pain that lies before me." He called this a "robust solution", but when I raised the question of the Section again, he said "you just don't realise the seriousness of your illness."

On the 22nd August Walter's first unsupervised Access took place. I found it harrowing; as Walter tugged him down the path, Gabriel turned round and shouted "mummy." It really upset me. And when he came to hand him back, there was soppy emotional goodbyes as Walter demanded a "kissy-wissy." I loathed witnessing it.

And my solution was "I'll just have to not care, - not care if he's damaged." Since Walter had come on the scene, I hadn't cared for Gabriel like I used to. "I can't afford to care"; it would mean too much anguish. However I was aware, deep down, that I had to carry on loving Gabriel; I was supposed to be loving him like God loves me.

My sense of outrage lies in this: - You can tell it's a male-orientated society; you can tell the legal system of the country is male-dominated! For it is so wicked, so unfair, so evil! You get a man wronging a woman, ruining her life; then she has to set up as a single parent and struggle away, only to find that the law imposes this man upon her for the rest of her life! The law should rather protect the woman from the man, but instead it imposes him upon her! This is what happened to me, and it happens to others.

Chapter 25
Nursery and Negotiations.

And so that summer drew to a close. Gabriel was due to go to Nursery. He started Nursery on 23rd August'89. In the first few months of his attendance a lot of negotiations continued between Walter and myself, with the aim of bringing the court case to a satisfactory conclusion.

Gabriel was very well-behaved when I first took him to Nursery; he started playing on the computer straight away and happily said "bye-bye Mummy", and I felt he had been left in good hands. And I had a liberated time by myself. However the very next day there was trouble with Walter. We were waylaid by him on the way home, and he said he didn't want Gabriel to go to Nursery. He harrassed me along the street, and I was very upset and emotional. The next day I told Mrs.Sanderson who ran the Nursery that she must never allow Walter to uplift Gabriel from there. And then the first Saturday he had Access he ranted and raved on the doorstep saying he wanted to "go back to the previous arrangement." It made me emotional for the whole day.

I felt how it wasn't fair that I was still suffering the same from Walter after all this time. I felt it was a "consequence of my sin," and my sin was enormous. My soul-friend Pater Leo said it was "my cross". I replied that the word usually means putting up with a burden, "not such a real, deep, penetrating pain such as this." *Pater Leo said this cross could make me "ripen, grow and become whole." I realised "we each have a cross to bear, and this is mine." I realised the pain wasn't going to lessen or go away.*

When I told Philip of my sense of sin, he said "we all fall short of our ideals, we all screw up." He suggested we did the handover with a third person, because I should arrange it to be with as little suffering as possible for Gabriel. We tried doing a few handovers with my friends. I felt that the essence of my pain was that I had to constantly hand Gabriel over into Walter's hands. And for a time I was quite bouyant in my suffering.

We had another Conciliation meeting at Walter's insistence. It was quite bland; he insisted that he had a share in Gabriel's education; I pointed out that, in achieving the unsupervised Access, he had got what he wanted; it was "open to review in the future." But we had a very emotional happening when I took him back to my house. He became full of uncontrollable emotion, his eyes welling with tears, as he broke into sobbing against the wall. He sobbed "you've made me suffer so much" and "I just want the three of us to be at peace." And I felt sorry for him, and agreed we should be friends.

After that, helped by my feeling sorry for Walter, I felt I had taken on and accepted the pain. And what I knew when I said Yes to pain, was God's love. And then the pain seemed to become a positive power.

For several weeks after that I had no contact with Walter, as the Saturday handover was done by other people. *I got a sense of well-being; I was better at caring for Gabriel. I found I could "take on his childishness", love Gabriel's childishness. I began to see him as "my companion."*

On the 24thOctober there was a case-conference about me; this was partly due to Vivien's suggestion that Gabriel should be taken away from me and adopted. But there was a positive, rosy and glowing report of me; and Vivien's idea was permanently quashed and vanquished. I was jubilant and relieved.

The next day there was a Conciliation service meeting, and we argued about the hours of Access and whether Walter would dismiss the court-case. I said I was willing to offer three hours, saying Gabriel was "too young" for longer, but Walter said the judge at court would give him a whole day, so he demanded four hours. We argued acrimoniously about it. I said he could have that whole day when Gabriel would go to school, and until then it should be gradually increased. We couldn't make an agreement. But after the catharsis we again went to the Pancake Place together, and I said the problem was "there's a lot of unresolved emotion between us."

The next day my solicitor Mr. Sutton said we needed "a joint minute" to tie off the court case, and I convinced him that we could progress to that by "mutual agreement." I said how every time we have a meeting there is a catharsis of emotion, so it progressively improves. So the next day I tried to settle matters with Walter by writing out for him a draft of a joint minute. We agreed that if we left it up to our solicitors, who have a vested interest in keeping it going, they would be writing letters to each other for months on end. We seemed friends.

The 30th October was the day of the terrible accident. Gabriel was run down by a car, and was taken by ambulance to hospital. Fortunately he came out of it unscathed, and Walter was always impressed by the fact, and grateful for the fact, that I phoned him from the hospital.

Not long later I received a letter from Walter's solicitor, demanding that he get seven hours per Saturday immediately, under threat of taking it to court. Now we had agreed that it be at present three hours, to be increased to six on Gabriel's going to school. So my reaction was to think Waltrer was sly, greedy, not to be trusted. I was disgusted with him; "what is the point of going through all that emotion to get agreements, if he does something like that! He's a slippery, slimy man!"

On the 15th November Walter and I had a meeting on our own and did our own negotiation; I made a successful agreement with him. I said I'd agree to put his name on the birth certificate if he would finish with the court case. And we made up this joint minute; three and a quarter hours immediately; from 30th April four and a half; when he goes to school six to seven hours; for Xmas and birthdays forty-five minutes those days with Access the following day; extra days of Access during school holidays. Having made this agrement we were very pleased with ourselves, and agreed it should be ratified by Netta Waterston.

A week later we met again, and agreed there was the problem of the birth certficate to solve, and the problem of joint care which should include Walter should I get ill. I was a bit distressed that he wanted these extra subjects in the agreeement. *But I felt at this stage that I was holding out acceptance and forgiveness toward Walter. I had accepted that I had to allow some kind of Access into our lives. The enmity and hatred seemed to have gone, and had turned into friendliness.*

On the 29th November we finally concluded an agreement, signed and witnessed by Netta Waterston, with copies handed to our solicitors. It was difficult; Netta insisted on re-grilling every item and Walter kept finding new objections. He asked what would happen if Gabriel were ill; I said "you can't get these things down in black and white; you'll have to trust me." But Walter said "If I don't get what I want, I'll take it back to court." Then he wanted agreement on what would happen if I myself were ill; I told him he would have more right to the care of Gabriel than Elizabeth and Helen had. The agreement was finally signed, and photocopied for our solicitors. We celebrated at the Pancake Place once again.

Then I had an argument with Walter about a week later about changing Gabriel's name on the birth certificate. I said when filling in the form, off-handedly, "you won't be wanting to change his name by any chance?" He replied "Oh Yes, I want him to have McKay as his middle name." I nearly hit the roof! "Over my dead body!" I thought it should be enough that he got proper Access and got on the birth certificate, without wanting to change Gabriel's name as well. I decided we mustn't fall out over it; I said "it's not fair you should insist on changing his name; you should give way this once; we don't want to spoil Christmas."

The 15th December was a crucial day for me. It was the day I had an accident on the ice, and whilst I was propped up in bed in the hospital with an injured spine, - with Coxygeal Sublaxation,- Philip told me he would be leaving his job. I realised how in my eyes there was no-one who could possibly replace him; he had been my best help and support since Gabriel was born. He said he would keep contact with me because he "cared about me." He got me home, after Dr.James had visited and told me it would be painful to sit down for some while, and I just felt that I couldn't do without him. He was so important to me, and we had come such a long way together. And I really loved him, and I thought how warm and earnest he could be; and I was so thoroughly miserable at the thought of going on without him. I thought how "cold" the psychiatric machine could be without the human warmth injected into it by Philip. All my life had been centred on his visits; "how could I survive without him?"

On the 20th December the Joint Minute should have gone to court and been ratified, so I celebrated with Walter with a bottle of wine. We also happened to open the bottle we put notes in when we first met each other; we smashed it. The note read "May what is between us be greater than what may become of us." We burnt it, saying "the past is dead, the future lies in front of us;" and we toasted "here is to a new future!"

Christmas came. There was peace and harmony between me and Walter, as we went to the Baptist Xmas service together. I was angry with him though later, for we had agreed that we should say the presents are "from Santa Claus", and Walter kept saying to Gabriel "this is from Daddy." And then he handed him a wrapped up present of a cardboard castle with the sweets missing, and I was really furious at the shoddiness of this, and was on the phone to my Mum about it. I realised my own aloneness over Christmas; my best friend Rachel had left and now Philip was leaving, and I felt I had no close friends.

In mid-January I had a meeting with Walter about what should happen should I get ill. My solicitor Mr.Sutton had suggested that, seeing Walter would have a strong right of custody of Gabriel if this were the case, it was advisable to enter into a formal agreement with him. Talking with Walter on the subject was very reassuring. I was relieved that he was not asking for 100% custody. He said he had never said that I was an unfit mother, and never tied to take Gabriel away from me. He said Gabriel just needed a secure place to rest his head till his mother was back. He said Gabriel didn't need a "substitute mother" as he should be seeing me. I agreed with him; Gabriel should be seeing me, not calling Helen "mummy"; I remembered how I had suffered when not able to see Gabriel in the hospital. It was very reassuring when he said he wouldn't allow anyone to take Gabriel away from me again!

(NB. This is very ironic, considering he then himself took Gabriel away from me for seven years!)

On the 17th January there was a big meeting in Helen's house, designed to work out a complete plan of what should happen should I get ill. There was Helen, Elizabeth, Walter, Philip and myself present. Philip wanted to arrange this for me, before he left his job.

I hated it and at first kept quiet, as they all started pontificating on my life as if I weren't present. It was agreed, there would be as few changes of home-base as possible for Gabriel and he should have as much contact as possible with his mother, the frequency of them to be decided by the "clinical team". I was thinking how this would be no better than the last time; instead of giving me a sense of safety this was making me feel more threatened by Craigdene than ever; I thought how I'd escape if I got ill. I was scribbling on a piece of paper, full of intense, black, bottled-up feelings. Then Philip asked me something, and my emotion just erupted. I was full of anger and hatred as I said it wasn't right that Gabriel should be taken away from me; I said how I was actively tortured in that hospital. Helen said how they sometimes didn't visit because I was "sleeping"; "you mean doped by drugs" I retorted. Elizabeth said how I had handed Gabriel over to her; "to look after for the morning, not to take away for seven weeks" I retorted. My bitterness over what happened the last time was apparent. They carried on to work out the details that Walter should be given 4 whole-day care periods a week. I felt I couldn't care less about the arrangements. If I were going to be actively tormented in Craigdene and deprived of my son by a "clinical team", "what's the point!" I said to Philip in the car afterwards, that if all my instructions last year had fallen on deaf ears, "what good are all your plans then!"

The next day Philip presented to me the new Social Worker who would be taking over from him, -Simon Mason. I thought how Philip had promoted so much healing in me; he was a "giant of a man," so who could ever replace him! I knew that my strength of feeling for Philip was like "a double-coiled twist of rope"; there would be nothing between me and Simon Mason but "a wisp of cotton thread."

Finally on the 23rd January I said farewell to Philip. I baked him a cake and iced it with cherries, as a present. He gave me a card which said "thankyou for teaching me so much about life through your willingness to share your experiences with me." Then it said something about hoping life would continue to provide me with "bouquets as well as brick-bats." He said to me very earnestly "thankyou for teaching me so much about illness." And I replied earnestly that it was by the pain I walked through that my sorenesses were being healed, and he had helped my wounds by letting the air to them. He promised he would continue to communicate; we agreed I would write and he would phone back. He kissed me on the cheek before leaving,- it was the only kiss he ever gave me. It was a very graceful parting.

Chapter 26
Blowing hot and cold.

In 1990 you could say I was "blowing hot and cold" about Walter; first I was friendly with him, then I was at enmity with him again.

In January of 1990 I went "green and New Age". I felt good about myself, starting a new Vegan diet, and I was liberated into a new life-style. I started working at the local health food store in earnest, having been promised a proper job there. After Philip had gone I had a bad time with the psychiatric service, because I didn't get on at all well with the new Social Worker Simon Mason; and I wasn't at all happy with that agreement we had made. Walter sided with me in these things, and this brought about an increase in friendliness between us.

When I talked with Walter, saying I wasn't happy with the agreement, - about what should happen should I get ill,- I found he objected to it as well. It had said that "the clinical team should decide" about Gabriel's visits. I said emotionally to Walter "it's not true that it harms Gabriel if I'm strange; it's not true that I'm ever too ill to see him." Walter said "I'm not wanting to be restricted by the clinical team." He promised he would bring Gabriel to see me every day in hospital. He claimed that Gabriel was upset the last time because he wasn't allowed to see me; *"in his little heart he thought his mummy was dead"; he should never have to go through that trauma again.* "Well said!" I thought, feeling that Walter was on my side!

It was only the second time Simon Mason came to visit me when he upset me very deeply. He didn't listen and he started pontificating about my illness and I hated his Craigdene mentality. He then said that he wouldn't let Gabriel come and visit me should I get ill, because it was not good for him to see me ill. I said "I disagree"; he replied "you have no right to disagree." I was so angry I threw him out of the house! I said "Right, I'm going, I'm going for a walk by the sea!" And so I got him out of the house. And I went straight down to Walter's, feeling he was my ally. He said how, in the event, he would insist that Gabriel should know his mother was there, and was alive. I felt he was my friend.

So now the court case was over with, I felt there was a new battle! It was against the health-care professionnals who were saying they would keep Gabriel from me should I get ill. I felt I really hated Simon Mason!

In March I had further talks with Walter and Netta Waterston, in order to hammer out a better agreement. Walter said how "Gabriel should know from day one where his mummy was"; it was mishandled the previous year. I voiced my opinion that Walter is closer to Gabriel than Elizabeth and Helen these days, as they are showing no interest in him. Netta Waterston hammered out a new agreement. Where it said "the clinical team should decide", she added that Gabriel should know where his mummy was. Where it said about taking things out of the house, she added it had to be a list of essential items. Where it said Elizabeth or Helen should have the home-base, she changed the order of preference putting Walter first.

Meantime the new senior social worker, Susan Cameron, insisted on having a meeting in order to "iron out the problems," and this took place in Dr.James' room. This was really because I was refusing to see Simon Mason. We pointed out the thorny crux of the thing being "the clinical team deciding the frequency of visits." Gabriel from the beginning should be visiting me. And they backed down and just agreed with us. I agreed to try working with Simon Mason.

Spring was coming and Walter and I had a nice time, walking among the daffodils in the spring sunshine, taking Gabriel on trips to places. *For a short while we were happy together, and I felt I had transcended the anguish, pain and rage of Gabriel's birth. But it didn't last long.*

Arguments soon resurged over the birth-certificate. Walter said he wanted me to pay the £7 to get a new extract of the new birth-certificate, saying "the other one will be null and void." Now I didn't want to give up the old one; I felt I had been forced into this. We had an argument about it. I felt I ought to accept the reality of the father's name on the certificate; I was trying to say Yes to reality, but it was like embracing a great pain.

About that time Walter started annoying me; he wouldn't leave when I wanted him to, and he made long sticky farewells. I felt he was encroaching too far into our lives. He was always wanting more and more time. I started feeling as coerced and bullied as ever, trying to steer round his bad moods. I finally felt I couldn't tolerate him any longer.

Then in May he turned nasty, threatening me on the phone. So we went back to another Conciliation meeting with Netta Waterston. This was a meeting of emotional nastiness. He said he wasn't happy

119

with the way I looked after Gabriel. He claimed he had to have a mid-week Access or it was "cruelty to Gabriel". I thought it ridiculous that he was demanding more than we had agreed after only four months. When Netta Waterston made it clear that he didn't have the right to a mid-week session, *he came out with the ultimate threat: "I'm taking it back to court, to apply for joint Custody!"*

I was horrified, and dashed away, overcome with anguish. I felt "I can't go through the pain of another court case; he's going to threaten that every time he doesn't get what he wants!" I was suffering the next day as I called on my solicitor; he said Walter could only apply for custody if he could prove I was an unfit mother; but he said Walter should be allowed five hours mid-week during vacations. I cancelled the change in the birth certificate.

We were waylaid on the way to Nursery by Walter, and he was threatening and bullying; he said if he didn't get what he wanted he would go back to court for Custody. So we had another Conciliation meeting. I said how "bullying tactics" wouldn't work, but how I was trying to be fair and keep agreements. I pointed out that if he took it back to court Gabriel would suffer too; "we need to go back to being friendly." Walter gave in and became emotional; he burst into tears. I said "you are daft," feeling sorry for him.

The birth certificate was a problem for me. When I got a re-registration form again from the Registrar's office, I came away saying "I don't want to alter my child's birth certificate." I came along the street saying "No, No, No!" *I felt I was being forced into it; "he could take me back to court anytime he likes, but altering the birth certificate is irrevocable!"*

I was determined to seek out a psycho-analyst, in order to sort out my feelings about Walter. We had yet another Conciliation meeting, in which we successfully got an agreement; Walter should have a minimum time every Wednesday, as well as the stipulated Saturday, and he would give me more time over the birth-certificate. We also agreed time in lieu for when we went on holiday.

At the beginning of July I took Gabriel for a holiday at Abbotsford Abbey, a Cistercian monastery in the country-side south of Edinburgh. When we came back from there we went on lots of summer day trips. I liked taking Gabriel places, showing him things and teaching him things. He was my companion.

And I hated Walter taking him away! I was convinced "it is a punishment for my sin in conceiving Gabriel." I was far from solving my own bitter feelings about it! My feelings were all to do with the conception being wrong. I thought how lovely it would have been, to conceive Peter's child; because I really loved him! "And if you conceive a child in love it is not immoral. The worst case is one like mine."

Chapter 27
A Sense of Liberation.

I was then liberated from all my torment with Walter by a visit to Rachel in Cairndale, in the mountains of Argyllshire, at the end of July, which was refreshingly beautiful. There I had an experience of self-transcendence.

I was pondering at Rachel's how wrong Gabriel's conception was. I wrote to Paul Thompson: *"Gabriel was born out of my fear, and my attempts to make life tolerable, rather than out of love; it dawns upon me how intensely wrong was what I did!"* Up until then I had always protested my innocence. Then Rachel's mother said to me: "you know the Lord has a special love for those in your position; he would love you more than anyone else in the room." I thought that was a lovely thing to say! And my thinking shifted on the issue. I used to think that I was innocent and God was unjustly punishing me; *now I thought how I was culpable of a great immoral deed, and I paid the penalty in terms of Karma, and God could still love me; God loved me especially, and I could redeem the thing by the way I loved my child.*

When Christ encountered the man who was deaf and dumb, and sang the words "Be opened," the greenness of the grass seemed to speak to him, and the sky turned a deeper blue; he felt the concourse of life flowing through him and outside of him as well; he knew he could communicate, was meant to communicate, and he could hear and speak clearly. It was like a door opened to him, a secret impediment in his being, flung open wide.

As soon as I arrived back Walter upset me at the handover, claiming that I'd upset Gabriel be "depriving him of his Daddy." *And I made the decision that day; "I'm cutting you out of our lives; you get nothing but what the law decrees."* I decided I wasn't struggling and wasting my life trying to painfully relate to Walter any longer. I transcended the old paradigm. I decided I'd just be clinical about it. And I decided to refuse to sign the birth certificate; "you are not the father according to the moral law of the universe."

I realised that the Conciliation service had been a great con-trick. I read through all the documents, and realised how sly Walter had been. *I decided to renege on all the agreements made by the Conciliation service. I felt I was enlightened about it all, and as if I were shedding skins. I felt as if I were "flowing with the river," accepting reality, resting in the law.*

I arranged a meeting with Walter and Netta Waterston, at which I was cool, calm and unemotional. I told him Walter it was the end of our relationship, and I told him he got what the law decreed and nothing else, and I told him all arrangements made with the Conciliation service were cancelled. Walter turned nasty and made threats, saying "I'll fight you to the last stand." But I felt he was a small mean man, like a wriggling worm beneath my feet; it was a triumphant day for me.

Walter accosted us along the street at the Llammas Fair. I said to him "you know as well as I do that you are not supposed to accost us along the street." He shouted at me "Nothing on earth shall ever stop me from recognizing my son!"

Meanwhile I had arguments with Simon Mason about my desire to destroy that modified agreement we had made about care for Gabriel should I get ill; I no longer wanted care to go to Walter. Simon Mason refused to destroy it at first, but he finally agreed that it was up to me to make any adequate arrangement I chose. So I altered the document to put back Elizabeth and Helen as the prime carers. I felt this was "one in the eye" for Walter.

Chapter 28
Accusations of Abuse.

Meanwhile Nursery began again. *Then on the 9ᵗʰ October 1990 Gabriel said things which seemed to imply that he had been involved in sexual abuse with Walter.* I made the allegations to the social workers, and an investigation was carried out, and I changed my solicitor to one who would fight for me, but it all came to nought.

What did Gabriel say which implied that he had been involved in sexual abuse? He said to me one night "I want to see Wally McKay; I've been a naughty boy." When I asked what he had done he said he had been playing with his "willy"; "I play with my willy and he gets all big, he gets all big; so can I see Wally?" It seemed to me to imply he was involved in sexual abuse; I was horrified and mortified.

I reported it to all the professionals, - Mrs.Bloomfield, Mrs.Sanderson, Simon Mason, Philip, Ted, Dr.James; they were all very kind and sympathetic, and they agreed that I couldn't allow my child to go somewhere where he was going to be abused. Gabriel had been complaining of a tummy-ache for ages, and I thought this was a possible explanation for it; apparently children complain of tummy-ache when they are abused. I felt disgusted and nauseated by the thought; knowing what Walter was like and how "sexual" he is, I believed that he was capable of sexually abusing a child.

After I had reported it to the social workers, they reported it to the police, who said they would have to carry out a criminal investigation. Accordingly Gabriel was interrogated by a police-woman called Beverly. When she talked to Gabriel, he said that he had a "sore willy"; and when asked who had made it sore he said "Wally did it." Despite this the police-woman said there was not enough evidence to take the matter to a criminal court; it could only be dealt with by the civil courts.

After the police-woman left, whilst I was bathing Gabriel, he said something else which seemed to indicate abuse. He said "mummy Wally scratched me." And when I asked where he was scratched, he said "here on my tum-tum," holding onto his scrotum. I was upset and enraged; Philip on the phone said I was right to be upset at the thought of Walter "nankipooing around" with my son. I decided that I would fight the issue, and refuse to give Gabriel up for access to the man.

When I went to see my solicitor Mr.Sutton, I ended up very cross with him, because he refused to fight. He was all "sweetness and light," but he said there wasn't enough evidence, and he just didn't seem to care. He went on about the "father's access rights" being protected, and having to continue these "supervised" till the child was older. I responded angrily "If he can abuse a little child he has lost all his father's rights!" My reaction was to change my solicitor! I chose Catriona McVeigh in Invertay, who was recommended to me by a friend of mine, as someone who would fight on my behalf.

When I phoned Catriona McVeigh she said she would take it on, so on the 1st November I went to see her in Invertay. I was thrilled by her, because she had conviction and passion. She said "I take the view that he has been abused," and told me how we could proceed. She said Walter couldn't have Access until the investigation was finished. I came out really happy, filled with a sense of hope.

On the 16th November there was a case conference, at which a lot of professionals were present. I said how I was convinced that abuse had taken place, and the reasons why; I said how I was abused when living with Walter. I argued that it would be helpful to my solicitor if they would put Gabriel on the "At Risk Register." I argued very eloquently, saying "If you are not helpful, how can I be expected to hand my child over to a man I'm convinced is sexually abusing him? If you don't help I'll have to move house and leave everyone I know behind, and go and live in limbo-land." Mrs.Sanderson from the nursery helped by saying how Gabriel had come out of his shell since Access had stopped. They made the decision that if the court should decide Access should continue, Gabriel would be put on the "At Risk Regsiter". Catriona McVeigh said this was the best result we could get.

It was at this stage, because Access was stopped, that Walter started accosting us along the street. In particular there was a frightening incident, when we were coming home in the dark from the nursery, in which he cruised beside us in his car, and then leapt out and took hold of Gabriel. I was distressed by this, and we had as witnesses two girls from the nursery who helped. Soon after Walter and his sister tried to kidnap Gabriel from the nursery. He kept cruising around the streets in his car, following us and frightening us. One day they came to the house, demanding "we've come for Gabriel." When I phoned the police, they told me that if Walter abducted his own son, it wouldn't be a criminal offence. And they said they could do nothing without an "Interdict." But Catriona McVeigh said she couldn't get us an interdict, as it "wasn't a competent court procedure." I felt under threat, and had a sense that the law was inadequate to help us.

Catriona McVeigh then phoned me one day to say Walter had claimed on a court document "she has had lots of sexual relationships with the many men who have come to her house." I was horrified, and replied to her that I had no relationships with any men since Gabriel's birth, when I had taken a vow of celibacy. I got very emotional about this; Walter was "fighting dirty."

There was a court hearing on the 5th December. Catriona McVeigh phoned me with the result; there was going to be a full "proof" on the 21st March, and there need be no Access up until then; it was accepted that nothing would happen if I didn't allow Access. Meantime someone called Joan McAdams was going to interview Gabriel and investigate.

Christmas day arrived, and Walter came to the door. I opened the door and let him in. This was partly because I had had a religious experience the night before, which made me generous, and partly because I felt sorry for the man. "Seeing it's Christmas day you can come in, provided you only stay ten minutes." He said "I'm innocent Mairi; I don't know how you can believe I could do such a thing." He came again on Boxing day, with a meek and sad face. I said to him that if he would stop accosting us along the street, I'd allow some kind of supervised Access between then and the 21st March.

However as he started coming to the door at the beginning of January, I began to feel he was unwelcome; "give him an inch and he takes a mile" I thought. He kept saying he was innocent; I began to feel sorry for the whole sorry business. This was partly because Joan McAdams meantime, who had several interviews with Gabriel, said she could find no evidence of sexual abuse. Catriona McVeigh warned me that without the evidence there was a good chance that the sheriff would restore Access.

On the 26th January I had along deep moving talk with Walter. We agreed that everybody had over-reacted about allegations of abuse. I said how I had been convinced of sexual abuse, but I wasn't any longer. I said how now I was "in a more accepting state of mind." Walter was moved to cry. I realised that the law had nothing to do with the human situation. I told him I intended dropping the court case.

After that I told Simon Mason I wanted to close the court case; I wanted to "lay it down". And I went to see Catriona McVeigh in Invertay, and she agreed to "cist" the court action, which would mean bringing it to a close. She said I should see what I could do by conciliation again.

Accordingly we had a Conciliation service meeting in St.John's centre on the 11th February. I felt I really suffered in that meeting. Beforehand I had thought "I don't want a relationship with that man"; but I realised I had to go ahead with it. In that meeting Walter was like a spouting firework of venom and bitterness and anger. He went on about Gabriel suffering from not seeing him. I said I was willing to restore the Access; I offered two hours of unsupervised Access straightaway , to increase to five hours by Easter. But he wanted five hours immediately, plus "a declaration of the vindication of his innocence." He wanted a public declaration of his innocence in court. We were urged to come to an agreement, as otherwise the meeting would be in vain; Walter suddenly accepted what I offered. He had been spouting like an ogre with hatred in his eyes; I felt miserably how Gabriel had to go between this ogre and my own loving heart. But the meeting produced a catharsis of feeling, and I felt sympathy for him, when he gave me a lift in his car in the snow afterwards.

Chapter 29
An Incipient Idea.

And so the court action was stopped and Access was resumed. However when Access started again, it again had such a detrimental effect upon Gabriel that he began whining and having tummy aches. It seemed to me that he was forced to see his father in a way that made him ill. I was awfully tired of looking after this 4-year-old child!

On the 13th February I was in a black mood; I suffered a raging pain in my mind that was analogous to an unbearable toothache; "I can't continue to look after him when his father makes him ill; I can't tolerate it; I can't hand him over and still love him; the only was I can do it is to cease to care about him." *I was going beserk with pain as the idea struck me from the dark depths; "I will get him adopted; then he will be out of this situation; then he might be happy and thrive."* I even transiently thought "it would be best if he died."

I talked with Mrs.Bloomfield earnestly about these thoughts the next morning. She told me I mustn't try and be free from my responsibility of looking after Gabriel; everyone thought I was being a very good mother; the pain I was suffering was part of "the pain of parenting." She said it was up to me to help the child to cope with the Access. A friend called Jan also helped by saying "he needs love from you, he turns to his mummy for love." I reflected to myself that "love and suffering go together."

But the idea of adoption now took root in my mind. I talked with Vivien about it because she had encouraged it when Gabriel was new-born. *She made the point that Gabriel was going to be hurt, harmed, torn apart, by the situation between myself and Walter all the time he was growing up; now out of love for him I had to take him out of the situation; I must "sacrifice" him.* She told me it would be "liberating" for all three of us. I agreed that I could see this would be a deep clean wound which would heal, as opposed to a long-term festering wound. Vivien averred that the upset to Gabriel would be a "healing thing."

When I phoned Philip, and Paul, and my Dad, to my surprise they were all in agreement that adoption was for the best for the child, although I had to make sure that I was doing it "for the right reason." And I also wrote to Pater Leo, saying how I could not continue like this; *it seemed a "pure white shining reason," to lift Gabriel out of the situation. It was time to let go of Gabriel now, I said, to save him from suffering and to make him well; a sacrifice had to be made, although the pain of my motherly feelings on giving up my son would be acute.*

I realised this was "mother's pain", our Lady's pain, that lies at the heart of the universe, - the anguish of the sacrifice of giving up one's son. It was a pain which began to make me feel wretched. I did not know at the time that it would leave me on the edge of insanity for many years.

But the idea of adoption, though fierce and full of conviction at first, began to strike with a terrible pain deep at the heart of me as I realised its painful self-sacrificial nature. My friend Vivien had been prescribing for me "the highest reaches of self-sacrifice that were found in motherhood." But what dawned on me was the regret that would remain with me the rest of my life. I believed it was the best thing I could do, - this pure white shining thing of lifting my child out of the situation which was so distressing him and making him ill, but that didn't mean to say I could do it. My child was my "companion"; I couldn't have borne such a cruel blow as to permanently sunder him from me. So my thoughts provided a reason for rejecting the idea: –

"How can I "save" this little child? Perhaps that's the point; perhaps I can't." I talked earnestly with his nursery teacher Mrs.Sanderson: "We can't know what the future holds. It is for God to totally save Gabriel, not for me. It is God's domain. I can do what I think best for Gabriel, but I can't totally save him; that is for God to do." I realised in my heart of hearts that I couldn't know which suffering would be "pernicious" for Gabriel; *"Why can it not be true that this suffering will be for Gabriel's "salvation" as I believe it is for mine? Who can say which suffering is pernicious and which for our salvation? Love and suffering lie together at the heart of the universe."*

Chapter 30
New Struggles and New Faces.

Having thought like this, having had the incipient idea of Adoption and then rejecting it as too painful, I found a state of mind which was like "acceptance," which I thought must be on the right road. And then my Mum on the phone confirmed me in this opinion by what she said; " He is your responsibility; you brought him into the world, so you are responsible for him till he is old enough to look after himself."

She imparted an even deeper wisdom the following day, after I became "hopping mad" by another example of Walter's meanness. "Make your mind up that Walter is not going to affect you," she said, "you mustn't get in a mood and pass it on to Gabriel; *Gabriel needs to see you as his best friend, he needs to be able to rely on you." And then an amazing thing happened that evening; Gabriel sat on my knee, kissed me and said the words "I love you very much mummy; you are my best friend." I was stunned by this, and promised myself that I'd strive to be a reliable "best friend" for my son.*

Then there was another case-conference at the end of February, in which Dr.James pointed out that Gabriel was certainly "going through a bad patch," due to seeing his father, whether directly or indirectly; he said it was clear that he was suffering. He said he had referred us to the child psychiatrist Dr.McSharry, hoping that in such a way we would get ammunition for the courts, if she affirmed that the access visits were detrimental to the child. It was also agreed that I would have a new social worker; I welcomed what was called this new "therapeutic input."

Meantime I was still finding it difficult not to get "hopping mad" at Walter's continual meanness. There was an occasion when he brought Gabriel back half an hour late, and said for excuse "he was eating his yoghurt." He was perpetually exasperating me. Philip put his finger on the cause of it when he said, "you feel he ought to pay for what he has done to you; he owes you for exploiting you; and when he's at his meanest, it raises all these feelings." Then one evening, just when the Gulf War gave way to "Peace", I had a deep talk with Walter, and he seemed to welcome the "therapeutic input," and I felt forgiving toward him, and felt there could be "peace" in my life. I realised for a few fleeting days that if this peace between us were not maintained, I could not have happiness.

Dr.James saw Gabriel about his tummy-aches, and we agreed that "even though it may be psychosomatic that does not mean the pain is any the less real"; he talked of "disfunction of the gut" and wondered whether to send him for tests to Strathwells. The next day I heard the good news that the new social worker I was going to get would be a child-care social worker called Steven Peterson.

It was about this time that I argued with Dr.McNeill that I wanted to stop my medication regime which was "prophylactic treatment." I said I wanted to return to my "natural normal self," able to return to my normal weight, able to have periods, and able to feel more mental awareness instead of struggling with sleepiness. I felt that my body was "frozen and unnatural". He replied that I obviously did not remember what I was like when I was ill, and refused to allow me to relax my drug-regime. (I think it was because I did indeed relax my drugs-regime that I became ill in July.)

I had another argument with Walter about shoes from the Clark's shop, that I'd put aside for Gabriel, which I wanted him to collect. And he refused to collect them and pay for them without myself and Gabriel accompanying him. And I felt how he just wanted to "get me involved"; how he wanted to go together "like mummy and daddy taking baby bear to the shop for some shoes." I really felt I hated him; I thought him "a frisky, encourageable, unruly, appetite-laden, uncontrollable goat."

On Mother's day I had a painful experience with Gabriel which really taught me a lesson. He got his fresh best trousers and newly polished shoes muddied in the middle of a field, with the result that I lost my temper with him and compelled him to go home. He cried out "Mummy please don't be cross; you're supposed to be my best friend," which made me rueful. Then in the evening, when I said I was sorry to him for always being cross, he yelled at me "you're not my best friend any more; you can't be my best friend ever again; you're not my best friend." I felt mortified that he should say this to me, on Mother's day of all days! But we made up again at his bedtime, *and I learnt from it that I had to see Gabriel as a soul-over-against me, whose respect and friendship I needed to earn.*

My first meeting with Dr.McSharry, the child-psychiatrist, went wonderfully well. She asked me a lot of painful and uncomfortable questions, about how I felt about Walter's fatherhood; I found myself bitterly averring that there's more to fatherhood than having trips to the park and being called "daddy." I said how the "child-care" was about the washing, the feeding, the clothes, the money, and the long screaming nights. Yet I was very pleased by the way Dr.McSharry said "the child has rights too." She repeated to me, professionally, what I had so long been arguing; ie. the father's rights should not have priority over the child's well-being. She said the evidence we were looking for was the child's emotional discomfort, and that we have to alter access so that the child became comfortable; supervised access was what she suggested. I was delighted, and thrilled with hope.

About this time I became friendly with a young man called Ben, and began doing decorating and home-improvements with him. When I next saw Dr.McSharry I explained to her how this "new fresh relationship" was doing me the power of good, and how I wasn't so "tied in a deathly knot" when this third person allowed feelings to flow and circulate. I waxed lyrical about the mystery of the "Holy Trinity," and was chuffed when Dr.McSharry said I had "a way with words."

Steven Peterson, our lovely new social worker, then stepped into our lives. My first response was to think that he had lovely gentle sparkling eyes and, as I told my Mum, "he looks like Jesus." When I said how Gabriel deliberately hurt me and did things to annoy me, he said "how do you want him to express his anger toward you?" and I didn't know what to make of the question. But I had hopes of the man, and believed he could help. However, the second time I met him I decided I didn't like the way he operated; he encouraged me to talk by asking questions, and then judged, dissected and criticized what I said. He kept applying "theory" to my problems with Gabriel, repeatedly saying "half the blame is yours." The man just didn't seem to be "on my side", and my net reaction to him was one of unease and dislike.

On Good Friday, whilst seeing a passion play, there fell into my mind some very intense unloving thoughts about Gabriel. "Let's scrap Gabriel, give him for adoption, and start again." I meant start again from marriage with Ben, doing away with this "ghastly mistake" of Walter and Gabriel. I realised that deep down there was something wrong in my life, which showed in anger toward my child. "I suppose the problem is that I haven't been able to love him." And that was due to the fact that I'd been unable "to accept and love his father's part in him." I thought how I'd just concentrate on trying to make him into a monk or a priest, as if that would exonerate me. "He is the cross I bear" I said to myself. I realised how I couldn't really love him because he was not a love-child.

On Easter Saturday there happened a horrible, violent experience with Walter. He brought Gabriel back carrying a trumpet. "I don't want you to leave that with him" I said, aware of the way its noise would annoy me. Walter replied "you are not considering his feelings," and we argued. And whilst we argued Gabriel broke off the end of the trumpet as he knocked it on the door. "How dare you break his trumpet!" erupted Walter, leaping in at the door. I was alarmed at his violence and said firmly "Please get out of my house." He yelled "I'm taking him away from you, I'm taking him right now." The adrenalin flowed through me and I screamed back "Get out of my house," launching myself at him and pushing him out of the door and slamming it shut. I was trembling after this, and Gabriel said something in childish emotion, taking Walter's part; "You pushed my daddy out of the door; poor daddy; don't you do that to my daddy ever again." It really broke my heart.

And so I had a horrible Easter, feeling that Walter was progressively taking Gabriel away from me, and miserable at the same time because I broke up with Ben. I felt mixed up in my feelings towards Gabriel, because of what Walter did to my emotions. I went through a real roller-coaster of a ride in my emotions towards my child, at one moment saying "let's scrap him" and in the next "I must be devoted to him." Sometimes I just wanted him out of my sight because of the emotions he caused. Then we went on another holiday to visit my friend Rachel in Argyllshire, and I came back able to handle my daily life with Gabriel much better, allowing him the freedom to switch on everything the way he liked. And, having met Walter in the local shop, I found I could handle him better too. So I felt I had transcended myself, transcended my sore emotions, for a time at least. I told Steven Peterson of my improved child-care techniques, and I related to him well and he was pleased for me.

But a few days later all the negative emotion welled up again. I had to see Dr.McSharry, and then I was shown out to where Walter and Gabriel were waiting to see her. As I sat outside the door I could hear Gabriel whining "I want to go out to my mummy" and "I want to go home." But when I took Gabriel home I found him very upset, like a wild animal, trying to bite me. When I tried to find out what was wrong he told me that his Daddy had upset him; "he made me cry". He told me as explanation "it was because I threw his hankie in the water." He had apparently thrown Walter's hankie in the burn in the swing park, and he had shouted at him and made him cry all the way home. I was upset, having said to Dr.McSharry that I hoped Walter wouldn't take his foul temper out on the child. *Having suffered so much living with him, I felt how unendurable was the fact of having the same vile temper now inflicted upon my child.*

Chapter 31
Fighting for Change.

*On the 12th April "something wonderful and lovely" happened;
Dr.James and Dr.McSharry came round together to visit me, and,
seeing how distressed both Gabriel and I were, they agreed that
changes must be made,* and they said these changes could be made
on the their authority. Two things should be effected: a system of
shared care or childminding should be set up, so as to relieve me and
take some stress off me; and secondly it would be officially arranged
for a go-between, so that I should have no further contact with Walter.
They considered this essential for the sake of my mental health and
stability, and therefore of Gabriel's welfare. *I was delighted that at last
someone was listening to me, at last something was going to be done
about it. A sense of great relief came over me; I had hopes that this
day was going to transform all of my life in the future.*

The very next day, as if to prove that such relief was necessary, I
became terribly upset again, as it was made clear that this theory
wasn't going to work in practise. Walter's sister came to the door
supposedly to be the third party to see to the handover, but instead of
coming instead of Walter, she came as well as Walter. I felt so
threatened by the two of them as they came up the path together,
demanding "bring him here." I slammed the door shut, saying this
wasn't "acceptable", but they rang the bell insistently, and Gabriel
became distressed. Then, feeling awful, but obliged to do this
"handover," I opened the door and handed Gabriel over to the sister
when I saw that Walter had retreated to his car. After that I was on the
phone emotionally to people, saying how Walter made it clear that he
wanted to get at me, to confront me, rather than have a third-party
hand-over of his child. I was aware miserably how once more Gabriel
bore the brunt of the suffering.

*But I still hoped that happiness and a calmer existence awaited me, if
only it could be arranged that I should have no further contact with
Walter.* When Dr.James came to visit he agreed that "he's obviously
trying to get at you." I said how it was supposedly solved two years
ago; he claimed he just wanted to "see him," to see his son; that there
should be so much trouble proved that this was not the case; he
wanted to get at me through the child. I told Dr.James that I didn't know
how much suffering I was letting myself in for when I left the man on
New Year's eve '85! He remembered it well.

I had a horrible day at the end of April, when my solicitor ditched me, and my social worker left me in the lurch as regards helping with handovers. My solicitor refused to act for me any longer, being fed up of my tales of harassments and need of interdicts; she said on the phone "I don't want to deal with this." She was all very eager to take on the case when it was a matter of "sexual abuse," but thought it trivial when it had descended to the present level of daily torment. I sat down benumbed by the news. And then, making a phone-call to Steven Peterson when he didn't turn up as expected, I was taken aback when he said he couldn't arrange for social workers to do hand-overs and get involved with Access, as Dr. James and Dr.McSharry had averred, and especially not on a Saturday. I was taken aback and quite benumbed at the news; all my hopes seemed dashed. I was so upset that I cried.

That Saturday I found relief by asking my friend Helen to see to the hand-over, myself going for a walk along the West Sands. I was distressed though by Gabriel saying he didn't want to go to Walter because "he might be nasty." On the following Monday I had painful experiences with both Steven Peterson and Dr.McSharry, because of their probing questioning. Steven watched Gabriel's behaviour and the way he lapsed into his squeaky mousie voice, and claimed that he was being "messed up" by his two parents. I pointed out that it was Walter who was the aggressor who sought confrontation. He told me "you can cope." *But I couldn't cope; I felt I was permanently on the brink of a mental breakdown.* When I asked what he was prepared to do for me, I found it was very little. He dismissed my "stress-related mental illness," which the doctors claimed made some relief for me essential, and said he would only apply for help for me on the grounds of being a single parent. I made the suggestion Philip had made to me, that perhaps if I myself found a child-minder to see to hand-overs, the social work department would fund it; he said that sounded possible, but I felt despair as the man left.

And then Dr.McSharry rubbed in more pain. I said to her how Steven Peterson had said I could cope and my illness wasn't relevant, and had put the onus upon me for finding the child-minder; and she said back in a way which non-plussed me, "what makes you so incapable of doing practical things?" She then asked Gabriel "do you like going with you daddy? Does he sometimes get cross?" And to my horror he replied "my mummy sometimes gets awful cross." She could see before her very eyes some of the difficulty between us; Gabriel gave me hugs which always ended up in his hurting me. And I explained how if in any way he got hurt, he turned on me saying "you hurt me" and tried to bite me. She said this was unusual, and then pronounced the following; all the child's insecurity, rage, confusion and frustration, which came out in this behaviour, are all caused because he experienced me in my rage. She said something had got to be done or he wouldn't grow up emotionally healthy, and our relationship was far too intense. I felt she then sent us off to cope on our own, whilst she went on holiday; *I sat on a swing feeling pained and miserable, thinking "just my luck to have a child with a behaviour problem," but aware that I had to take on the responsibility of loving him.*

At the end of April I went to see my new solicitor in the form of Angus Gourlay; my friend Agnes, herself a solicitor, had recommended him to me. I told him the whole story of my harassment from Walter, and asked him of the possibility of obtaining an interdict; I believed Walter would take heed of the law of the land if I obtained an interdict forbidding him to approach me. His sympathetic reply was, "you've had a lot of hassle from this man for a long time, haven't you?" I replied a simple and earnest "Yes". He agreed to act for me, and invited me to fill in legal aid forms, with the result that I felt the meeting a complete success; it seemed that he was sympathetic and understanding and believed in my cause.

Also at the end of April I managed to find a child-minder who would work on Saturday morning, from the list of child-minders presented to me by Steven Peterson. Steven had told me that this, paid for by the social work department, could only be a temporary and short-term arrangement. I went out to Fernhill to visit her, and thought her nice; I explained to her the whole situation and she seemed happy with it. However the next day Steven made me cross by his attitude toward it; he said he wanted to negotiate with her to knock the price down, and asked me how much I was prepared to contribute; he also intimated that it would only be for two months. I felt frustrated with the man. *However, as the arrangement began to work, and I wasn't confronted any more by the enraged Walter, I became happier and more balanced. Things started going better.*

However this didn't last long, before Walter deliberately sabotaged the arrangement. When I arrived at the childminders one day, to collect Gabriel, I was horrified to see Walter's car at the door, and I saw him in the child-minders house, remonstrating with the woman. The child-minder told me how he had said to her "I am not leaving Gabriel with you until Mairi comes back," and she was so alarmed that she called the duty social worker to defuse the situation. I was upset, and didn't want an emotional scene in front of Gabriel, so I left him in the house, whilst I went out to the car where Walter was still remonstrating with

136

this social worker, and said "you are distressing the child-minder whom I have employed; would you mind leaving the premises?" And I also said "You've done this deliberately, to get a confrontation with me." I was awfully embarrassed when I went back to the child-minder, because I felt that this had caused her so much hassle that she wouldn't want to do it again; I thought what Walter had done to her was disgusting. When I got home, after dealing with a very upset Gabriel, *I felt how this "nauseating little man" seemed to have power over me, power to wreck my life, in a never-ending way.*

The System cannot know the God which surrounds it, for its puny might of self locked Love out, afraid of the Time-span which comes upon men suddenly, afraid of the Creativity, and of the dark Void.

Chapter 32
Despair and Agony.

In a despairing fashion at the end of May I felt my troubles were never-ending. Walter could sabotage all the efforts I could make to improve my life, and to live a life without being tormented by him. I appealed to Dr.James and Steven Peterson and my new solicitor Angus Gourlay to do something about Walter's behaviour, but it became clear on discussing it with them that there was little they could do. Angus Gourlay wrote a letter to Walter's solicitor on his dictaphone about that Saturday's incident, but he confided in me that it didn't really jeopardise the Access. I tried to be positive, thinking how life had generally improved for us and how the Spring was here.

And then I had bad news that the child-minder refused to offer us the help anymore, because dealing with Walter was too much hassle. I felt closed in. I began to get very angry with Gabriel for petty reasons. I became aware that I was taking it out on Gabriel, because I was subconsciously aware that he was a "little bit" of Walter and therefore I couldn't tolerate him. When I told this to Dr.McSharry she said I needed "a break," so she arranged for Helen to look after Gabriel for a few days.

Meanwhile I was having more difficulty with the social work department. I had found another childminder, but they had talked to her behind my back, with the result that she declined to do it. Steven Peterson, together with his superior, didn't appear when they were supposed to, and I was hurt when this superior said to me on the phone, "there are children in the country being abused; you and your son are not important, and you can wait!" I was upset that these childcare social workers, unlike the Craigdene social workers, were taking no cognizance at all of my mental health; they didn't seem to realize that my illness made me vulnerable to stress. *I was finding I really couldn't handle this 4-year-old child with the stress that Walter was putting me under; but they took no notice.*

I began to feel complete despair, as I saw that the "wonderful idea" of keeping Walter out of my life wasn't going to work. And then the social workers approached me, saying that their work with me was "done," and they would have no further involvment with me after 6 weeks; they said the arrangement with Walter and childminders was "the parents responsibility." I was shocked, as they hadn't effected anything; I thought they were pathetic and useless people.

And then Nicholas Lawson, Vivien's husband, stepped in to help with the handover. But on the Saturday that all came to nought. When I arrived to collect Gabriel, Walter's car was outside the house; I waited twenty minutes before I became angry and emotional enough to risk confrontation by knocking on the door. Finally I did so, and Nicholas handed over Gabriel to me, saying he was having a talk with Walter. I was hopping mad, feeling this was really "treacherous". I took Gabriel home seething with emotion, and when he said "mummy please don't be cross with my daddy," something in me snapped. I yelled "he is not your daddy; can't you get that through your thick head; don't you ever use that word again in my house!" *I was so full of violent emotion. I recognized how my emotions sprang from a wound in my being.*

The 30th of May was a very painful day, as Steven Peterson reported to me what Walter had said when the social workers had a meeting with him. He had claimed that I was "not a fit mother," and that I was making Gabriel into "an emotionally disturbed child." He claimed that I was damaging Gabriel because I was saying bad things about himself, turning the child against his father. The social workers had insisted that the damage to Gabriel by his two warring parents was a "shared responsibility." Walter had apparently raved on about me being to blame, and said he wanted a "written declaration" from me to say I wouldn't stop Gabriel from calling him "daddy". I was of course upset by all of this; and then Steven said I could help Gabriel as he grows up by giving him "a reasonable interpretation of his father." *At this point something in me snapped, and a great cry of "No" rose up inside of me. Lots of painful memories came to the fore, in particular the way I'd said to Walter "you could only be the child's father if you were my husband, and you were not." The thought surged up in me; "As far as I am concerned, truly, and in the sight of heaven and hell, as well as human law, he is not my child's father!"* Steven was surprised that he seemed to have silenced me; I replied "you have just touched some sensitive raw nerves."

The next day I was justifying things to myself; I said to myself how I did not say "nasty things" about his Dad to Gabriel; I just said nothing; the only thing I did was to take Gabriel to task for calling Walter his "daddy", because I believed he wasn't a daddy in any right meaning of the word; far from being a genuine father he was "an usurper." Meanwhile the storm-clouds were gathering about Gabriel's birthday on the 5th June, about how long Walter was to see him, and whether he should hand in birthday presents to him, or keep them for use at his own house. Walter was beginning to make a great fuss over the issue. However I wrote a letter to say how Walter should keep the child's bike for use on the Saturdays, as I was giving him a scooter. So in the event Gabriel's 5th birthday passed by unmarred.

Gabriel sometimes came back very upset by Walter. One day he said how Walter had said to him "I want to have my son." And he had apparently replied "No you can't have your son because he belongs to mummy." He came back deeply distressed by this, repeating "Daddy was nasty to me." And I busily reported this to all my friends, as proof of Walter's possessiveness, and as proof that he was "directly distressing" Gabriel. This war went on endlessly, with no end in sight. Dr.McSharry said that I should encourage Gabriel to tell me these things and herself these things, so that "a picture could be built up." I told Dr.McSharry how my solicitor-friend Agnes said how really the child has no right of influence in the matter until they are aged 8 or 9; this is awful as meantime it was a matter of "imposing the man on the child." She replied that it required "monitoring" over a long a period of time, and she herself wasn't prepared to do it.

On the 12th June I howled with pain, and cried for hours, when I received a letter from the solicitor which revealed Walter's bid to take my child away from me. I howled so badly I thought I was having a breakdown; I reached out to everyone who might help me, but when they failed, finally spoke on the phone to "good old Philip", who tried his best to comfort me. *The nub of my endless pain, which seemed to throw me in contact with a cosmic agony, was this; "I can't stand watching Walter take Gabriel slowly away from me."* The letter was like a declaration of intent; Walter's intention to take my child away from me. Because of my apparent grief my support-system kicked in and people came round to help me; first Dr Miller, whom my parents had phoned, then Mrs. Bloomfield, then the CPN's Mary Bellmore and Ted; none of them were much help, not understanding this "mother's pain" which was so afflicting me that I felt at the heart of some cosmic agony.

It was in writing to Pater Leo that I got to the heart of the matter. I wrote how I had been trying to accept this access as reasonable and controlled, and now Walter suddenly surges up in this uncontrolled, uncontrollable way, with his great lust, desire and greed, saying "I want all of him, I want half his waking life, I want to have him." I wrote how it causes me "endless mother's pain" and how "we ought to be able to limit our own pain." I meant "I have a right to say I am not capable of treading this path of pain laid before me;" I was screaming to Pater Leo across the miles for him to help me in my pain.

And then I contemplated on this pain, and thought how it was like some sharing in a cosmic agony, Christ's agony on the cross. Then I reflected on whether I had a right to limit that agony. Then I remembered deep within my soul how some special agony was demanded of me, how suffering was my vocation. I remembered how I had once averred "you must understand the suffering to understand the love." It dawned on me that some special agony is demanded of me because some special instruction in love is given to me. The worst pain known, -mother's pain- was inflicted upon me until I knew God's own agony, - the agony of love. I could understand that.

Chapter 33
A Vision of Freedom.

The following day, the 13th June, overwrought by the sense of suffering as I was, I really "lost it" with Gabriel; I practically beat him up. He had bitten me painfully on the thigh when I was on the phone, and I lost my patience with him, so I locked him up in his bedroom. And there he went on a rampage, tearing to bits the new poster I had put up for him of a little fawn, and taking the dried flowers from the vase at the window, and trampling them to bits on the floor. *When I went in and saw what he had done, I really "lost it"; I smacked him all over, I practically "beat him up". Then I slammed the door on him and locked it. I had never lost my temper with him like this before, and I don't think I have ever done so since.*

I then yelled to people down the phone "why didn't somebody help me?" When I finally got around to yelling at Philip, he told me very soberly that I was jeopardising everything and at risk of losing custody of my child; if the social workers thought he was "at risk" with me, they might remove him from me. At this sober thought I calmed down, and realised I'd better not let anyone know what really happened here. So when a GP came round, and then the social workers, I played it down, and pretended nothing serious had happened. It was horrible, because I realised that the trouble was, if I told no-one what happened, I wouldn't get helped. The social workers claimed I had said on the phone that I was "psychotic" and that I was intending to give Gabriel my psychiatric tablets, in order to "kill him off." I was horrified at this untruth, and did my best to fend them off. *I felt how useless this "support system" was, in that instead of helping they placed more stress upon me than ever by being a threat.*

Things eased off after that dreadful day; Helen kept taking Gabriel off my hands for a while. I was trying to come to terms with the fact that Walter was asking for so much more in the law-courts. I remembered how Walter used to say he "just wanted to see him"; and now he wanted "to have him, to possess him, to take him away from me." *The pain just stared me in the face, no matter what practical things I did. It just seemed that that the uncontrollable, which we had tried to control, would be out of all control in the future. I was trying to come to terms with enormous pain. It felt like God's flaming spear piercing my heart; the pain was ineluctably mine.*

After a few days I went to see my solicitor Angus Gourlay in Kirkcraig. We agreed how unreasonable were Walter's demands, especially the idea of residential access, of Gabriel staying overnight with him. Angus Gourlay said he thought Walter was being particularly difficult in order to make me upset. He composed another letter on his dictaphone, whilst I sat miserably; I tried to find out what would happen next but he gave me no clear idea. But he said the court could always vary the provision for access, making it more favourable to Walter. Whilst I sat miserably on the bus on the way home, with the rain pouring down the windows, an idea pieced me out of the blue with great pain; - *"I never gave my consent for this child to be conceived; therefore he is only half mine and brings suffering with him. I have locked myself into suffering by being so immoral."* Such misery and pain were mine, as I had this thought, looking at the landscape through a wet window.

I realised more about my pain a few days later. I realised that, after all the pain I went through to get away from the man, I still had to relate to Walter through my child. *And all that agony I went through, of being distressed by Walter whilst emotionally dependant on him, Gabriel would have to go through too. And I ached at the thought of it. It would happen all over again through my child. He would do it again to the child who was a part of me.* The pain of that for me was *"like a scream in eternity."*- -

I thought miserably how, if I had only known all this at the time of Gabriel's birth, I would not have kept him! I would have let him go for adoption far sooner than letting this be done to him; it was a big mistake! *I thought how I couldn't endure it because you want to save someone you love from the suffering you yourself have been through. How could I endure to "hand him over on platter" to be hurt and harmed!* But it was my own fault for being "one flesh" with the man!

At the end of June I took Gabriel for a holiday to Iona. It was a marvellous holiday which really set me free. At first I was bothered by Gabriel's babyishness and clinging to me and reversion to his old "poohs in the pants." But he was given his own "childcare worker" who looked after him whilst I could attend the thought-provoking sessions offered. And we quickly felt liberated from the stifling suffering of KirkMichaels. In my contemplation I began to wonder if being the mother of an unwanted child who brought me pain was indeed my vocation. I began to think it wasn't; if I had remained chaste my life would have been whole and I could have been there for other people, instead of expending myself on an unwanted child. I realised that my "vocation" was to remain childless. I began to realise that I was clinging to a home and material goods in KirkMichaels; I wished I could stay there on Iona. I made enquiries about staying on the island, but a window of opportunity did not present itself. The warden of the Centre told me that to try and live on Iona was a matter of trying to "run away from my pain." I disagreed with him; I felt that I could be set free. So I had a talk with the New Age character there whom Gabriel said "looked like Jesus with his dressing gown on"; he had long and flowing reddish locks, and wore a long multi-coloured robe with bare feet.

I asked this Jesus-looking character "Is it true that you can recognise the call of the voice of God by the fact that it requires you to leave behind all you cling to?" I explained that, though I felt the called to live on Iona and abandon my home in KirkMichaels, people were telling me to go home and "face my pain" there. He agreed and we agreed together that you cannot fail to recognize that "silver-toned voice", and that we are "free to change our own lives." *And I felt that night that I was set free to realise that I was free; I could say "I know the Way." It was a complete revelation for me. I had needed to go to that island to realise that I was free; I had known the Way to be set free. "The Way is to know that your soul, your innermost being, is free."*

"You became free when God touched the centre of your soul; always that centre remains free: always you know the way to it; it is through the Door found open on this island, and open in your own will. Keep touching that centre and you are free, able to change your life, transcend pain, to be a part of a world of becoming. You know this Way, you have hold of it in Me."

It was a vision of freedom. The night before I left, watching magnificent sunset-skies, I was aware of how the visionary power of the island could burst apart the smallness and selfishness of our lives. It was as if the holy spirit was gushing there. *So I felt I was no longer bound in pain by Walter in KirkMichaels. "I live under God free, and now that I am free I would not again be bound!" With this revelation residing in my heart, I travelled back from Iona.*

Chapter 34
The Cool Concept.

When she awoke the Coolness of the Concept was there; she could go outside the System, to find God in the Void. "Madness waits upon that path," she heard the whispering; but her own voice rose clear; "I desire God with precipitation, as He desires me."

"There is nothing but the System," said the System -Server; "beyond the System is only the Void." "You are wrong" she said, "for I have seen God; there is God in the Void." "It is your madness speaking."

And so I travelled back from Iona exhilarated and full of the conviction that my soul was free; but when I first glimpsed KirkMichaels I thought it a place of muddiness and sickness which would soon close around me.

The first day I was back I wrote letters to all my soul-friends speaking of what I'd realised on the island, and saying I felt called upon to leave behind my home of comfortable security in KirkMichaels in order to embrace a new life. But on ruminating about it, I saw there was a difference between interior freedom and the external reality; I could keep myself interiorly free by constant visits to Iona. I realised "all I need to do is to continue to realise that I am free." But quite rapidly the reality of KirkMichaels closed around me, when I had to go shopping and make visits to professionals like Dr.McNeill and Dr.McSharry. And very quickly I realised I couldn't give up the security of our home here. This was the reality confronting me, rather than just "dreaming". But it was more important to be liberated inwardly, than to physically leave behind my pain, and Walter, and my home. I had the realisation that I could be more free, opening up my home to others and opening up my life, being a "flexible living spirit"; "I must be new."

I had lots of fresh ideas; I wanted to start an "Iona Friendship Circle" in my house, and thought of letting it out whilst I tried for "a long winter let" on Iona. I found I was much less threatened by Walter, because I didn't feel so afraid of him; I felt I could be interiorly free of what had bound me. I had this amazing and growing feeling of being fluid and being able to change. I even talked in a friendly fashion to Walter, trying to arrange that he should give me £10 a month for Gabriel's clothes, and that the Access could increase to an extra hour on Wednesdays when Gabriel went to school; it seemed a lovely healing conversation and the enmity between us seemed temporarily dissolved.

The following day it was all ruined between myself and Walter when he exploded with temper at the Donkey Derby. Walter happened to meet us there, and to my dismay started to go round the attractions with us. Then he put Gabriel on a donkey, but he wouldn't leave go and ran trotting along beside him. I was annoyed, as it ruined Gabriel's first ever donkey ride. So when Walter then stickily asked if he could make more agreements with me, I said No. And he breathed venom in his foul temper in a moment, shouting "Right it's off, I'm not keeping to that agreement." I felt sickened to my stomach, and went off in the other direction, trying to absorb the healing energies of the place by walking barefoot on the grass. I was later reflecting on how you couldn't "deal" with a man like Walter, because he had no centre to be true to, but only oscillated in violent moods; " I don't think he has a soul." I came to see that Walter was not worth dealing with. Another thing I realised that same day was that I wanted Gabriel to go to the Woodend school rather that the Catholic school called St.Winifreds that I had arranged.

After this particular day I seemed to be getting faster and faster mentally in that I was writing lots, but never stopping to write down my oontomplative prayers *I was going too fast!*

I kept getting "bad vibrations" from things, and making plans to live in Inverlang, and starting to sell my university books to students. I decided I was going to "disburden myself of my possessions." I was going to redo my will; I was trying to open new bank accounts. I started buying all sorts of things at the shops. I was going too fast and my thinking and judgements were becoming haywire.

I started to act on certain rather bizarre principles; such as: "if it is a present give it to someone else", "anything that will come in useful for Gabriel keep", "I'll teach Gabriel, but not play with him". I decided that I had to "leave behind" my old soul-friend Pater Leo, and give to my friend Ailsa his letters. I decided that a chance encounter with Forbes the ferryman in '81 made him "my true husband", whom I should marry. I decided that all my friends had "something wrong with them" and I had to leave them behind. I was planning to give away as "leaving presents" every thing I possessed before Christmas; then I would leave without telling anyone.

The next day I started writing from an even more bizarre mood; for example "I encountered Nicola and gave her a Wedgewood dish, and told her there was someone I might marry.- - I gave Shiona a hatpin. I bought batteries from a man to whom I nearly gave a television. - -I bought from the Fiona Finlay Art shop a lovely exercise book for Gabriel, telling her he was Walter McKay's son. - - I couldn't get rid of the antique, the small gold box, I took into town." I was also opening and closing various bank accounts. I said at the end of that day's writing, *"It is the day I have realised "Don't go too fast for other people."* *It was the right thing to say, because my brain was racing like anything,* and the following day the CPN Ted and Mrs.Bloomfield, and Dr.James all came over to see me, presumably to check out my mental health. Dr.James insisted on reading the page I'd last written, *and presumably he didn't find it very sane.* *Presumably nobody thought I was very sane.*

I said to Dr.James, "those of you who are not manic, be envious of those who are, because you miss your own selves."

For the next thing I knew, sometime during the next day a whole host of people, of nurses, came rushing round my house banging and knocking on the doors and windows. What did I do? Fear and adrenalin rushed through me; they had come to "take me away" to the dreaded hospital. What did I do? I hid, crouching down, in the one corner of the hall where I couldn't be seen from either the front or back windows. They were yelling "we know you are in there; come on out." I thought I was safe, hidden where I was; they couldn't get in at me. However I was wrong. Steven Peterson broke in through the bedroom window; then he went to the door and let the whole troop of them in. What did I do? I threw myself on the bed, and pretended to be unconscious, or just coming round from sleep, as if that were an excuse for not hearing them. But it didn't work as a ploy; they injected me with the dreaded largactil, and carried me off to the waiting ambulance.

"I'm opting out of the System, and trying different paths; only in the Void and not in the System can God be found." "Tell me more," tempted the System-Server, watching her cynically. She spilled what she knew; "Through the Time-span which is present I may enter the Door; for the Present alone is power, being everywhere at the same time." "Tell me more," tempted the System-Server. "I know the Way" she said, "I know where the Door is; and by my own Light-Energy I can hold it open." And they took her to the Asylum.

Chapter 35
A Crazy Awakening.

The following day, waking up in Craigdene with Largactil in my system,- in the newly built Morlond Ward,- I was still determined to write my journal, but what I wrote came out weird and nonsensical: -

"The day of "bring me peace Lord as I tread in the quagmire" became finally real. Gabriel was taken away from his mummy, just like a man foretold. And I know he remembers that day when he was sickening in the quagmire, his mother rescues him before dying herself. I found those stories of "Dumbo" and "Bambi" very harrowing. I see now what Gabriel means when he says "Don't get lost mummy." I shall never forget the way he was desperate and sore, trying to come after me on the road to Strathnaver; and his little face was hot and red-raw; he seemed sore all over. So when we had sorted things out for packaging, we went home."

Although this shows plainly some of the grief of my separation from Gabriel, and his being upset, it also shows a lack of ability to think rationally; I jump quickly from subject to subject, in a way that prevents the whole from making sense; I think they call it medically "flights of fancy". All these things happened, and were connected in my brain, even though they can make no sense to the reader, because there is no obvious connection by time or meaning.

But there was a connection for me. "Dumbo" and "Bambi" were picture book stories I used to read to Gabriel, and they are about a young animal losing his mother, or trying to rescue his mother. The plea of "don't get lost mummy," was a fear Gabriel expressed regularly when I temporarily disappeared into the back garden, and he couldn't find me. And I am obviously comparing the crying anguish, that day, with another day when he was trying to keep up with me tearfully on the road to Stathnaver when we were visiting Rachel. And it was that day there was something about packing before we went home. "Treading in the quagmire" was something I'd heard of in the Baptist church, in relation to the "slough" in "Pilgrim's Progress."

The rest of that day's writing continued in this non-sensical way: -
"I thought about Janet,(the nurse who gave out the tablets); she gives what she has surplus; that's why I can't take what she gives. - - I thought about Jesus; the feelings between us are so strong that it is hard to be pleasant with each other. - - I realised today that I have my green one. Then I realised with a shock that they had pulled out of selling cabbages. It was a very good birthday party.- - I've decided I

was going too fast for the dancers; I thought I'd take my body and touch the only silkier, and go barefoot. This time I quickly pinched a few things and was off again."

After that I only wrote sporadically, though scribbling away manically, with big writing in multi-coloured pens. I organised it as follows: "Black = Current, Green = Vision, Red = Religious, the heart, Blue = Water". Then I pronounced "There's current in the water, but there isn't water in the current." I then decided "Let's make everybody laugh in the religious novel. It is a religious comedy; nobody has ever done that before."

I decided it was my purpose to write a novel: - "My books are more precious to me than my son. For he is an accident in my life, whilst my books are my purpose.- - Or, my purpose was my books. - - His birth an accident, unpremeditated, unplanned for. - -"God's plan Mairi!"- - For my books came first, but my purpose is infinite."

I said to Dr.McNeill who was prescribing me lots of extra drugs: - "That's the trouble with freedom and privacy; it can never be guaranteed.- - Just remember me when you've given me more that I can take.- - You have to get more privacy here before you leave.- - We've done this before; I gave a book for you to read and you spat it out back at me. Now therefore, you are only permitted one page."

I said to a nurse called Simon when I came in very wet from a walk with him: - "Nearly drowned of course when I jumped off the pier, and I can't swim. I do act out my own novels. Now I know what it feels like, ie. to drown. But now I am alive, and I live for evermore." *(NB. This was very ominous in that about a year later I tried to commit suicide by drowning myself.)*- - "I am always getting way-laid on the way, that's why I haven't got up the mountain-top yet."

I made plans for my novel: - First of all, "I could make my novel much more fun if we did away with black because there is too much of it." (I meant everything I had written in my journal-writing in my "current" life up till then.) "Get onto the interesting bits.- - Dead bodies never litter the streets."- -I decided I had to work out my characters: - "Elizabeth Drummond, student nurse, eyes blue. The kind nurse who had been nursing him, compassionate with eyes of blue. - -Liz, Lizzie, a real character and not ficticious." - -"There's nobody going to hurt you Mairi, whilst I am here." "My name shall be Mairi Best. (My Grandad's name was George Best.)- - If ever you can't believe I'm telling the truth, you my friends, tell me so. - - If a child is meant to come along, sent by God, then he will. That is vulnerability for you; capability to be wounded. Here we adjourned."

I had a conversation with Lizzie about a couple of small oil paintings of Iona: - She said "I always wanted to go to Iona; Iona paints a picture in my mind of tranquillity and peace." "Having a painting is not the same as having a vision," I replied, "the reason I return to Iona is my vision."

I decided the scenario would be a spaceship, and I'd call it "Starship Morlond." I decided on the characters from the patients in the sitting-room, which was always very heavy with smoke. There was a "Navigator," an "Arthur Dent" character, a "Captain Angela", a "Princess Mairi" as heroine, etc. I kept popping in and out of this sitting room, asking them questions. *I asked the crew of the "starship Morlond" if they wanted to go to Mars. They said they didn't want to go to Mars; they wanted to go to Barbados. A few days later I intimated that really the "navigator" of the starship wasn't in charge of the destination; but secretly the author could make it go where she liked. There came a shout of "So you're not going to bloody Barbados!"*

I hated the smoke in that room. So one day I went in and complained: "I don't see why the only room here should be a smoking-room; let your body breathe." The reply came "it doesn't say any thing about it in the bible." I said "Yes it does, and I know the bible off by heart." Then coming back a few minutes later, I said *"It does say in the bible, thou shalt not lust after thine own pleasure, and I should think cigarettes come under that heading!"*

Chapter 36
Craziness Tranquillized.

"I am detained here by my pain."

For some strange reason, - I think it was because I had not received a letter from him for ages, and then when I phoned him another strange monk answered,- I suddenly became convinced that Pater Leo had died. And I howled my head off! I wept plenteously with a terrible grief. "Now I know he has died; he really has died; il est mon pere, he was my father!" There was a nurse who comforted me in my crying. I said "You must always tell me the truth after that." I wrote "it was total exposure."

There was a joke about the two nuns in the dark room. - "They were developing themselves." I later added "They were silent because they weren't there."

I thought I was writing Zen Koans: - "Death isn't so bad ; it is the dying that hurts." "You are spreading your love around, with a thick butter."

Somebody said to me, "You've written all these books; could you write a book about a pack of cards?" I replied "There's more wisdom in that pack of cards than there is in the bible. My Grandad used to say that."

"Our navigator is flying us due East.- - Towers, small stone straight streets, ruins, harbour, pier, sands, sea, off where the seagulls hide.- - We have a very sceptical navigator here. - - Our Navigator has just nipped off to bed!"

"Denise, young and pretty, short dark hair and grey eyes, joining Starship Morlond. Peter, the hero, young blood, knight in shining armour. Glyn, alien on board, going a different direction. - - Why don't you know there is a God? Have you never met him? Never seen him nor any evidence of him? Will you be happy if I prove it to you, to your understanding?- - I know I can eat nuts, but I haven't the money to pay for the bloody nuts!"

"Brigit, stowaway, unknown quantity, she'll provide the excitement. - I don't know where I am going; do you know who is in charge of this starship? - - Must we go hungry? I've been preoccupied with my son. Could you speak English? - - I decided Brigit could be the Navigator, seeing she wanted to be. - - For a novel, all you need do is to create the characters, then the novel creates itself.- - Princess Mairi- you are a part of me, you are my alter-ego.- - Sometimes somethings are best seen from a distance!- -End of first chapter."

And in her madness she uttered these words;
"I know where the Door, the Ultimate Time-Span Is;
I shall hold it open with my left foot!"

All this I wrote when I was "High", - "high as a kite" as a doctor once called me! But my mind was soon dragged down in the mud, by my being forced to take medication, - dreadful things like largactil and haloperidol, that make you feel dreadfully ill. What happened when this stuff was forced on me was recorded in this poignant manner:-

-"I do act out my own novels. Don't interrupt or you will disrupt the whole flow."
(I was manically scribbling about the Starship Morlond)
-"You are overwrought; we will give you an injection."
(They always threaten medication in Craigdene, when you get emotional.)
-"Red; that sounds like the wrong novel ."
(I realised the danger I was in.)

"Do they feed us at 12 o'clock? So this is the zoo!"
(I was desperately trying to deflect attention away from myself, but the ploy didn't work. They gave me oral medication, but I held it under my tongue, and they forced me to open my mouth as they dug about with a spatula. Then realising I hadn't swallowed it, they then held me down and injected me with the largactil.)
-"You have no more power over me; your power has run out."
(I shouted this as I leapt up. But very quickly the drug had effect, and I could barely utter things with slurred speech.)
"Vow; I do not speak again! So, he took my voice from me at last. I am dumb, as was always meant, but I hear. You have sent me through to my own world! Well done you idiots!"
(I felt that my creative state had permanently been torn away from me; that I had been pushed through into the "Void" of my own inner world.)

Someone said to me in concern, perceiving how ill I was:
"What have they done to you?"
I could only utter a strange nonsense about how I had been violated:
"Open my mouth , and show - - toothless."

Chapter 37
In the Dark Room.

I was yearning, aching with the wait. The nurse I called "Superman," because of his similar looks to the film-character, had assured me that Dr.James was coming to visit; I waited for hours, within the cage-like walls of the "Goldfish bowl",- the dreaded room upon which all the mental might of the nurses was focused, the glass windows and doors allowing vision into every single corner. There was no escape from being watched. With a lively soul-fire I had fought with every ounce of my will, every shred of my being, every trick imaginable, to get out of that room, just to see someone, talk to someone, to put an end to the "solitary confinement."

But then this thing had happened which was like a kind of death, like a rent in the depths of my being. I had once more come out, dressed in the hospital pyjamas, trying to get along the corridor, past the smoking room. But Chris and another nurse were talking in there, and saw me. Again came the boom of "Get back to your room Mairi," and the twist and pushing of my arm, which horridly hurt my shoulder. I went toward my room, but trying to show my strength of will, immediately came back, saying to Chris; "I'll do anything you want me to do, but please don't hurt me anymore." His reply came cruel; "Another word from you and you'll get an injection." It broke my will; it smashed up my psyche.

And now, when it was too late, my doctor, whom I had for years adored, was supposedly coming to visit me; it was also the doctor I blamed for getting me locked up. It seemed to me that because he had come to read my journals the day before the psychiatric "system" had rushed in to take me captive, that he was to blame. I was brim-full of emotion. And then I was told by "Superman" that he apparently wasn't coming after all, as visiting time had passed. My overflowing emotion, which I knew I mustn't express to anyone in the ward as the result would be the forcible administration of more medication, was breaking inside me like waves on the shore. I felt wetting her hair would help; it would "earth" some of it. I stood under the shower, and then tied a hospital-style blue towelling dressing-gown round me, pulling it tight round my waist.

Suddenly he was there; I became conscious of him, before the words were told, - "Someone to see you Mairi." I was shown into the doctor's room which was next to the nurse's station. I had wet hair and bare feet and was naked but for a dressing gown, and the bottled-up passion was flashing from my eyes. He sat in the chair in the semi-dark room, and I stood before him like a tower of streaming energy; "How dare you do that! How could you so betray me! They have broken my will!"

He protested "it wasn't me, it wasn't me who got you hospitalised." "You're lying to me, you had read my journal!" He was taken aback by my spitting out of enormous anger and energy. "And don't you remember I thought you OK? Mairi your memory doesn't usually fail you."

My anger didn't let up; it was bottomless. "They have broken my will," I yelled again. And then a howl of anguish leapt out of me; "You can do anything you like to me, I can suffer anything, but how dare you put so much suffering on that little 5-year-old child who happens to be my son?!" He was overcome, and responded with affection; "Mairi I haven't done this to you, I've never done anything to hurt you."

He seemed overwhelmed by my completely uninhibited passion. I wasn't aware of anything but that passion; not of my hurt shoulder, and not of my nakedness underneath the dressing-gown; this was the powerful appeal of an intense psyche to another psyche. He grabbed hold of my arm, as if to contain my intensity. On the instant my rage relaxed and I gave in my energies.

The memory of that Passion of mine in that dark room was something that dwelt in me for years afterwards. The moment lived in my consciousness, compelling me, making me yearn, making me want to beg him to come and talk with me about "the gap which opened up in my psyche." The memory of the moment created a bond between us.

Chapter 38
Out of the Goldfish-Bowl.

The windows of Morlond Ward when it was first built, and when I came to be contained there in 1991, opened fully in both directions. By 1994, not only did they not open any more at all, but also the handles had been taken off, so that the "inmates" couldn't even imagine that they could be opened. I was told that this sad change was due to me, due to my many escape attempts!

I was in the "goldfish bowl". It was called this humorously by certain nurses because it was glass all the way round to such an extant that the unfortunate inmate could be viewed from all angles at all times, if the curtains were left open as was generally required; and this room was situated just opposite the nurse's station, so that the inmate could be observed at all times whatever movement was made. This was ideal if that unfortunate person was on "red", - which meant constant non-stop observation. The other "observation statuses" were "amber" which meant observation every ten minutes, and "green" which supposedly meant you didn't need to be observed in this oppressive manner. I had done something supposedly so wicked, like refusing to take medication, that it merited being put on "red" in the "goldfish bowl". This room, be it noted was originally built as the "baby's room", in a mother and baby unit, the mothers' room being next to it; *only an intense psychiatric unit like Craigdene's Morlond ward could so pervert its intended usage.*

I remember how every time I came out of this room, trying to get out of the psychiatric prison of minds, constantly watched, trying to get dressed in suitable clothes that would allow me access to the dining room for breakfast, or to get out to the telephone, or just to get out to see and speak to someone, I was told by bullying nurses "Back to your room Mairi." It was said to me over and over again, until I tragically felt my will had been broken. But I was determined to escape from this place. I had a travel bag, so I packed it the night before with all the clothes I wanted to keep; the ones I didn't want to keep I left in the wardrobe and drawers. I wasn't sleeping, hardly sleeping at the time, so I lay in my bed waiting,- waiting patiently till the early morning, when I thought I might catch the nurses off their guard.

It was light, about 6am; the nurses were busy drinking coffee and joking, their backs toward me. I sneaked out of bed, and put a couple of pillows beneath the covers instead, so that it would look like a body. The window I had left open a little the night before, so it wouldn't make a noise in opening. I kept my head down near the floor, so I couldn't be seen. I slowly pushed the window wide open, and shoved the travel bag out of it; I heard it plop to the ground. I was already dressed, as I had gone to bed with my clothes on. I took a look at the talking nurses; they were relaxing before their early morning wake-up routine; they weren't looking. I quickly sat on the window-sill, swung my legs over, and jumped to the ground. I pushed the window closed behind me, so they wouldn't notice it. So I was out! That was the easy bit, I thought ruefully; the hard bit was to get away from the area before the search parties could find me, which was difficult, as the hospital was in the country.

I thought the best way to get past the other wards and units was to stride manfully along with my bag over my shoulder, as though I had a right to be there; if I acted suspiciously, I would awaken suspicion. So I strode out along the road acting as though I were a nurse going off duty. I breathed a sigh of relief when it worked; I reached the main road. I was scared; I knew that if the nurses found me missing they would alert the police, whose cars would come along the main road. I wondered how long I had before they would discover I wasn't in the bed. I walked down this road, till I came to the sleepy village of Nethercraig, ready at any moment to jump over the wall, if I should hear a car coming. I got onto another road, and then another road; I hid for a while in the garden of a large house, trying to calm myself down and think what I should do next. It struck me that, before the countryside should come alive with police cars crawling around looking for me, I should take my chances, and accost a car, and try to get a lift to the nearest railway station. I walked through a wood to the next main road, then decided to put this plan into operation.

When I put my thumb out to hitch a lift my greatest fear was that I might discover it to be a nurse, coming to the hospital for the morning shift. But a guy stopped for me, and I pretended to be a person who had come out jogging, and carrying washing in my bag. It seemed to work, and I got a lift to Kirkcraig. I had a small amount of money; I got a ticket to Edinburgh, and got on a busy morning train. I was busy thinking on this train; where should I go, and what should I do? I knew I had to hide away for a whole month if I wanted to get off my section; I had brought a Halifax cashcard with me, which I had secreted away at the time I was supposed to yield up valuables. I wondered if I could use it to get some money out. I thought it might be better to "hole up" somewhere reasonably close to my home town of KirkMichaels, rather that going to Edinburgh or beyond, so I decided to get out at Inverlang.

My feelings of fear were subsiding, by the time I got out at Inverlang. I made for the town centre, and there got £200 out of the cash machine. I wasn't thinking clearly about how this money was to last, because the next thing I did was to buy clothes in the shops. I had this idea that I wanted to completely replace the clothes I was wearing, partly to "slough off" the hospital, and partly so I wouldn't be recognized. And because my feet were very sore, due to bad-fitting foot-wear, I also bought some new shoes. Then I got changed in some toilets, and threw away all the old stuff. Then I set off looking for somewhere to stay, walking for miles and miles, looking for "Bed and Breakfast." When I eventually found somewhere, and the landlady showed me a room, I thought she thought I seemed suspicious. There was a burly ageing overweight taxi-driver down the hall, and he made overtures to me. Later that night he knocked on my door, and I rather stupidly let him in. He lay in my bed all night and kept making love to me. I felt I didn't care, and let it happen; this was partly because I felt my will had been broken, and partly because I felt, as I always do when manic, that sex would somehow miraculously cure me.

In the morning I felt I had to leave that place, because the landlady was suspicious; so I went off on the hunt for another "Bed and Breakfast" place. My feet by now had become incredibly sore, because the new shoes didn't at all fit me, so I also hunted out the local hospital, thinking I should go there to have my sore feet dressed. Somehow I didn't think this an idiotic thing to go to an "A and E" centre for; I was convinced I needed medical attention. At last I found another "B and B" establishment just round the corner from the local hospital; so I booked in and then went to complain about my feet. The nurses patiently applied ointment and bandages to my feet, and when asked for details about myself, I told them a pack of lies. Somehow they seemed to believe me, and I felt relieved to get out of the place. They told me they these new shoes were so terribly badly fitting, that it would be better if I went barefoot. Accordingly, I walked barefoot, though tenderly on the concrete, from the hospital to my new "B and B" place. I think the landlady was suspicious about me, because of this and my obvious distressed state of mind. She tried to draw me out in conversation, saying that she understood about psychiatric illness. I paid her £40 for two nights stay, and went to bed there in a strange attic room. I opened the attic window and gazed out at the stars. *I found I could lay in bed and gaze up at these stars; and I felt then at last calm and safe, as if there were no-one pursuing me any longer. I felt so calm and safe.*

157

Suddenly there was a knock at the house-door and I heard commotion downstairs. I didn't think it could possibly be anything to do with me, because I was feeling "safe". Then the landlady knocked on my bedroom door, and told me I was wanted downstairs. I went down, wearing just my nightdress, still confident that it could be nothing to do with me. And then I saw two policemen confronting me, and they asked my name. I gave them a completely false name, believing I could fool them, and still thinking they couldn't possibly be looking for me. And then one of the officers talked for a while on his walkie-talkie and said "Yes she matches the description." He then said to me "get dressed because you have to accompany us down to the station." Meanwhile the landlady was being incredibly nice and motherly to me, and said I needn't worry, and she would come with me.

So I got ready, went with them, and I was still convinced there was no way they could know who I am, if I denied it. I felt that, once having reached that "safe point" under the stars, when no-one could know where I was, I was invulnerable. Once at the police station, they put me in a room with a bare table, where this maternal landlady comforted me, saying everything would be alright. Then a policeman came in and said in a very direct fashion; "you are Mairi Colme aren't you?" I said "No, No, I'm not." And I kept on denying it, until finally an ambulance team arrived from Craigdene, and they said "Yes that's her!"

So I was torn away from this deeply understanding landlady, and shipped back to the hospital, where I was once again put in a room and "observed". How did they find me? I wanted to know. How did they know I was in that particular "Bed and Breakfast" place? Elspeth, one of the nurses, revealed to me the fact that she had spotted me whilst driving her car through Inverlang, and the hospital had alerted the police to the fact that I was in that area, and so they had searched through the local "B and B"s. I thought that motherly landlady who was kind to me was really wonderful; I saw her again, when she came to visit someone in the hospital, a few weeks later, and she gave me a £5 note. I was sounding her praises, when a nurse called Jim told me a different version of events; he said it was this landlady who phoned the police, because she could tell I was psychiatrically ill. I was absolutely appalled by this, as it rocked my faith in her kindness. I recalled how she had taken £40 off me, for the stay; *had she then shopped me to the police, and later shown me this pretend generosity of giving me a £5 note? The whole thing left a bitter taste in my mouth.*

I once said, "Life is a mixture of blood and shit. The blood comes from God, and the shit from man."

158

Chapter 39
Cured of Distress.

What happened to Gabriel, you may well ask! Well Steven Peterson, the social worker, on that day when all the nurses trooped into my house, took him away and handed him over to Walter! And after all those years, when I fought and made agreements, to keep his time with the man down to a minimum!

There was an event a few days after my admission which I shall never forget. Walter brought Gabriel to visit me and I took the tender 5-year-old Gabriel into my room, and he told me frantically, with scorching tears streaming down his cheeks, "Mummy, don't leave me with him, that nasty man, he's locking me up, he's locking me up in a room with the spiders!" I knew he meant locking him up in his bedroom to force him to stay there and sleep there at night; I had always allowed him free access to come out, free access to me. And then Gabriel said something awful; "Mummy, if you don't kill that man, I will myself get a gun and kill him; mummy you've got to kill him for me!" I was horrified at this coming from a 5-year-old child, and affected by his emotion and frantic tears, and went out of the room to get a nurse as a witness. But Walter and the nurses blamed me for upsetting the child. It caused me such pain; "I needed a witness and you all zilched me out!" *And Walter folded the child away from me, like he did for years into the future, vowing that he was not going to bring him back.*

When they didn't come back, and nobody brought Gabriel to see me, as they did on my last admission, I became increasingly distraught about it. I thought the only explanation was that he was so distressed that they couldn't bring him. I made desperate phone-calls to everyone I knew, asking them to go help Gabriel. I felt something terrible was going to happen, unless somebody got help to my child. But he was left with his Dad, and no-one helped.

In mid-August I was very distressed that I couldn't see Gabriel on his first day at school. It was such an important day, for which I had prepared for so long; it was awful to miss such an important day. I remember making a flurry of phone-calls from the Morlond ward phone trying to insist that he be taken to the school I had decided on; but he was taken to St.Winifreds, the school for Catholics and problem children, and not the Westgate which I had decided upon. I was outraged and hurt. I remember desperately appealing to Dr.McNeill, *to please let me out, for that one day, so that I could see my son go to his first day at school. But Dr.McNeill forbade it.*

Meantime I was taken to Ward 6, the lock up ward, which is supposed to be for "behaviour modification," but is really there to prevent people escaping. What provoked this move was an incident when it was discovered that I still wasn't taking medication. They insisted that I ate my lunch after my tablets so that I couldn't secrete them under my tongue. And I was getting quite befuddled by these tablets; I remember saying, holding up the salt, sugar and Lithium Carbonate, "I can't tell any more which is salt and which is sugar!" So this horrid nurse said I'd get an injection to calm me down; at which frightening point, I ran away, in my night-dress, out of the back door and out of the patio, and down the steep hill of grass toward the road, intending to "escape." But Steven Peterson's car was just coming along the road, and he leapt out, accosted me, and forcibly took me back to the ward. Whilst in the car I pleaded with him that I couldn't stand it any more in Morlond Ward, because it was like a "prison of minds," in which you are always being watched, and he promised to do something about it. And so the next thing I knew I was packed off to Ward 6.

But I was quite glad to be in this "lock-up Ward," because everything was so much simpler than in Morlond ward; the nurses were "bigger and gentler". Things were a lot simpler; you knew were you were. And here I had another Doctor, and not Dr.McNeill, who had been enforcing the dreaded Lithium down my throat; they gave me instead the standard tranquillizers, and a drug called Lorazepam: on these I came down from my mania fairly quickly and easily; with the result that I was taken back to Morlond Ward as "cured" in a couple of weeks. Meantime I had met Matty; I remember how we became acquainted by writing to each other on different coloured pens on the margins of newspapers. Then we started going for walks together, when we were first let out, and I felt that had fallen instantly and deeply in love with him. I remember we were talking about marrying each other, and I wrote him love-letters. However when I moved, back down to Morlond Ward, the nurses would only allow limited access to him, and I began to realise he was "ill", because by that time I was well.

I remember coming down the hill and grass in bright sunlight, accompanied by a nurse, on the move from Ward 6 to Morlond Ward, feeling really well, and telling this nurse that I felt like "squashed oranges." By this I meant, not the bruised fruit, as she mistook it to mean, but feeling fresh in your mind like when drinking fresh morning orange-juice. I remember feeling the dismay on entering Morlond, because I knew it would be going back to Dr.McNeill, the Lithium, and the "prison of minds" I knew it to be. And so I was back in Morlond Ward, no longer manic, by mid-September, when I began sanely writing my journal again.

When Christ drove from the wildly-possessed man his demons, he was left sitting at his feet, feeling like a calm mill-pond on which the sun shone, purged of everything savage and fierce, bowed and newly human, with the tender awareness of a new-born infant. And so he was redeemed from destructive power, sitting there in his right mind.

You become mad by embracing the pain of reality. Madness is not inescapable. Some personalities have such a flaw in them that they are urged to embrace what they know will drive them mad. But there is always a way back, for those brave enough to take it.

Chapter 40
Recovery and Anger.

As soon as I came round and was no longer manic, and was writing again, the emotion that possessed me was a great anger. "How dare anyone take my son away from me and hand him over to Walter! How dare Dr.McNeill do this to me and my son!" *I felt as though I had indeed "lost" my son, because the love and trust he used to give to me he would now give to his father! This was an enormous pain to me; that I had indeed "lost" Gabriel, lost him to Walter.*

The Beloved; "The Soul-Hater is not my husband."
The System-Server; "To the Soul-Hater I will give your child;
for he is the child's father, and your husband."
And the Beloved's soul screamed.

But Philip on the phone told me I needed to fight, to get to see my son. In my despair I was imagining marrying Matty, and going far away to live, leaving the problem behind. But Philip encouraged me to fight for Gabriel's visits to be reinstated, saying I needed a regular visit with my son and needed to keep in contact with him. On a few odd occasions I managed to speak to Gabriel by phone; he cried and wailed and said that his daddy was "locking him up." And I just felt how acutely he was suffering, and all my motherly instincts came to the fore, and I ached to get him back.

Dr. McNeill wasn't helping. Though I was well again, he said it would be weeks before I'd be let out; he said I must be still "ill" because I wanted to marry Matty. So I changed my story and said he was only a friend, but Dr.McNeill said I was "changeable" and therefore ill. I pleaded with him that my 5-year-old son was suffering and needed his mummy; but he said I couldn't see him bar once a week, probably in Walter's company. The pain of it surged though me. I pleaded that for years I had given Walter access on his own, and so deserved the same, and he replied, "That's different; Walter wasn't ill and you are!" I was mortified. I was debarred from seeing my 5-year-old son because they said I was ill, but how could I ever prove that I was not ill? I felt I was going to be there forever! I knew weeks of suffering stretched in front of me; "when shall I ever be free?"

Near the end of September I was allowed my first access visit with Gabriel, for half an hour in my own house, supervised by the social worker Greta Christie; it was made amply plain to me that I would only be allowed to see and speak to Gabriel when overwatched in the same room with her. My pain and misery were complete, because above all I wanted to be alone with Gabriel. However in the event Gabriel chose a solitary moment with me to tell me that Walter upset him and kept getting very cross; "mummy can I come back to live with you?" It really cut up my heart to see how Walter made my child suffer as he once made me suffer. But I knew I couldn't tell the truth, or I would be accused of putting these ideas into Gabriel's mind, due to my mental illness. I thought how one day I would pay them all back, and take Gabriel far away. - - However a few days later I was allowed to go out with Walter and Gabriel, and I saw with pain how the love and trust Gabriel once gave to me he now gave to his daddy. I felt grief-struck about this. "Have I lost my little boy?"- - Then Walter told me on the phone that he didn't feel any "warmth" from me, and so he wasn't going to let me see Gabriel.

However the Access visits with the social worker continued, and I felt a lot of love and affection for my son, and I felt I couldn't abandon him; I would have to fight and struggle for Custody back. And then my social worker, Steven Peterson, returning from holiday, explained to me that I still have full legal custody of Gabriel; when I came out of hospital the full custody should be returned, and my arrangements with Walter would then be voluntary again. I was immensely relieved. Then right at the end of September Dr.McNeill said we were "moving towards discharge", and I was immensely relieved about this as well. Steven Peterson then had a talk with me, telling me I had to alter my attitude to Walter, and had to allow him generous access times when I got the Custody back, saying I shouldn't fear him like I did, as he had no real power to bully and coerce me. But I thought how far he was from understanding the situation. Then Walter started threatening and bullying me about money, saying that unless I gave him £100 for looking after Gabriel he would create trouble with the DSS. I eventually gave in about this and paid him the money.

Then as I began to have more outings with Walter and Gabriel, and to have "Passes" to KirkMichaels, it dawned on me that the "reality" of my life lay with Walter and Gabriel. Reality didn't lie with Matty, with whom I had been having romantic walks and talks. I realised that my relationship with Matty must come to an end once I left the hospital; it was essentially a "hospital relationship" and I could see that he wasn't well. So I tried to become friendly with Walter, realising that, after I'd spent 5 years trying to minimise his influence over my child, he had now entire power over him; the love, affection and trust my son once gave to me, he now gave to him; essentially I'd lost my son to the man. I was left to sort out the mess, and it seemed to me the only way I could proceed was to get friendly with Walter; it seemed to me I had to "throw in my lot" with Walter and Gabriel.

Meantime I was very angry with the support system which had allowed this situation to come about; I felt especially bitter towards Dr.McNeill, who still deprived me of my freedom and kept me in Morlond ward though I was completely better. I remember thinking, walking round Kirkcraig, how hundreds of people along the streets were more "mentally ill" than I was, and yet I was stuffed full of tablets and locked up in a mental hospital weeks after I was fully better! I was very upset the day Dr.McNeill reviewed me, because he said he wanted me to be "stable" for a far longer time before he let me out; he said how after being so completely "well" for several weeks, I "might have a relapse," which I thought absurd. I argued back that it wasn't fair to keep me in hospital after I was 100% well, as I should recover and recuperate at home. But, though he admitted that I was now 100% well, he wouldn't let me go!

Chapter 41
A Dismaying October.

For the whole of the month of October the horrible situation closed around me; on the one hand I was forced to sleep and stay in the hospital, making hour-long bus-rides into KirkMichaels every day; and on the other hand I had to handle Walter every day, cajoling him into letting me see Gabriel, getting painfully and messily involved with him. I kept thinking how he was a "nasty piece of work", and I didn't want anything to do with him, but Steven Peterson kept urging me to make a relationship with him, recognizing that we were "the parents of the same child." Meanwhile Walter was in his element, controlling my seeing of Gabriel, continually insisting that I showed him "warmth", and trying to bully me into having a "shared custody."

Meanwhile Matty was bothering me, constantly coming round to visit me; I wasn't interested in "relationships," being too busy fighting for my son, so I finally and cruelly told him in no uncertain term to "get lost." But then I began to fall into the trap of relating to Walter; he insisted on going everywhere with Gabriel with me; he had a right to do this till I was discharged from the hospital, when the Custody would revert to me. I found it gruelling; part of the time he was "as nice as pie", the other half of the time he was threatening and bullying and demanding "warmth"; it was impossible. Basically Walter was demanding that I become "romantic" with him when he had me over a barrel!

Meanwhile I was being tormented by Dr.McNeill, to whom I had to appeal for Passes; he would promise me them and then not give me them; he would offer me a few days pass, only then to say I had to come back afterwards. I felt I was living in two places, and spending half my life on a bus. Finally I was given a whole week's Pass, and told I could have Gabriel back. The handover of Gabriel now loomed before me; Walter had said to Steven Peterson that it would be "over his dead body", so I was apprehensive, and full of miserable expectations. However it all went smoothly, thanks to Steven, who was a real help, and Gabriel came back to sleep at my house. However the price I paid for it was that Walter wanted to get "sexual" with me, and always wanted the three of us to be together and go places together.

But the temporary "liking" between us soon wore off. On one occasion we went to Stuart Palace together; Walter was so very bad-tempered that the whole excursion was ruined for me. Gabriel kept ringing a doorbell, though we told him to stop it; Walter suddenly slapped his hand, and his face turned black as thunder. We agreed that myself and Gabriel should go round the gardens, whilst he went on a guided tour round the house. But when we waited for him at the exit, he didn't turn up; I became very worried because I didn't have the money to get ourselves back home, but we eventually found Walter in a morose mood. He complained all the way back in the car, saying he had been "rushed." By the time we got home I felt fed up of his ill-temper.

Finally at the end of October I was put on "trial leave," which meant I was still sectioned under the mental health act, but was on a long-term "pass." That very day Walter was horrid to me; I came in, talking about what had transpired at the hospital, and then noticed his dark and moody countenance; "what's the matter Walter?" I asked. "You never greeted me; there was no hug and kiss," he said, "you are so very cold, and I can't stand people like that." I was dismayed, hurt, close to tears, and he continued, "I've shown warmth to you, and now you make me feel as though I've wasted my time." *I thought what a horrible reception to someone who has just come out of a mental hospital!*

We then went that day to Cameron Park, letting Gabriel ride there on his bike, and there was more unpleasantness. Gabriel threw a paddy; Walter glared at him and said "he is in one of his moods"; my reaction was to cuddle him. Walter said "you're making a mistake; you are ruining everything I taught him; he's disturbed; I know what it is caused by," meaning it was caused by me! I felt completely miserable. In the evening, after I had bought and cooked a meal for us, Gabriel again was difficult when getting him to bed, and Walter again said that I was to blame for his "disturbed behaviour". It was several hours before I could get him to leave; he was in a foul mood; and I was left feeling shattered and bitterly unhappy.

In the next few days Gabriel showed much disturbed behaviour; he kept repeating, for no apparent reason "I'm upset"; it seemed he was copying Walter's behaviour as well as his phraseology. And he also kept repeating "help me, please help me." When I put him to bed he kept saying "Please don't lock the door, please don't shut me up in the dark." I found out by this, on questioning him ,that Walter did indeed lock him up in his bedroom at night, as I believed he did when I was manic in the hospital.

This is the state of affairs in which I was left by the Psychiatric system and by my so-called "support system." My son Gabriel I found "spoilt" due to his stay with his father. And I myself was inextricably, personally involved with the man I hated, with whom I had fought all these years to free myself from, to liberate myself from because I found him soul-destroying. And I was left right in the middle of this messy and sticky situation by the system which was supposedly on my side. It was impossible; pain circulated through and through me. But I tried to be brave and strong, and to carry on.

Chapter 42
A Defeated Rut.

Carrying on, when left in such a problematic situation, was difficult. It now fell to me to get Gabriel to school in the morning, which wasn't easy. I had Walter always trying to interfere and invade into my life. None of the professionals were any help. *And I felt bitter over what had happened to me, - that in my hour of weakness, my son had been handed over into the hands of my enemy!*

I decided it was time I "owned" my illness and tried to understand it. When I went to see Dr. James he replied to me that no-one did "psychoanalysis" in Kirkshire, as psychiatrists didn't believe in it. I put the argument forward that I didn't see the point of drugging myself up, so as to allow no "quality of life", when they don't seem to work any way; he strictly said he wouldn't allow me to come off the drugs, and they had allowed me a two and a half year stretch without being ill. I said I wanted to live without drugs and experiment with "flying and crashing". He said I couldn't do that when I had "responsibilities," ie. a child to look after; I replied that in 5 years and 2 illnesses I had never come anywhere near hurting Gabriel. "What about your threat of throwing him into the sea?" he replied. I was mortified; I had only said that to Ernest to see if he was gullible enough to believe me, and 3 years later I get it thrown back in my face as an argument why I'm not allowed to come off drugs! Dr.James also used the argument that I didn't realise how very "ill" I am when I get manic; "you do things in your illness which would make you blush." I felt very pained by this. I felt he was being ungracious.

Then I went to see the parish priest, saying to him too that my illness should be handled differently, and that I need to come to own it and understand it. I spoke of the "loveliness" of the generosity of my state of mind when I was manic. I did things I didn't normally do, because freed from the usual bonds of the mind; for example I had washed all of Gabriel's baby toys and given them away to the babies that I knew. I compared this with Van Gogh who gave away all that he had and went to live with the miners. I said how "madness" in the past was venerated as being something to do with the divine; nowadays, because it is labelled as an "illness", all rights and freedoms are taken away from the mad person and they are treated as though they are subhuman. I said how I have a better memory of things this time and I could see how there is no great distinction between when I'm well and when I'm mad; it is the same me. I said how I wanted to understand my illness.

A little later I went to the Citizen's Advice Bureau complaining how I had no "Rights", and because I was a manic depressive all freedom was taken away from me. I couldn't stop the Lithium which was giving me dreadful side-effects and I couldn't change my psychiatrist. The lady read out to me what she had found out about Section 18; if after 3 months the patient refuses to take the medication, the psychiatrist must obtain a second opinion from someone appointed by the mental welfare commission. I heard this with great dismay, as it would be easy for Dr.McNeill to obtain a second opinion; all these doctors hung together. I felt more helpless than ever. I went to see another minister about it, complaining about how I was forced to take Lithium, and was hurt terribly when he replied "What do you expect me to do about it?"

It was because I felt so maltreated and misunderstood by doctors that I kept my relationship with Walter open, because he gave me a lot of sympathy. We occasionally went places together and occasionally had tea together. Also at this time I began to relate to someone new called Maggie, whom I met taking her two kids to school; I quickly found her very dominating, and judged her to be rather "schizophrenic" in lots of ways, but she became my friend.

I began to get on really well with Steven Peterson, as he tried to pull me out of what he called my "defeated rut." He told me of what I did in my illness with some liking of me. He said I was very changeable, seething with wrath at one moment, then giggling like a school-girl; sometimes I seemed in great mental pain. It seemed to him that when I was ill "the mask dropped", and it let out all the aspects of my true self. He insisted that I stopped thinking of myself as "a failure", he said I used my illness as an excuse. He said that at the end of the day I wouldn't say "I didn't do it because I didn't try," but I would say "I didn't do it because of my illness."

Meanwhile I was very chagrined by the difficulties Gabriel was having at school; he didn't seem to "listen" apparently. I kept trying to be friendly with Walter, but he kept sulking and being bad tempered. I was really getting into a rut in December, between difficulties with Gabriel and difficulties with Walter. I felt Gabriel wasn't being appreciated by his teachers, who dealt with him in the wrong way. And I hated Walter's moodiness, and the way he demanded kisses from me in a way I found obnoxious. When I saw Steven again he was very helpful and kind, telling me that he would try and tackle the teacher problem in the New year; and as for Walter, Steven told me that submitting to kisses in this way, so that he shouldn't turn nasty and moody, was downright "abuse" and that it was a violation of my integrity and I had to say No to it. I said how I submitted to it for Gabriel's sake, because if Walter turned nasty and moody, he would take it out on Gabriel, as he had done in the past. But we agreed it must be stopped, because I couldn't go on like this.

When I confessed to Dr.McNeill my problems, trying to be open and honest and expecting sympathy from him, he was really horrid because he sided with Walter. "You are so very inconsistent," he said, "one minute you say you love the man, and the next that you hate him." I protested that he tormented me when I was in his grasp, "and I just want him to leave me alone." Then Dr.McNeill said "Heaven only knows what the poor child makes of it; he must be bewildered by the adults in his life." I thought that a cruel thing to say, and left bowed down with sadness.

On the14th December, when I tried to tell Walter that I didn't want to be kissed by him, it was a horrible experience. I tried to talk to him about the subject when Gabriel was having a bath. I started by saying we could have "a friendly relationship" without kisses. He replied that "its just a little way of showing affection, a sign that all's well between us." Then he started attacking; "you surely can't go on like this, - without a sexual relationship." He implied my life would be worthless and miserable without one, and especially without one with himself. When I said how many people prefer to live their lives in celibacy, he ranted and raved at length about how my life was "miserable and worthless", and he scorned and scoffed at me. Then he averred that, as I was remiss at offering a kiss at the door, it showed "insensitivity, vulgarity, and low culture." I was pained; and he went on; "I used to have respect for you, but I don't now; I wouldn't want you anyway." When he left I was angry that he had so insulted me in my own house! My feeling that night was "I'm not going to slave away making meals for him, when he doesn't even respect me." I had this awful feeling of being despised by him, which made me miserable all the next day. I then had the strength to tell my friend Patricia that I had to get him out of my life; *"I must re-establish some form of integrity and self-worth in my life; I can't go on living a lie."*

There was a three-day silence. A minister suggested to me that I try "a middle way"; I replied that such a thing wouldn't work with Walter; *either he would have a sexual relationship in which he dominated, or he would take up a position of hatred and enmity; he didn't know the meaning of "friendly relationship."*

170

On the 18th December, just a week before Christmas, he was still bullying and coercing me; it was when he returned Gabriel, and I didn't intend opening the door to him, but he said "you must let me in because I want to speak with you." He started off by saying the last Saturday was "my fault" for not showing him affection, and I made him "upset", and I didn't think of other people. I protested "and were you thinking of me when you heaped all those insults on me?" He said it was me who was "insensitive" and I should be doing the apologizing. I felt like the worst kind of whore, and who can't stand up for herself, for her respect and dignity. And then I felt how he had power over me and could "turn the screw" by two remarks he made. He said "I'll see him on Friday, because it's my right isn't it?" and he said "you are making me a Christmas dinner aren't you?" I was powerless to reply, for it was understood that he shouldn't see the child overnight because it caused distress, and the Christmas dinner I felt completely bullied and coerced into. I tried to say No, but couldn't, as I couldn't bear him turning nasty; I wanted to say "in the light of what you think of me I don't want to make you Christmas dinner." But he left without my saying it, and I felt stunned and sickened.

That night I wrote a letter to Pater Leo, explaining how I have become enslaved to this man in the same way as I was when I lived with him 6 years ago, doing my best to "please" him in order to stop him turning nasty; "where's my integrity, where's my sense of self-worth?" And I explained how if he turned nasty "Gabriel will be the one to suffer." I told him how I am being "forcibly kissed by a man I loathe. I can't go on like this." I told Dr.James about it and he said "women have been struggling in the same way for millions of years."

On the 21st, just a couple of days before Christmas, I made some kind of breakthrough by having a good talk with Walter in the freedom of the outdoors in the swing -park; the freedom of the open air gave me the ability to stand my ground. I told him that if he were making it clear, as he did the last Saturday that he had no liking of me and no respect for me, then affection and kisses had no place in our relationship, and neither did Christmas dinner. He said that he didn't mean to say those things, but was "emotionally upset", so wasn't responsible for them. He said "Jesus wasn't responsible for his actions when he was emotionally upset", and this made me angry. We shouted and strutted and kicked up the gravel for some time, but finally I won the battle. I made the point that if we returned to a state of enmity it would be he who lost out, because he would forfeit all the extra arrangements which are over and above the legal requirements. This won the battle for me, and he agreed he would stop the demands for "warmth and affection." He nearly burst into sobbing, saying everything had been going along so happily, and he didn't want a big upset just at Christmas. We came to an agreement about Christmas dinner; that I would invite him for a meal at tea-time but it wouldn't be a "Xmas dinner", and he would come about 4pm on the day.

However, on Christmas Eve I had a massive spiritual experience, finding "the Truth in my soul". And as a consequence I refused to let Walter come in on Christmas day.

Chapter 43
Xmas Truth in my Soul.

Crushed and confused as I was, unable to stand up for myself, living a lie, allowing myself to be forcibly kissed by a man I loathed, having lost all my integrity by the gruelling torment the system had put me through, I clung in my mind to the one memory I had which was beautiful and true. Feelings circulated through my mind of Dr.James and that moment in the dark room. I realised then that I had to "sort out my own soul and find Truth in it." I realised that I must acknowledge the persons whom I love, like Matty and Dr.James, and find honesty and truth in these relationships. *"It is in those places where I love that I shall find honesty and truth, where I shall find the truth of my own soul."* For *"Love is Truth, and Love is the God living in the soul!"*

There was a buld-up of intensity approaching Chrsistmas as I got opened up Dr.James. I confessed to him how I'd had sex with that man in Inverlang when I had escaped there; His reaction was "It is a good job you have a guardian angel looking after you." I felt we had touched a vein of integrity between us. And after that, the day before Christmas Eve, I thought a lot about him, so carefully, choosing a card of VanGogh's "Starry Night", I applied my pen to the paper: "I feel so deeply and sensitively toward you that it is hard-going to speak to you. Can I talk with you? Please can you find time in the New Year to talk with me further about my "madness"?

On Xmas Eve I took the letter round, intending to say "it's something important so please don't open it when you are busy." But to my surprise he led me into his room; I trembled with anticipation as he opened and read it. "Mairi" he said, meaningfully. "Yes," I responded, drawing myself to attention and looking straight up at him. *The moment exploded in my soul; in that moment, beyond the bravery of broaching the subject, I dared to directly face the bright reality of another soul, assenting, brave enough to encounter the "Wholly Other" of God. In that moment there was Truth steaming into my soul!*

Short and sensitive words followed. "You must remember that I am you doctor." "And how could I forget it?" I replied. He intimated that he would indeed try and come to see her, but "it must be platonic." "I'm very good at platonic relationships," I replied, mentioning my best friend being an Austrian monk. I mentioned a few ideas about Van Gogh, how he pursued the Truth of his soul, despite his manic illness. With earnestness and passion I continued: "I've got to find some Truth in my soul; I cannot go on with things denied, hidden, brushed under the carpet. I have realised that if I am going to find Truth anywhere, I must find the truth in my own soul, through my loving relationships. And if I deny my loving relationships, I deny myself." I looked up at him, close: "One of the biggest - - is You, You!"

When Christ released the woman from the power of Satan, from being bent double for 30 years, she felt as if the gaze of his warm, soft compassionate eyes had made stone icicles fall and dissolve from her innermost being with a wholeness and rush of joy, so that she stood tall and straight; as if his voice singing through her had set her free.

What I felt on leaving was beyond me to describe. And from that day, that moment when "Truth streamed into my soul," I was endued with the power to change my life, and be true to myself once more. I felt that "Truth came down," Truth was born within me, that Christmas Eve!

The revelation I had that day had indeed the power to change the rest of my life. I felt I was "standing up" at last, and would have no more of the lies, deceptions and dishonesties which sprang from a fear of the truth. I realised the first thing I must do was to "own" all of my past experience, to own my madness.

I had written to Matty. I explained to him how I had to let go of him in Craigdene, had to sacrifice him, because it was the only way I was going to be let out of the place and get my son back; I explained how Dr.McNeill's attitude was that, as long as I wanted a relationship with him "I must be ill", so with my mother's feelings toward my little child, I had no choice. Writing this letter was me looking back at last on something very painful, and owning it and coming to terms with it; I sensed how I had been "tortured." I asked Matty to forgive me for hurting him so much.

What to do with Walter?- that was the question on Christmas day. I realised he was the prime source of the lies and dishonesty in my life, and I didn't want to relate to him any more. When I awoke on Christmas day I felt beautiful, full of "the Truth which lives within me" as I did when I was young. Then I thought about Walter and what I should do with him in the light of this new Truth; I had promised he could come at 4pm and have a meal. So I phoned him, said how the lies and hypocrisy in my life emanated from him, and I how didn't love him, said I wasn't having the "pretence" of inviting him in on Christmas day. His response was to turn to predictable threats; but I felt that I had on "the armour of Truth."

The result was that I had Walter standing on my doorstep with hatred streaming out of his eyes; he handed in Christmas presents which were mean and worthless. The next day, Boxing day, I reminded him he should bring Gabriel back at 4pm, the stipulated time, but he didn't bring him back till 6, and I was really worried; I even phoned the police, concerned that Gabriel had been kidnapped, but they refused to help, saying it was impossible in law for a father to "kidnap" his own child. Eventually, two hours later, he was brought back; apparently they had been on a long walk along the Willow Braes in the cold and the dark. I felt Walter was starting a new ploy of dominating over me by making me worried as a mother.

I did some reading of the stuff I wrote when "mad", and realised I was more true to myself then; the rest of my life seemed to be all inhibitions; I realised that "when I am most myself I am called ill." I said "no-one can make me afraid of my madness any more." I thought of all the men in my life that I really loved, feeling I had to shed my inhibitions. "This is where I will find truth and salvation in my life; in those places where I love."

Matty came to visit me, and I felt that our carresses and kisses were the expression of the touching of two souls; I felt really good after he'd gone, because I felt I'd been true to myself, true to the me which is deep down. Meanwhile Walter was spouting things at me, and threatening to upset Gabriel, but I felt that he had nothing to hurt me with. *I saw how he liked to think he possessed me and owned me, but I realised that he had no claim on me; "for I never said yes to him, never committed myself to him, never married him,- he has no power over me."*

My New Year's resolution was: *"I will be true to myself from now on."*

When Christ healed the blind man, and a brightness of vivid light penetrated to his soul, in that moment the world seemed to come alive and call to him, vivid and real, impressing itself immediately on the senses and soul. So he opened his eyes, and could see a new world which was his and responsive to him, which could laugh and sing and cry with him.

Chapter 44
A Threat-System.

When I resolved on New Year's Eve to be "true to myself," I knew that in doing that I would be "beautiful". I said to myself, listening to Beethoven and with a lighted candle, "Keep true to that Truth, Beauty, Love you see shining within." I rapidly found that in freeing myself from my enslavement to Walter, that my heart was opened to a springtime of love. I decided I would "follow where the love in my own heart leads."

And I decided I would "stand for truth" where that last hospital admission was concerned. I remembered how we had an agreement that, not only was Gabriel on no account to go to Walter if I were ill, but also that visits to his mother in hospital would be "as frequent as possible." Now why was that agreement so openly and flagrantly flouted? *And something else,- Gabriel thought I was dead; they allowed him to believe that I was dead! Walter took advantage, and Dr.McNeill was culpable! I decided I found it "unforgivable"!*

I was now better able to handle Walter. One night, when Matty was in the house, he came to the door, and fell into a jealous rage; "Who have you got in there? Is it that man you knew at the hospital? I'm not going to have my son associating with mentally ill people." I said I could be friends with whom I liked. He wouldn't get off my doorstep, so I said that if he didn't go I'd call the police. "You can call the police if you like, but I'm coming in!" But I pushed him out, outraged that he had tried to force his way into my house; I felt how it proved that his purpose all along was to dominate over me.

I received a reply-letter from Percy Gerard, whom I got to know in an earlier manic episode in Norwich. I had said to him that I was going "to write, to write the truth," so that everybody should know the torture that goes on in mental hospitals. He wrote positively and enthusiastically; "I would love to see you write the novel that is in you; use your manic-ness as a gift, as a creative force." I wrote back that I felt ringed-round by foes rather than a friendly support-system, but I must be "true to myself and true to my madness, for my madness is like a friend." I said I felt he was like "a warm light-giving candle of a friend in a wide darkness." I really admired Percy Gerard; he was a fine rational, sophisticated, intelligent, refined gentleman; Walter on the other hand was brutish and goatish and believed in emotion and the impulsive will. I felt how ironic a card life had dealt me, placing the man I admire so far away and the goatish Walter on my doorstep!

I at that time read through what I'd written when supposedly "ill" and decided such things couldn't be written by a "mentally ill" person; I saw that I had been "like a solitary ship on a sea of pain." I realised there was "a Truth I know in madness;" it is a deep-down touching of the self. I realised that in the painful path out of madness I had to take to myself all the pain I had denied in being mad. I decided I'd talk with people about what I'd said when considered mad; "I will search out the truth in these matters; people think I will not ask because I am embarrassed; but not any more, now that I consider my madness to be my friend, and do not fear it." I owned my madness for the first time as a friend "whom I must honour, love, learn to understand, and never betray and never deny."

When I saw Steven Peterson for the first time after the Christmas break he told me to be careful of writing such truthful letters as I'd written to him; "be wary of how other people may respond to you." I happened to tell him how Gabriel complained that his Dad "punches him in the stomach", and he was instantly galvanized into a social -worker reaction, saying he had to investigate it; I moaned that we had been through all this before. But I tried to deny Walter access to Gabriel that day, as I was instructed, and he resorted to his usual threats. He came back later, banging on the door and shouting through the letter-box; "you'll be sorry, I'm taking the case back to court and this time I won't stop." He wouldn't stop banging on all the doors and windows, frightening both me and Gabriel. But I was pursuing a "vein of truth" and I found that night the introduction to Clare's poetry which spoke of a "disorder" similar to mine, more interesting than Walter's antics.

My support system now became worried about me, because I was delving into my own madness and searching after truth in this way; they although I might be "getting ill." When I went to see Dr.James, and started talking about "Truth " and poets' madness, he said suddenly "I am worried by you." After that I became rather scared, because of what happened the day after the last time he said he was worried about me; I had been confronted by the dreadful sight of the Craigdene squad coming. I went back and promised Dr.James that if it would make him happier, I would shut down for a while this pursuit of truth into the realms of madness. I was left feeling glum; it wasn't fair that everyone should be threat to me just because I spoke the truth in an uninhibited way. I felt I had to get out of the place, out of KirkMichaels, as it was a "dangerous place" for me. I felt pressurized on all sides, forbidden to go into what fascinated me, ie."madness", and forced to go into something I wanted nothing to do with, ie. my relationship with Walter again. I was losing my sense of freedom.

I nearly went off somewhere that weekend, as I felt scared, but I decided "I'm not going to run, I'm going to stay put and face it." I felt I couldn't tolerate this, fearing every time I spoke the truth in an uninhibited way that the Craigdene squad were coming after me! When I saw Dr.McNeill he kept saying, insultingly, that I was always changing my mind, so it was difficult for anyone to judge if I were getting ill. Then he entirely sided with Walter; "No doubt his banging on the door is his understandable reaction to your changing your mind yet again!" I felt how I really loathed him; I realised that if it ever came to a Custody case in court, I hadn't a hope of being backed up by him! The next day I told Walter I wasn't interested in fighting him; I thought how Dr.James and Dr.McNeill were a far greater threat to me than he was.

I thought to myself that I wasn't going to fight against Walter again, as Steven was insisting, when I would end up unsupported. *For 6 years I had been trying to protect my son from that man, and look what happened; at the end of the day I was left unsupported, and finally "they handed Gabriel over to him on a platter!"* I began to feel how everyone in my support system was a "bastard" because of their arrogance, even Philip and Dr.James, because they "labelled me as manic, as if that wrote off any truth in what I did or said." I hated what I felt as everyone's arrogant attitude towards me. I found out from my CPN Ted, that essentially the reason why I was hospitalized the previous summer was because I had chucked him out of my house; I was angry about it, for I knew how I was being "true to myself" when I chucked him out. I felt a "straightjacket" on my spirit, in that I couldn't be "true to myself" without grave danger. It was then that I formulated the plan of going to live elsewhere, perhaps near Percy Gerard in Norwich. I thought of saying to Ted, "it is not you and me against my madness, it is you against me!"

Steven then told me that he wanted to launch " a full-scale investigation into Gabriel's welfare"; he said that teachers shouldn't be getting annoyed with a child of that young age. I nearly replied "But it was OK to let Walter for a long time distress him by locking him up!" He said that it needed my co-operation; there was the veiled threat that if I didn't co-operate they might take Gabriel away from me; I thought secretly how I would refuse to co-operate. The thought was in my mind, *"It is not a support-system, but a threat-system!"*

I went for a walk with Walter along the shore, and we had a "friendly talk." I said how my turning him away on Christmas day was a matter of "being true to myself", and apologized for it. I said how futile it was to make a show of being true to myself when there were so many enemies and so many threats "out there." I said how as parents we were threatened by the establishment and the System. And so we must stick together and be friends, because "the threat is not from each other but from "them"."

The lame foot which had been bothering me since coming out of hospital, the very painful heel, was now examined by a psychic healer. She said that it showed that there's "something basically wrong with my understanding"; it stemmed, she said "from intense hatred and negative feelings which had been buried." I realised it was true that my lame foot "expressed a hitch in my psychical being." I decided to search for a psychotherapist.

When I saw Dr.McNeill I talked with him about VanGogh's suicide, which I had been reading about. He took a blood-test as usual, to check I was taking as much Lithium as he prescribed; "can we reduce the tablets?" I simpered, saying untruthfully how drowsy I felt. "No not yet," came his hateful reply. I came out feeling rotten because I had been untrue to myself. *I felt what a long way I'd come from Christmas, when I felt it great and glorious to be "true to myself"; now the System had got in motion again, and I had to be untrue to myself because it threatened me!*

I wrote a letter to Percy Gerard complaining bitterly how I couldn't be "true to myself" in this place; "everytime I am most true to myself they label me as manic; they only think I am normal when I am placid." I made a list of all the things which caused me to be labelled as "ill"; when I was uninhibited, or aggressive, or said anything mystical, or when I changed my mind or said anything uncharacteristic. "Perhaps this is because they think that normal people don't think and feel in this way; I don't know; all I know is that it is unbearable." I said how angry I was that Dr.McNeill recently renewed my section, and asked if he knew whether that would prevent me from moving away from the area. "I can't live under this kind of tyranny at all."

I wrote a letter to Pater Leo saying how I wasn't free to be true to myself anymore, because I couldn't express myself in an uninhibited way, or speak truly, without being under threat. "It is a whole System that is against me, that breathes down my neck like a monster. Such a tyranny is exercised over me that I am screaming out for the freedom to breathe and be myself. When I was true to myself I flowed with love inside; now that I am untrue I feel frozen with negative feelings."

179

Chapter 45
Turning Mystical.

So I decided that night when I wrote to Pater Otto that the answer could only be that I should cease relating to the world, ignore the world, "and plunge myself into the love of God instead." I decided I'd devote all my energies into reading and writing of the love of God. *For what I needed was "Air"; and "Love is the air I need to breathe, to restore my soul."*

"Why did you go mad?"- "I was making flights into the Void."
"Why?" - "I was seeking God there."
"Why?"- "Because in the System which enslaved me, He was absent.
        I went mad because I was looking for a God who was absent."

And so I lost interest in the world and began to "plunge myself into the love of God instead." Instead of wasting my energy battling with the support system, I turned myself to a mystical investigation of my understanding of God; "there are no mental health sections in the rarefied atmosphere where God's love lives!"

I earnestly began to read the many mystical texts I possessed, I delved into the lives of the artists, musicians and poets who had trodden the path of madness before me, and I began my mystical writings. "Writing must be my Raison d'etre, as painting was forVanGogh." I began to explore the Book of Beloved again and realised it was my task in life to be exploring God's love; "all my life and all that I ever write are but efforts to elucidate and understand that revelation of God's love." My direction should be "ever upward, ever onward, into an understanding of that rarefied atmosphere of God's love."

I no longer felt the "tyranny of the System." I felt that the love which made the streams flow and moved the stars was also smiling from behind my eyes. I realised how mistaken I had been at Christmas about loving men; "all those people my heart flooded out towards, and not a single one has responded." My friend Maggie at this stage tried to persuade me to "fight" against Walter, but I replied it would be "a waste of time, of effort, of soul-energy, of my life itself; it would be a waste, full-stop." I found that the way to stop fighting was to be "centred in peace and love." Meantime I was seriously engaged in writing my mystical book; I was full of ideas for it; it was becoming quite exciting. I felt fully alive in my creativity, feeling that I was "sharing in the creativity of God."

Percy Gerard finally wrote back to me, and I was delighted. I felt how he could replace Philip as my soul-friend, for Philip was annoying me by forbiddingly saying that being creative was "dangerously intensifying." I had realised that Philip had done me harm, by turning me away from my own mysticism and creativity for over 5years; "he had betrayed the love within me, and enslaved me to the System." I felt I had taken "a mighty big wrong turning" for the past 5 years; I had been "ensnared by the System"; I had not been myself. But in my reply to Percy Gerard I said how now, with eyes turned away from the world toward an understanding of the love of God, "I am Myself." I had remembered my vocation; I was breathing now, after feeling asphixiated, and my book had begun. Percy said that writing a book was like "giving birth to a 10-lb porcupine." I replied that it wasn't, and I was speaking from experience. I said he shouldn't compare the ghastly experience of giving birth, which wasn't creative at all, and which allowed outside interference, to the creativity of writing, when you have a sense of being mastered by a power greater than the puny powers of self, and which is joyous, always personal and pure.

I wrote all the more after that. It brought about a great peacefulness of mind, because directing my energies to an outflow. I obeyed Percy's advice to "stay cool" when the CPN Ted came to my house and construed my quietness of mind to mean anger. This annoyed me and I felt I didn't want any more of this System monitoring me and intruding into my house. Percy's concept of "coolness" was that you should "appear to conform whilst retaining the integrity of the essential you." I found this helpful.

At this time I wrote to the "Westwood clinic" to ask if they would take me for Psychotherapy, saying that people's reaction to my becoming manic when reality and my mind snapped apart, was to lock me up and stuff me full of mind-sickening drugs; "there must be another way, a more sane, kind and humane way, to deal with that snapping apart, or an understanding which can prevent it from happening."

But the person I was really seeking Psychotherapy from was Dr.James.

There was a lot of embarrassment between myself and Dr James, whilst we were learning to trust each other; he didn't trust me because of false conceptions he had, and I felt couldn't trust him, because I doubted whether he had helped to hospitalize me; we needed to talk, to thresh out some truth.

In January, determined again to ask him to visit me, I went round to the surgery with a mixture of yearning and apprehension. I said to this marvellous man who represented to me "the Wholly Other" the words I had rehearsed: "Let me say first of all, thankyou for what you did for me on Xmas Eve, for my encounter with you gave me the power, the ability, to find the Truth within me for which I was seeking." He challenged "What do you mean by Truth?" I talked on a bit about the truth I was delving into about poet's madness, and how creativity is linked with the manic state. He said suddenly "I am worried by you." He was pottering about with needles, when I gathered up the courage to say "I thought you were going to come and see me?" He told me rather crossly that I was "capable of causing a great deal of embarrassment," and questioned my platonic friendship with Philip, and declared I was a danger to him and his profession!

It was a Saturday morning and I had been eating a cream-cake when he came to the door; I was self-conscious due to the fact that I had cream round my mouth, but I talked passionately of how wicked it was that the law-courts granted Walter such Access rights, and he replied "I usually take the fathers'side, being a father myself, but in this case I don't." I felt a warm cosiness, believing that he was on my side. I thought how I could not view him as an enemy; he always charmed me into believing him a friend. "I am glad to find you so very well and so very rational," he said. "Well that's nice to hear, especially coming from you." I wanted honesty and truth from him, so I asked: "Had you judged me manic the day before they rushed me to Craigdene?" He assured me "No."

I really wished that I could have a deep and honest talk with him. There always seemed to be so much we did not say, so many memories brushed under the carpet. I felt so attached to the man; it made me believe in lost souls seeking each other through reincarnation. I felt he was wary of me because I was a threat to him; he had lots of misconceptions about me. But I felt he knew everything I had suffered. I needed to talk things out with him.

Chapter 46
Negative Energy.

Then I found out on enquiring that the certain document in which it was agreed that Gabriel should not go to Walter were I ill, had gone missing. It had conveniently gone missing from 7 different files! I was angry, for it was supposed to be an important document; I felt angry against the System, though realising that this was "a waste of energy".

I became passionate at this time about the fact that I wasn't really "ill" in my last bout of mania. I went to see a minister who had seen me when I was supposed mad; he said how it seemed to him just "an over-emphasis on perfectly reasonable things." I happened to find out from Dr.James that the day before I was carried out by the Craigdene squad, he had seen me, and he said "you were slightly excited but you weren't manic." This made me moreangry than ever about it, in that 24 hours later, without anyone else seeing me or examining me meantime, the Craigdene squad were sent to get me; they didn't check up! The day after finding that out, I was seething with negative emotion; I was convinced that they had put me into hospital without my being manic. I felt how precarious my existence was; I felt that in that place life wasn't worth living. I felt that if Dr.McNeill should renew my section I'd protest by non-co-operation and refuse to speak to him; Philip warned that if I tried that, Dr.McNeill would lock me up in hospital. My negative emotions against the System thus became stronger than ever.

I felt how this mass of negative emotion was crippling my life and crippling my capabilities. I realised that this anger was only crippling myself; it was futile and going nowhere. I realised how I must somehow allay the power of these negative emotions because they could do me no good.

And then one night I phoned up my friend Helen, whom I blamed for sending the Craigdene squad round; I yelled at her and blamed her, and her response was "you don't sound very well at the moment; you are aggressive and that means you are not well." I yelled at her "I will pay you back!" However having put the phone down I realised what danger I was in. Maggie and Louise came galloping round like the cavalry, providing me with the emotional stability and security to talk for an hour with Dr.James.

I blazed my anger at Dr.James, telling how I was tortured in Craigdene, locked up there when I wasn't manic, and how I was so mangled and crushed that they broke my will; it was a "death of the soul" when my will was broken, so broken that I felt I had nothing left to live for, and so was willing to throw my life away with that man in Inverlang on momentary comfort. *I yelled "Don't you remember that howl of anguish that I let out in that dark room with you?" I was conscious of the other people in the room, as I yelled about that moment; "Don't you remember how I accused you in that room! Don't you remember my anguish because they had broken my will! Don't you remember my Passion!"* I knew he remembered it. Finally when calmed, I said "I trust you." *And then I saw that I needed to face the howl of anguish in my own mind.*

That document I sought finally turned up, and I discovered, not only did it say what I thought, about choosing other carers rather that Walter, but it also gave some authority to my parents. I phoned my Dad about it, and he said he gave Steven Peterson "permission to do what had to be done." To me that sounded like an echo of him telling me to have an abortion, and I was angry with him. I said how I'd given him some authority over my child, and in the event what he did with that authority "was to hand my little son over to Walter on a platter!" I was angry about it.

Then I had a talk with Sean Maddison, the Mental health officer who had helped to section me the previous August. And I found out from him that everything I had said could be reasonably understood and explained in the present; the only "bizarre idea" he said I'd intimated to him was that I was "holding the door of heaven open with my left foot." I explained to him how this was a fundamental idea in a book I had written twenty years earlier; I explained how the universal grief of the world was to me expressed in this idea that I was given the lowliest task of holding the door of heaven open for others whilst denied bliss myself; I explained how it wasn't a "bizarre" idea, and it couldn't show mental illness if it were currently understandable to me. Then he let me know that my admission was mostly the CPN Ted's doing; "it was due to you wanting a reduction in medication." I was appalled; "I was considered ill because I dared to rebel, dared to say that I should have power over my own life!" I deemed it worse than anything that happened in Russia!

The next day I felt that I had to expurgate some of my emotion, because "if kept buried, it would have power to kill." I wrote to Percy Gerard about how I was "put away" because I wanted to take some control of my own life; I was "nullified out of existence." *I said that what I couldn't bear was that so much suffering was put upon my little 5-year-old son, and I found that unforgivable. Gabriel told me that Walter*

184

was *"locking him up"*, and we had a legally binding agreement to say that he should not be handed over to his father. And I kept saying to people "please go and help Gabriel," but everyone's attitude was "you are considered mentally ill, and therefore nothing that you say can be true." No-one even went to check up on Gabriel, and I was powerless to help him, and he was allowed to believe that his Mummy was dead; it must have seemed to him that no-one was ever going to come and rescue him. *"The people who in their pride of power took my freedom away also put that degree of terror and torment upon my little child."* I could forgive anything done to me, but I couldn't forgive this torment put upon this tender 5-year-old son of mine; I found it unforgivable; *"I hope that everybody roasts in hell for it!"* I felt that this was a crime which was "screaming out for redress and revenge." I realised that it was the "energy of hatred" that possessed me.

I felt I needed help because of this seething "energy of hatred" within me. It wasn't "a thing directed from me with will, but something that erupts from a rent or wound in my being"; "it leaps out". I realised that the thing that would do me good was to "let out my howl of anguish."

185

Chapter 47
The Norwich Experience.

I knew another section was imminently to be imposed upon me; I felt angry that I wasn't worthy of being counted a citizen; it would "nullify me out of existence"; I would have no freedom and no rights; I wasn't even allowed to vote. Philip pointed out to me that, if it were true, as Sean Maddison said, that I was hospitalized because I was wanting to reduce my medication, the detention was illegal. I was determined to get a hold of the detention order, to find out what it said, and to seek redress.

Steven Peterson visited me, and when I blamed him for handing Gabriel over to Walter when it was contrary to that signed legal agreement, he started threatening me. He said "We have power without your consent to refer it to the children's panel, and because of your psychiatric history, that might not turn out in your favour." He was threatening to take Gabriel away from me and put him into care! I managed to see him out of the door by saying unemotionally and serenely "I am not interested in you or the System you are part of." *When I saw Dr.James afterwards he told me to "stop stirring it," because otherwise people would think I was ill, and "there is no redress, there can be no redress!" When he said that I must "go along with the System," as the only way to get free from sections, I said with the energy of trueness to myself, "I won't comply with a System that is evil."*

I had a deep moment with Gabriel. He had recently been getting very emotional and blaming me for his emotion, saying "you made me upset"; he had learnt this behaviour from Walter. But one day he suddenly said to me "I love you very much mummy;" and I replied "I don't know what I'd do without you, life wouldn't be worth living without you." And we clung to each other like two souls on a whirling raft.

Maggie was being a help, strengthening my will in my fight against the System; but where she went wrong was in telling me what to do, and she had some very weird ideas. Percy Gerard was also being a great help on the phone; he said he was moved by the pain I lived in; he said all I could do was to "live life as quietly and sanely as possible," until they would let me go. When I asked if I could possibly come and live in Norwich, he welcomed the idea. And so I felt a sense of the fresh air of freedom awaiting me somewhere.

Then one day I had a childcare social worker visiting me, to ascertain whether it was necessary to start "an investigation." Maggie was with me, and she said things which made this man suspicious. And the upshot of it was that he declared it was his legislative duty, to "launch a full investigation, with or without my co-operation." I was upset, and sobbed and got a terrible migraine; *I felt how the threat was real of having Gabriel taken away from me, and said to myself how I'd "go to the ends of the earth to keep him with me." I cried out "I can't live under such a threat."* A friend called Gail came and told me that I must "stop fighting", because I was "at breaking point"; this alarmed me, because it was dangerous to let any one think that; it was like one more threat. Looking out of the window into the dark I decided that I would flee from this place, and I phoned a friend who was a lawyer, and ascertained from her that the new Mental Health act could be broken by being free of its grip for one month; I wondered whether I could "outlast its power."

Then I was thrown into real bliss for a few days by finding out, from the "Scottish Association of Mental health", that it was true that if I stayed in England for 28 days my section would be broken. And Percy Gerard volunteered to be the person who would help me to do it. I had such intense phone-conversations with the man; he was willing to hold out a helping hand to me, willing to share in the complicity. I was thrilled by my new plan of abandoning my home in favour of an ideal of freedom; all I needed to do was to keep out of Scotland for 28 days and I'd have cracked it! I was in veritable bliss at finding this out, and by the complete help offered to me by Percy.

My hero-worship of Percy soared; I thought he was the most wonderfully humane person I'd ever met. I then found out that the person who might help me to stay away for the month would be committing "a criminal offence" and might be jailed; I was absolutely astonished when Percy said that despite this risk to himself he would still help me. I was intending to "escape" illegally, but at the end of the day, before leaving, I notified Dr.McNeill; he hadn't renewed the section yet, and I thought I might dissuade him from doing so by acting responsibly.

Before leaving for Norwich, the last week in February, I had a really nasty argument with Walter. When he demanded to know where I was going, shouting "I demand to know were you are taking my son," I refused to tell him. He turned to threats; "One day I'll be taking him on holiday, and I will leave you to worry by not letting you know where I am taking your son!" The argument really sickened me and I thought how wonderful it would be if I could finally get away from the man; if we went to live in Norwich he wouldn't get much Access and we would be free after all these years of torment.

So we set off on the train to Norwich. After a horrid journey, I was shocked on meeting Percy to find he looked "an old man," and he had a wife. For a few days things went fine; he let us stay in a "Halfway House" which he had jurisdiction over; he took us for a run to the local villages including Walsingham and I found I could have a good talk with him, and I showed him my writings; and I really felt that perhaps Norwich held out to me "wide horizons and unguessed possibilities." Then things began to go wrong; the schizophrenic who was willing to do a house-swap with me changed her mind; I had a bad time with the Council's Housing department, who weren't very eager to let me move to Norwich, and when I visited a Women's Refuge where I would have to stay for a long while, I really couldn't stomach it. I realised that everything really depended on how much help Percy was willing to give me. But I was quickly completely disillusioned by Percy. I had this "dream" that I would be invited into his kitchen, sharing meals, reading his books, playing with his cats, etc. In reality he carefully parcelled out his time to me, not committing himself at all; he gave me 40 minutes of his time in his office, and there he said I had to accept the fact, the designation that I was "recovering from psychiatric illness". I was angry at this, feeling he hadn't believed me or sympathized with me at all. "No we are not coming to live in Norwich" I said to myself. And we set off home.

I was so glad to be home. It had been stifling in that city of Norwich; I loved KirkMichaels in comparison; "the sea, the sky, the fresh beauty of the place." I loved my home, and felt I would never again think of giving it up. I realised then how fortunate I was to live in such a place; I decided I would never again delude myself into thinking "the grass is greener on the other side." I had pursued a dream that didn't exist; from then on I would love and appreciate what I had, and be prepared "to suffer and learn in what was my real world."

When Christ faced healed the man with the withered arm, it was as if the man felt the warm waters of a green-growing oasis lap around his body; he seemed to touch something which gushed through him like a fountain of life. His desert-life was inundated by a blessed warm flood, and he believed the green things of his life would begin to grow again.

Chapter 48
Crusading for Truth.

And so having learnt a lesson from my Norwich-experience, and glad to have a home that I loved and the fresh beauty of KirkMichaels to live in, I decided to keep my feet planted firmly in reality, and "to suffer and learn in what was my real world." I would stay in this home, taking on board my suffering here. One thing I realised was that I had to "tackle my reality" in the shape of Walter.

I then found out, by letter, that my section had been renewed. I was so very angry. I had argued with Dr.McNeill before going to Norwich that he shouldn't renew it, saying I complied much better under a situation of persuasion rather than coercion. So, angry to find he had renewed it, I walked to the hospital and shouted at Ted over it; I said it was "coercion by fear" which was an "abuse of the law." It was contrary to the British belief in freedom and I was going to appeal against it. Accordingly I found out the name of a solicitor specializing in Mental Health Law, called Julia MacBride, and had a fervent talk with her on the phone about this section infringing my human rights.

I then went to keep my appointment at the Westwood Clinic in Edinburgh, hoping that they could help me to express "the howl of anguish" that remained inside of me. But it was useless; they sat there listening to me completely impassively! That was no good! So I went round to the surgery again at the beginning of March, to appeal to Dr.James again, and said what I had to say, trembling like a leaf. *"Look you know me; you are practically omniscient about everything I have ever suffered; I need to talk with you; it is you I need to talk things out with."* I said of the howl of anguish inside of me, which needed to be let out; *"you know what that howl of anguish is, because you heard it."*

Dr.James explained that such "Psychotherapy" would need a lot of time and he didn't have the training. He thought and then said "You are right that we have been through a lot of suffering together; and I've learnt to be a good listener in my job as a doctor." But he said he wouldn't want to be "a crutch". "It's not a crutch I need," I replied " it is someone to help me to face and come to terms with the howl of anguish in my own mind, in order to control these energies of hatred and anger which leap out." These energies were like a monster chasing me which I must turn round and face. I explained how all the other times in the hospital I had come through whole and resilient, but this time they had broken my will. I reminded him of the nurse Chris and his treatment of me; he replied, "Perhaps you attracted the man." I pondered on this strange thought.

He then said "I've certainly lost a lot of sleep worrying about your future." I was touched; it made me feel that I was special to him. "I'll certainly try," he concluded, and he agreed a time to come round and see me, and I felt I was special to him. And I went out with bliss bursting its banks, until it became like pain.

When I saw Dr.McNeill I had the energy of anger in me, but kept my cool. I told him I was appealing against the section, saying it would deprive me of the right to vote, which was a right and freedom which everybody in the country enjoyed; I said it wasn't justified and I would have my say in a court of law. He seemed perturbed and replied that he did it for the sake of the ease with which he could put me in hospital should I become unwell. I said back that if I were unwell he could section me in the usual way; I said "you are arguing that you so abuse the law for the "ease" of doing something to someone against their will; do you think that is acceptable in a society that believes in freedom and human rights?" And his reply came "Yes I do think it is." I felt how much I hated him! However I came away a bit glad because, on my asking, he said it was acceptable for me to get my medication from Dr.James rather than Ted, the CPN; I would be glad not to suffer the constraints of the latter breathing down my neck. Philip told me that Section 18 was used very sloppily, and if I challenged it, it would establish case-law; *so I felt I could "strike a blow for freedom" for everybody; I felt like Spenser's Red Cross Knight, crusading in the cause of Truth.*

There was a certain lie which had grown monstrously out of proportion. Years ago, in the hospital, I said to Helen's husband Ernest, to test if he were gullible, that I had thrown my crucifix into the sea, off the end of the pier, and "could just as well have thrown Gabriel into the sea." Now, years later, everybody had got hold of this story as a true utterance. Dr.McNeill came back to me with a really sick version; "you thought Gabriel was evil and so you were intending to kill him by throwing him off the pier; that's why you threw the crucifix away as an action against evil." I was horrified to find my utterance come back to me this way. I was determined to fight against such a monstrous lie, to campaign for Truth.

I felt a lot better after I'd decided that I was crusading for Truth, for I realised that I could do it with a "coolness", a calm strength, an incise energy, which wasn't like the heat of emotion. *I was determined to strike a blow for the freedom and rights of everyone suffering under Mental Health law in Scotland.*

190

Finally the Tuesday night arrived when I had a marvellous talk with Dr.James, our first "psychotherapy session,"which established Truth between us, sorting out Truth from untruth. All sorts of untruth lay embedded in his mind; his belief that I had a sexual relationship with Philip and therefore said he "abused" me, though the whole thing was platonic and mystical; his belief that I was "promiscuous" in the hospital, and also with that man in Inverlang; his belief that when passionate with him in that dark room I was "as mad as a hatter." I explained away all these things, saying that when manic the masks fall away, so my expression of feeling in that dark room was not less real and true, but more real and true. He listened to my protestations, though the whole process made me blush. I said I wouldn't be using him as a crutch; " I want to find Truth in relation to you, for I believe you find Truth in you own soul in relation to the Wholly Other." I told him of the brilliance of my experience on Christmas eve; "the Truth I find in relation to you liberates me." I said how for years I hadn't gone to see him because I liked him too much; and I wondered why sometimes he seemed cold and insensitive. "Let me tell you something Mairi; sometimes I draw back from you because you are so strong." I thought it a lovely thing to say, and blushed with pleasure.

For days afterwards I felt a great release of energy which set me free with its healing power; I felt liberated, re-born out of Truth, "I have a new fresh strong soul to face the world." Then there was a brief period, up until the Spring day which was Mother's day, when he regularly came round to do psychotherapy, and he kept making me blush and I dwelt on what he said with pleasure. I longed to say things back to him, such as "Your hand is in my being and it is a mastering hand" and "I need you like a need water and air." I told him "I've always been sensitive towards you, because sensing that you are involved in my life in some incomprehensible way."

The next day, I had a special and marvellous day in Edinburgh, to meet my solicitor Julia MacBride and to rendez-vous with Philip. I felt so good about myself, like a modern liberated woman, inwardly free and beautiful and strong and true. I found Julia MacBride sympathetic and liberated in her thinking, as I explained to her the abuse of Mental health law by Dr.McNeill; it was used for coercion by fear, for the ease of readmitting me. After seeing her Philip picked me up in his car, and we went to a cafe together. I felt I really loved him, for our friendship in its depth and strength could never be equalled. His constancy and care in the 3 years since he'd ceased to be my social worker were astonishing; he told me how he really "cared" about me. We talked about everything in this café, with such a rapport and sense of fun.

And then we touched a deep vein when I told him what that "secret" was that I had kept from him back in '88; it was that I had begun a period after 5 years without one, and the release of the warm red blood was as if God were touching my womb and healing me. Coming home I thought what a marvellous and faithful friend I had in Philip.

Chapter 49
The Adoption Decision.

For some time, ever since he came back to me from Walter, I had been having serious difficulties with my little Gabriel, for he seemed to have caught some "emotional sickness" from his Dad. He was always having paddys and pointing at me shouting "you made me upset." I felt I couldn't cope with him any longer; I did all the daily tasks to care for him, but my heart wasn't in it any more. I felt that the something I had put in his heart, be it love or truth, wasn't there any longer; the love-bond between us wasn't there any more. I couldn't afford to love him when I had to keep handing him over to Walter in a way that damaged him.

Then on one occasion, the 12th March, he threw such an almighty paddy that I said to myself "he is beyond my help." I knew how Walter had been locking him up in his bedroom, for the slightest misdemeanor or to make him stay in bed. I had never locked him away from having free access to me. I felt that 5 years work of love had been undone. I felt that the only way forward to heal Gabriel was to have him adopted; it was the only way to give him a chance in life, the only way to protect the love within his soul. I had been through this several times over,- the idea of adoption,- *and I had always given in because that umbilical cord between mother and child was too deep and strong; but this time I thought I could do it.*

I reflected ruefully on how I used to believe, was led to believe when Gabriel was new-born, that the System would protect both me and the baby. Then I discovered that the people I asked for help used the authority of the System to hand my child over to Walter "on a platter"! *Walter was like an ogre I had escaped from, and I asked the System to protect us from the ogre; and the System took the child who is the tenderest part of me, and handed him over into the same ogre's power! That is why I kept saying "on a platter"; "my son is like a morsel to eat for the ogre"!*

I reflected ruefully on what suffering I'd gone through because I am "forced to relate to a man I loathe because he is the father of my baby." I reflected ruefully how, if I were not always striving to do "the most loving thing" my suffering would have finished ages ago. The only solution now it seemed was adoption, as it could sever myself and my child from Walter forever. *It would be very free-ing; Gabriel needed to be free, and I needed to be free. The main thing was that it would allow Gabriel to be healed and grow up with a chance in life. I thought it was so ironic that I could only sever myself and my child from Walter by severing my child from myself!* I always knew that, even when pregnant; I knew I had to sever myself from the baby in my womb before I could ever be free of the man who was destroying my soul. And then I gave birth to it and loved it, and all the way along tried to do the most loving thing, making things worse for myself. *And now I saw the only way to protect my child's soul from being destroyed, was to make a decision as in the "Caucasian Chalk-circle."*

The story of the "Caucasian Chalk-circle" runs like this: - A mother who had abandoned her child then takes her case up against another woman who had brought up the child and loved it; the child was made to stand in a chalk-circle in front of the judge; and he told the women to each take a hand and tug, and the true mother who had "the strongest love" would succeed in tugging it out of the circle. It happened that the woman who really loved the child let go, so as not to hurt it. Then the judge said to that woman "I see that you really love the child, so you are the true mother." In the same way I thought to myself, I had to "let go" of Gabriel. *"For true love doesn't tug; it lets go"!*

It was true that for myself I couldn't stand by for years watching Walter's emotional domination over my child. I loathed the way he kept repeating to him "Do you love your daddy? I want to know if you love your daddy?" I couldn't stand watching it; he was robbing my child of the freedom in his soul. My intent wasn't to "throw him away", because he was damaged, as was true of some of my Adoption ideas in the past; it was to give him "a better chance." And it would be a better chance for both of us; it would free us both to be whole persons. In a way it was like my breast-feeding for the first week of his tiny life, before it became unbearably sore; *I could say that I'd given this child the best start I possibly could, and now it was time to free both myself and him.*

In the Baptist service one day, looking at Gabriel, I thought how I would be able to bear giving him up because "I'll still be a mother." I realised that the essence of my reason for doing this was that I "couldn't bear to watch," to watch the child I loved grow up into a crippled, sick, inadequate adult. *I'd rather do without him myself, in order to put love and life into his soul.* I thought how hopefully I'd see him again at the age of 18, and hopefully I'd find him a whole person. I decided I would keep this Adoption decision to myself for one whole month, to see if "my purpose holds", before speaking my intention to anyone.

That night when contemplating I said "Yes, I have decided for it." I realised that giving up Gabriel would be for me "a manner of death." But all my life I had been "trying to die", because I knew that was where God's love was to be found; and I believed that "out of death comes life." Through the Book of the Beloved God spoke to me with the words, as regards all my suffering, "Forget it now, lay it aside"; *and I felt I could do that, and there would be "a bright new life awaiting me on the other side." I felt God was saying Yes to me. I would embrace the point where God wanted me to die, and it was here; I would be "rushing into His love."*

Chapter 50
The Purpose Holding.

Having made my decision for Adoption, as the only away of giving Gabriel a chance of growing up with a free and loving soul, I realised after another few days that it also signalled the end of my binding to Walter. I was very glad; I would finally be able to "walk on."

I had very strong memories one day of Peter, whom I loved before I ever met Walter, and who I felt honoured me, rather than using me to satisfy his lust. I realised it was true that Gabriel was not "the child I wanted," not a love-child. And I had spent all this time looking after this child, and stuck in a relationship I couldn't break because of him. Walter had thought that by using me for his lust he could dominate over me forevermore. But I'd had enough, and at last I was breaking the connection.

I became even more aware of the "sickness" Gabriel had imbibed from his father; it was a whole sick way of relating to the world which he learnt from him; it came from his father like a contagion. I felt so angry that after all my efforts to protect him, the System had allowed it. I could see it happening before my eyes, but I said to myself "I'm not willing to watch"! Because of this I realised I had ceased to "care" about the formation of Gabriel's mind and character. The System had given over the most tender part of me to the ogre and then given him back; but he wasn't "the same child"; I felt he had been damaged inside too deeply for me to heal. *The System had put me in the situation of slowly watching my son's soul being destroyed and I hadn't been able to stop it; but "you cannot make me watch!"*

Listening to the dawn chorus one morning I had a clear perception that I should no longer fight the world with the world's own weapons and ways; I would no longer try to prove in a law-court that I was "sane"; "instead of trying to break the chains, I'll wait until they fall off ." I thought that after all this experience of the world, I'd like to "return to my origin, to my innocence," and become a nun. I decided I wouldn't try and explain my intentions to anybody.

That day Morag Weston, from the St.Johns Adoption society, came to discuss things with me. I was glad to hear from her that nowadays, if a child is placed with adoptive parents, the mother does not have to be totally deprived of contact with him. However there was a "knotty problem"; it was also true that the father would have "access visits" to the child; this would be nigh impossible to prevent unless it could be established that contact with the father was positively harmful. I realised that I would need the help of Dr.James in this, and it was a matter of "taking a risk"; if we went ahead with it, telling social workers I couldn't "handle" Gabriel, it might not turn out OK. In addition it bothered me considerably that the only acceptable way of getting a child taken into local authority care was if it were abandoned or the parent unfit; there was no "alternative theory" of the mother sending forth the child in the hope of a better life. However I was told that it might be possible for me as custodial parent to place Gabriel with anyone I wanted some distance away. I felt there was hope in this, but I needed it to be argued by Dr.James in the courts that the continuation of Walter's access would be a bad thing.

That day Gabriel happened to have a most awful paddy, howling at me "mummy help me, why can't you help me, I need you to help." *I felt he was "beyond my helping", but I quietly and consolingly urged upon him what I always kept repeating "Always remember your mummy always loves you."*

A great tiredness now came upon me, because I had been through hell to make such a hellish decision; I saw that giving up Gabriel was the greatest thing I'd ever do in my life. *In doing this my true love of him, my desire to do what is for his welfare, was greater than my connection with him, that umbilical cord which people call "love". Therefore in giving him up I loved him more than I have ever been able to love him before. I would indeed be "yielding him up into the hands of God."*

I phoned Percy to ask whether, if he were placed in the Norwich area, he would extend "a helping hand" over my son, and he said he would, and I felt very grateful and glad. I felt that in that way I would hear about Gabriel, and the wonderful thought came to me that I could always write to him, and I could in that way carry on a "soul-friendship" with him. I believed that Walter's possessive love would wither and die through distance, but my "mother-love" would subsist, and transmute into a soul-friendship. *I was positive that "my love would subsist," and endure beyond parting.*

I was determined to go away for a bit, and not take Gabriel with me; I wanted to do some clear thinking and establish myself on my own to see how I felt. I had a good talk with my friend Henry Maple, saying whilst rocking Gabriel on my knee, "Do you think I'll ever recover from it when I've lost him?" I said how afterwards I wouldn't want to stay in KirkMichaels any more, because I felt an isolation from the whole community, because they didn't support us. I said how after making this decision on my own "things could never be the same again." *This giving up of my son for adoption, this yielding up of him for love's sake, would be the greatest act of my lifetime; it would be "the sacrifice of my motherhood."*

At this point I felt that all the emotion which for so long had grasped and ruled me, had been tamed and brought under control. I felt "the ruling, mastering hand of God upon me." I realised by reading a book I had written in my youth that when at that age I was full of wisdom and unsullied by the world; and since then I had "fallen" into the world of experience, of emotion, and had surpassed the limits of it. So now I wanted to "turn again," to revert to the way that I myself had enunciated; I was going to revert to the "Master" in my heart.

Then one day I was really outraged in perceiving how Gabriel was also imbibing from Walter some of his perverted ideas of sexuality. It was quite innocent when I used to make Gabriel giggle by attacking his "tickly bits," his thighs; but Gabriel told me how his Dad had taught that he could excite himself; I thought this "sick". There were all sorts of little things which were evidence of Walter teaching him about "sexuality". I knew it was Walter's "religion" to believe that the highest form of spirituality lay in sex. I felt he was sickening Gabriel's very soul, his ability to relate, that he was jaundicing his innocent apprehension of the universe.

Then events overtook me. It came to Sunday 29th March, Mother's day, which was one of the most catastrophic days of my life.

Chapter 51
The Abandoning.

Mother's day, Sunday 29th March '92, saw the catastrophe which, it seemed to me at the time, signified the end of my relationship with my child forever. "I have lost my son," I sobbed in the church, after having a "tug-of-love" battle with Walter at the church door.

I had walked with Walter as far as the Catholic church, and he was being insistent that Gabriel stayed with him whilst I went away, then right at the church door he grabbed hold of the child's hand and insisted that he went with him, instead of going into the church with me. I felt it was descending to the lowest of the low; *"how could he do that, making my child a tug-of-love object in front of a church-door?"* He forced the child to choose between me and him, and I let go, and went in alone. And I howled and sobbed my heart out for the whole of Mass, feeling that my tears were commingling with its sacrifice. I felt that Gabriel had made his choice, by not letting go of Walter's hand; I felt it was the "final separation between mother and child," and in a sense, in truth it was!

Afterwards I went round to Henry's house and cried on his shoulder; I felt that my decision for adoption had not hit me emotionally until then. That separation of mother and child, because Walter tugged him away, was so symbolic. And I couldn't easily get Gabriel back. Walter later came to the house with him, demanding to come in and talk with me, and I said I just wanted my child back. Walter took him by the arm, shouting "you've had it, you are going to lose your son, you are not getting him back!" There was a physical tussle, and Walter ran off with him. I was anguished in the extreme, and I phoned the police, saying that the man had "abducted" my son. The police came, but they weren't a help; they contrasted the "rational father" with the "emotional mother" who had been "mentally ill", they actually commented "we can tell who is the loopy one here"; and they believed Walter when he claimed the child was afraid of me. It looked for a while as though I wasn't going to get him back, but I did in the end, in the evening.

I talked with friends on the phone in the evening, saying how irrevocable and very symbolic it was. *Walter wouldn't let go of his hand, so I let go, I wouldn't tug. For I had understood that "True love doesn't tug, it lets go." But I wouldn't have any more of these "tug-of-love scenes"; "I am letting go of my child's hand"; it was crunch-point, time to give him up; Time or else God had caught up with me!*

I was pained to discover that, after all the free access between me and my child, that night Gabriel wedged the door shut, so I couldn't get into his bedroom; I felt he was lost to me, his heart closed against me. I had a wee talk with him that night, saying I wouldn't be looking after him any more; he said that I didn't love him, and I replied *"I do love you Gabriel; it is because I love you that I am doing this; I'm not having you as a tug-of -love object between me and Walter, because it is destroying you. It is because I do love you, and perhaps when you are older you will understand that."*

My plan that night was summed up in one word of Christ's- "Abandon".

When Christ called to Matthew the tax-collector to "Abandon and follow," his hands instantly loosened and slackened, all his hardness melted and slipped from him, there could be no more clutchings of the coin; he stood naked in his sensibility, and abandoned all that he had known for the image of softness which had melted him in this Man.

The next day was a day of endless struggle, and I let it be known at last that my intention was Adoption. I wondered whether if I just "abandoned" Gabriel and went off, he would be put into care, or whether trying to arrange something with an adoption agency would be a safer course. I talked endlessly with everyone, saying how my "true need" was to go away for a bit; if I could have "a break" I would fight for Gabriel's welfare and future when I came back. But the solution was dropped "like a gift into my lap", in that Maggie phoned and volunteered to take Gabriel. I felt how all our struggling is in vain because "the solutions come as gifts."

The next day I had a very painful talk with the police who came round to see me. They said they would do nothing to help me to protect Gabriel, or to keep his father away from him. When I said that Gabriel was being "abducted" from his custodial parent by a man who was emotionally harming him, they replied "the only thing that counts in law is a black eye" and they washed their hands of the matter. I went totally cynical about the police; I saw that if I left Gabriel with Maggie they weren't willing to help.

I had a marvellous deep talk with Dr.James; I spilled out my soul to him, telling him at long last of my adoption decision. He replied graciously, "I will do my best to make it happen as quickly and easily as possible, with the least suffering to Gabriel." He said he said he was a bit worried how some things I said implied I had ceased to love Gabriel; I said these were just "pangs of pain" escaping from me, but that the adoption decision had taken place in the higher reaches of my being where I was "the deeper impulses of will and love."

Then I accused him once again of doing something he didn't do; I accused of him of playing a part in my last hospital admission. This was because Philip told me that it was a fact that Dr.James had been involved in sectioning me the previous summer, and it was a shock to me, because I had said "I trust you" by accepting his own version of his innocence. "I find it a painful fact to accept, and I presume it is a fact." It was an excruciating moment, because he said No, it wasn't true; he had not come to section me but to see how I was out of genuine care. I was mortified, and wanted the floor to swallow me up! I grasped his arms and wrists; "Oh I'm sorry; how could I do this to you again? Forgive me!" He said back with grace, "That's OK. I know you now; we are friends; you can say what you want to say." The words dwelt in me with precious intensity.

I wrote him a letter then; "I want and need to trust you, but the things the world tells me, the things everybody tells me, leave me stricken through with doubt. It matters to me that I trust you, that I trust myself into your hands." *I told him how I have "a desire to trust him" and I would never doubt him again; no-one would ever shake my faith in him.* So when Steven Peterson came round on the 1st April, threateningly, and said that Dr James "would betray you, as always," I was adamant; "No-one at this stage will shake my faith in Dr.James."

That day, the 1st April, something hellish happened, which had me "running scared." Steven Peterson came, threatening that unless I tell him everything about my "adoption decision," he would send me back to hospital, which he had power to do as I was still under section18. And so I was forced to "open my heart's holiness." *And when I'd told him it all, he said that I just wanted "to be rid of Gabriel"; I felt that having opened my heart, he had trashed it! It felt like a "rape," like a violation of the sanctuary of my house and the sanctuary of my heart.* I felt this was insufferable, that I would not tolerate it. And then he said that the psychiatric System "had concern for Gabriel's welfare." And by that he didn't mean concern for Walter's damaging of my son, or how he could successfully be adopted; he meant that they were concerned that I might do something to harm him. It came home to me with a shock what had happened when they had "concern" the last time; I had no chance, do choice, not a hope in hell! My backside was actually aching with the fear of injections; I realised what danger I was in.

And so I realised that I had to think about "the preservation of my free soul." After Steven Peterson's club-footed interference, I had little choice. I couldn't handle the situation, and I was laying it down. *My child was beyond my helping, and I couldn't "steer a course" for him anyway, so I felt I must "make a choice for my free soul." There had come the time at last, that I should "yield him up" completely.*

I decided to go off, initially to my old friend Paul Thompson's house in Edinburgh. That morning I took all my packed bags together with Gabriel in my friend Nicholas Lawson's car, and we went round to see Dr James after delivering my son to Maggie. I told Dr James that I was "temporarily abandoning the situation." He was initially cross with me, saying I was endangering myself. I found out from him that Steven Peterson had been round to see me because he had heard about my well-guarded adoption plans from Dr.McNeill, who had heard about them from Mrs.Bloomfield, who had been told about my sobbing in the church; I was appalled. He suggested that he try to persuade Dr.McNeill to lift the section, so as to take the pressure off me. I said "bless you", seeing at the same time his eagerness to help me and his essential helplessness. I told him how my trust in him never wavered when talking to Steven Peterson; *"I trust you utterly, I trust you completely."* I said to him on leaving *"I entrust my son into your hands, I entrust everything into your hands."*

Saying Goodbye to Gabriel had been dire. When I had left him in Maggie's hands at her flat, with her two kids of similar age, he cried and clung to me. I felt I might never see him again. I tricked him, saying "it's OK I'll be back tonight", knowing I wouldn't be. *I had a knowing that I was abandoning him; I felt I had to do it to raise him above the situation, to put him in a safe place, and ultimately to get him adopted. I had a knowing that this was a separation for a long time. I felt I couldn't leave him any physical thing to remember me by, but I had left something in his heart; - my repeated words which I had taught him; "Always remember, my mummy always loves me." Leaving him was heart-rending.*

And so I left; my friend Louise delivered me to the railway station, and I told her to assure everyone that I was "just going away for a bit to think." I knew otherwise. I found I couldn't stay in Paul Thompson's house, as I felt under pressure there, so I wrote a farewell letter from Glasgow library, to Dr.James. I wrote that he shouldn't allow anyone to think that I was going off "manic", because I certainly wasn't; I just wanted to go off alone somewhere in order to think. I said I hoped no-one would hunt for me, for "I don't intend to be found, in any state, let alone a certifiable one." I said I just wanted to "find my own space" somewhere; *"Abandon is the best wisdom I can attain at this moment."* I said I was yielding up my son into God's hands, and into his loving hands at the same time; I said he should not allow Gabriel to think I had abandoned him because I didn't love him. And then I thanked him for the good he had done me. I enclosed with this letter a document I had signed which said; "As far as is in my power I yield into Dr.James' hands all of my authority, rights and power as a parent," saying that he should be the only person to speak for me.

Through being "mastered" by you, I got the secret of dying, of how to totally self-yield to God. And that was why I had to go, not letting anyone know where I was going, lest I should be prevented. You wouldn't have allowed me to go if I had admitted, "Well I've found the secret of dying, so I'm going off to die!"

Then I went off on a train, heading for Southhampton. Travelling on the train in the darkness I thought how I would go and seek the wisdom of my soul-friend Pater Leo, and how I wanted to impart to Dr.James the fullest possible knowledge, and how I would contact Percy Gerard in Norwich as he might be able to help. And I thought how I would like to kill Walter, and how I must keep a "free soul," if I wanted to have any say in my son's future.

- And then my journal-writing ominously falls silent.

"My fight for Gabriel can't go on. I knew right from the beginning that the only way to cut Walter's soul-destroying relationship with me was to sever my connection with my child. I knew at his birth that the wisest step would have been immediate adoption, but I took the child up to love because I believed that was what God wanted of me. And now 6 years later I have given up the child in the ground of my will because I believed that was also what God wanted of me. To my credit I did not extinguish the child's life, even in the face of great suffering; I did not leave him as a foetus, "a dead thing" on Walter's doorstep. Rather I gave him life; I spent 6 years, feeding and clothing him and nourishing his soul. I have nourished him with 6 years of life before I ultimately leave him on Walter's doorstep."

"But it is not because I don't love him, but because I do. To my credit I have not given up my fight against Walter because I couldn't stand any more of it, but because I could see it was damaging to my child's soul. I took the fight to its limits. That was its limits, when Walter wouldn't let go of his hand on the church doorstep! For the suffering of it was

tearing his soul in two; I saw it in my child's face! And I knew I had to give him up, had to let go of him, and ultimately "abandon him on Walter's doorstep"! It is the only way to "cut the Gordian knot" of this soul-destroying fight between me and Walter; to give up my child's connection with me!"

(NB. At the time I wrote "Having taken on board the agony of all this, you don't expect me to now say "I want him back," do you? No way! The mistake and sin of relating to Walter, which I have so dearly paid for, is now over; the connection is cut!" But little did I then know, that I would have to go through the agony of fighting for my son's access to me for the next umpteen years!)

Chapter 52
The Scarborough Experience.

What I needed was entire Aloneness. All my life people have been preventing me from attaining my end, claiming that when I went into the Void, letting go of that reality in which men live, that I was mad, and bringing me back into that reality by the force of drugs. But in my best moments I always knew "The persona of my madness knows more than I do." What madness means is a transcending of the present reality in which most men live. "Only in the Void, and not in the System is God to be found." In my book, the Beloved goes out of the System into the Void in order to comprehend the Star-love; this she does out of her inability to understand her suffering or to reconcile it to the Star-love she once received. And so in the same way, I kept "opting out" into madness, like a moth attracted to a candle-flame.

So I had "abandoned the situation." I had left Gabriel in a safe place, left him with my friend Maggie. It was as if I had put him in a high safe place, safe from the deep swirling waters which surrounded me. I felt that now I had made the tug-of-love war come to an end, and now no matter how much myself and his father fought, and no matter whether I got ill or not, Gabriel was now safe from it all; I really hoped he would go for adoption. I believed that he would.

So there I was in the middle of the night, on a train heading for Southhampton, feeling that I had done the best thing, and that now I was free to go away somewhere and think. I wasn't manic at that point, for I knew what I was deliberately doing, but I rapidly became manic in the succeeding days. I was "running scared," fearful that I would be pursued. I had taken the last night train out of Glasgow, eager to get out of Scotland, so that my section would no longer apply, (for I was still under Section 18 of the Mental Health Act), but it had occurred to me on the train that I could possibly find a refuge on the Isle of Wight, where I used to be a nun long ago in my youth.

The train hit Southhampton, and the first thing I did was to find a B and B place where I could leave my luggage. After a wee rest on the bed I came down the stairs, and the most amazing thing happened,- I found the landlady talking to someone who was a Craigdene nurse! At least she was the spitting image of a Craigdene nurse, and dressed in a nurse's uniform! My reaction was one of complete terror; I thought she had come for me! I ran out of the house and along the street in terror, convinced that I had been "found", and that the police and an ambulance would be after me. I didn't slow down till I'd reached a shopping mall. I ran into a large store, and peeped from behind the door to see if I was being followed. I saw a clump of four policemen talking together not far away. I thought they were looking for me. Then two of them separated off and came my direction. I was so very scared, and I remember I jumped on an elevator, convinced they were coming after me; and then I pretended to look at hats, just praying they wouldn't come up the elevator!

I walked a long way that day, trying to find out about the boats to the Isle of Wight, and trying to avoid the police, but eventually I went back to the B and B for my luggage and got a taxi to take me out of the dreadful place. I spent a lot of my precious money on getting this taxi driver to take me out into the country, to a point further back up the railway line. Then I got a train to London, then swapped stations, and got another train up North. I felt I was really "on the run" with the police seeking me nationwide. So I was trying to think of a place familiar enough to me, to give me a good chance of staying there for a month; I hit on Scarborough, the Yorkshire seaside resort on the East coast, as I used to go there as a child on holidays.

So the train pulled up in Scarborough and once again I sought a B and B; by now it was late at night, and I had difficulty finding a place, though there was a whole row of them along a street on the North Cliff, because most had no vacancies, and to some of them I thought my story sounded suspicious. At last it was a suave lady's man to whom my plight appealed, and he gave me a room for the night.

I couldn't sleep. I spent all the night scribbling notes to Dr.James; I felt that at least I could make my writing legible now that I was no longer on a lurching train. In the morning I was very polite to the landlord whilst he gave me breakfast, spinning the story that I had come to sort out my "novel" as I had brought the manuscript with me. I set off to the other cliff, which I knew better, walking along by a choppy sea in the bitter-cold wind. It took hours to reach the part of the town I was familiar with, and I sought a B and B there in vain. So then I walked miles all the way back again, getting so very cold; I wasn't enjoying myself.

The next night the landlord came into my bedroom with his master key; I repelled his advances and became determined to leave. I was aware how badly I needed somewhere to stay, as my money was running out, so having reached the other cliff, I went into a pub, to see if I could meet someone, throwing it all on God's providence. By now I was possessed of the recklessness that goes with being manic. I thought it would be significant if my name could be guessed; "Rosemarie" this guy said, and I thought it significantly close to my own name of Mairi; I told him how I needed somewhere to stay. What followed was horrid. I remember that he had sex with me on a stone floor, which hurt my back. I remember how after that he took me to his flat, which had nothing but a bed, a kettle and burnt-out black walls. He made love to me over and over again, whilst I was becoming progressively manic. I talked to him on and on, never-endingly, whilst desperately needing food and drink and sleep and medication. He kept locking me in that flat whilst he went off to work. Then he would bring fish and chips back, but I talked so never-endingly that I never got the chance to eat them. He made cups of tea, but I never drank them because I couldn't stop my manic talking.

Days and nights were passing; I realised, somewhere in the back of my mind, that if I didn't eat and drink and sleep, I was going to be found dead in that place. It was brought home to me what Steven had once said, that you could die of being manic. I tried to tell this guy; "look you have got to do something, you have got to get me to drink, or get a doctor to me," but all he cared about was the endless sex we were having. Then one night I blinked my eyes fast whilst I was looking at him; and I tell you, it was the face of the devil! I was scared out of my wits. I realised I had to get out of there, that this was an evil power that had hold of me. I got dressed whilst he was asleep, and then insisted with all the manic wiles I knew, that he take me out of his flat that morning. It was freezing bitter cold, and I only had on a blue flowery dress, and no underwear. Once away from his flat I started screaming along the street, "Help, help, Police!" Having earlier shunned the police, I realised I now needed them to save my life.

Scared by my screaming and shouting, the man ran off down some steps; I sat down on these steps for a while, then realising how very cold I was, I realised I had to attract some attention. I remember going along the main promenade where quite a lot of people were, shouting "Help, please help me," but I couldn't get anyone to take any notice. The nurses in Craigdene afterwards sincerely believed that I was "found naked dancing in the sea," but this wasn't true. I felt close to dying, and was desperately trying to keep alive. I came across a window-cleaner up a ladder cleaning a shop window; I felt I was being offered a way back into life, as this was a golden chance to gain attention. I shook his ladder, shouting "Will you marry me? If you come down you can marry me if you like." The shopkeeper came out, saying that if I didn't stop this dangerous behaviour, he would call the police. "Wonderful" I thought, "if he calls the police I'll be warmed and fed and have the attention I need." So I carried on shaking the ladder.

When the police finally came in their car, I told them they should arrest me, because I was an escapee from Scotland's Mental Health Act. *But though I knew this was a way back to life, I had no idea of the harsh initial torture and then the long months of suffering which would follow by taking this path; I had no idea of the ghastliness awaiting me.*

The police treated me horribly; they didn't warm me and feed me. On the contrary they threw me into a horrible bare cell, with one foul-smelling blanket, and left me there, closing the slat on me, for hours and hours. I needed food, drink, medication, and they just left me there for ages whilst they made "investigations". I remember sitting there rocking myself back and forth in my misery. When they finally opened the door and let me out towards an open police-van door, I verily skipped with joy thinking that I could only go to something better, I was "going towards life." *But I was mistaken; the only thing I got was injections in my backside.*

I was taken to what I presume was a psychiatric unit in Scarborough. At first I was put into a large open-plan reception room, where I espied on the floor my back-pack which had my manuscript in. I made a mad leap for it. I was asked "Is that your bag?" I feared I was going to be locked up, and to somehow save my bag from a similar fate in my manic away of thinking, I replied "No it doesn't belong to me." Somebody picked it up and tried to open it. And I leapt upon it shouting "It's mine, it's mine, I own it!" They were taken aback by my violent behaviour. Then I attacked somebody who had a cup of tea, because I so desperately needed to drink myself. They then gave me a cup of tea, and because it was too hot to drink, I threw it back at them. Seeing they found all this contradictory behaviour unacceptable, the next thing I knew, they had given me a tranquillizing injection in my backside.

The injection was the dreaded Largactil. I have always been super-sensitive to this drug, suffering horrible side-effects; my tongue becomes so slow and slurred that I can't even speak. I suppose I needed it at the time, to bring me back from the brink, - the brink of madness or hypothermia, the brink of death; I needed to be brought back into life. I remember how Dr.James said he had phoned to ask how I was, and was told I was "soaking up Largactil like a sponge." They gave me so much. I remember they had me in this large high room, with a large expanse of window looking out over Scarborough, with a bed in the middle where I just lay whilst they gave me endless injections of Largactil, or the liquid syrup. I remember I used to go to the door, and try to say "Is there anybody there?" hoping for some food or drink or human comfort, and there was one nurse called John who was nice to me. I don't think they were deliberately unkind to me; they just didn't realise how desperately I needed drink. *I remember thinking how terrible it was that I had expected, by getting caught, to get warmth and comfort, and someone to help me drink a warm sweet cup of tea, and this I never got.*

I don't know how long it was before I was returned by ambulance to Craigdene, probably a week. Things were marginally better there, because I got longer periods of consciousness between the drugs, until finally they gave me them in tablet form and I was able to spit them down the toilet again, as I usually did. Dr.McNeill enjoyed wielding his power over me again, now that I was in his ward. I told him tongue-in-cheek how it was a good idea to remain on a section because you get automatically "brought back to the point of origin," brought back home. He believed what I said and kept repeating for years afterwards that I had said how it was a good thing to remain on a section.

I also weaved this tale for him about what the whole experience had been like spiritually or psychically. *I said I had "been in the sea," - I had meant the wide sea of death, of the eternal waters which encircle our limited human consciousnesses, but he believed I meant the physical sea. I said I had been in the sea, struggling against the tide, against the huge waves, and I was being pulled out and pulled down, but I caught and clung to the bars of the railings along the sea-front, and so managed to rescue myself. Because he was told that I had been found wet due to the rain and cold and half-naked along the promenade, he seemed to believe this story, though to me of course the whole story was an allegory.* I meant that I had got so manic, so cold, hungry and thirsty, that I had had a brush with death, that I was close to yielding up my consciousness on what I had discovered was a "wide sea"; I had had to fight to stay alive. And the railings I had clung to I likened to my trust in Dr.James; for thinking about him, hoping to see him again, had helped me to fight. Dr.James understood all this mysticism, but Dr.McNeill's opinion was that I was "a danger to myself and others," needing to be locked up.

Spring and Summer came to Craigdene, and there I remained, languishing in a cage.

Chapter 53
Cliff Mysticism and my Master.

NB. This knowledge is dangerous because it has the power to drive the soul "mad". The knowledge of God's love is dangerously close to madness; I know this better than most, as my own being has always been close to madness. It is indeed like a tight-rope or a cliff-face, and therefore not something to be recommended to anybody else! My knowledge of God's love I have attained through madness. But God forbid that others should have to go through "madness" to know His love!

Something happened to me, on those Scarborough cliffs, which was like a nuclear explosion in my mind. I had understood something fresh and new and mind-blowing about the nature of Death, because I had been close to Death. And my Psyche came out of it fresh and new and young. But something dire had happened to me, and I had got stuck in a world of unreality, a life "between the two worlds," a mind-set where the only person with whom I could henceforth communicate was my doctor, my dear Dr.James whom I loved so dearly, whom I took as my "Master."

I tried to explain to him in my writings, what had happened and how much I loved him: - "I expended my life, my monetary ability to stay alive, because I realised that out on the streets of London or stowed away on night trains, you would not be able to read my writing; so your claimed inability to read my writing was going to cost me my life! I put my communicating with you above the value of my own life; my love of you condemned me to death. And so, because I wanted to touch you, love you, communicate myself to you, I have sacrificed my life for you." I felt I was given only one week to live, on those Scarborough cliffs. *And what I did to get back to him was one of the most noble and self-sacrificial act of my life-time; the bravest act perhaps. I was willing to go through the horrors and tortures of the psychiatric system, by throwing myself on the mercy of a policeman, in an attempt to get back to him.* I wrote, "I swear I shall be true to you, but that does not mean I may not have to let other things master me,- fire, water, blood, earth, air, and lust. But I will walk through it all with the hope of seeing you on the other side."

And there on the cliffs of Scarborough I had this total loving-devotion to him as my
new-found "Master," with a new understanding of what is meant by the term; for I was fresh and new, baptized into the waters of death,

my soul revitalised, alive with fresh new knowledge. "By "Master" I didn't mean at all everything I thought I knew by the word. It was as if God mastered me through him; as if I wrote "your hand is in my being and it is a mastering hand," and then realised that his hand and God's were the same thing. I realised the German word for "mastering" (beherrschen) comes from the word "Lord", and when you yield to God then He is "Lord" over you; to "master" never did mean to "teach." So I was asking Dr.James "Will you be my Master?" meaning would he let me yield myself to God's love through him. One thing I wrote on Scarborough's cliffs which I think beautiful: - *"I have only one desire, which is my heaven, one pure intent of my single loving soul. It is to be so known, mastered by you, that I am so yielded up to you that I no longer exist."* It is like the little mermaid yielding herself into being sea-foam out of her love's intensity and purity!

What really happened on those Scarborough cliffs? I wrote: - "Swift sweet Death is beckoning fast.- -There is no need to throw myself into the sea; I think I can die of my own accord. - -To die, to utterly yield up the self; I can do it now; whether I can do it over and over I am not quite sure." Then I laughed and cracked jokes all the way along the esplanade at the idea "it is easy when I can't swim." For the point is, in my enlightenment I found that *when you truly die, and utterly yield up the self, then the eternal waters throw you back out again, into a fresh new reincarnated life! When I died I was re-born. The waters won't let you die. For a living soul is bouyant.* It is so obvious and so true. For a moment I suppose I had a choice; of not coming back, of remaining there, in the bliss of the eternal arms of God. *But the life that was within me, which I suppose in that moment was my devotion to Dr.James, made me surge back upwards into life. So it was as if I "gave up bliss for him";* "I sacrificed what I have attained in attaining it."

In this struggle which is our life, God is waiting for us to give in; it doesn't matter to whom we give in, as long as we give in. In the same way, once knowing the way to bliss, it doesn't matter for whom you go back, as long as you go back.

I had a fresh, new, young knowledge, and was yearning and desiring only to get back to Dr.James. I wrote, - "I beg of you, put me somewhere, give me the ability to go somewhere, anywhere in the universe on whatever planet at whatever distance in the future, to encounter you, and I shall be there. Put me in a place or enable me to get to a place, where you can come upon me, where you can find me, know me, master me. For you are my Master for this incarnation."

Looking back, I can see that all my life I'd been getting into ecstasy and then being forced back by other people into reality. On this occasion I had transcended everyone and everything when I got away to be by myself "on the mountain-top," on that lonesome cliff; and I had reached my end. I had embraced the point where I could die into God's love; I had entered the realm where I could hear the laughter of God.

At the very beginning of June, still in the hospital, having gradually weaned myself off the heavy medication, and feeling I had passed beyond the realm of soul-destroying suffering, I started writing again "to create something beautiful as an act of obedience to my Master." I wrote it to Dr.James, so that I could keep silence when with him, and just let him read it. I found it hard to relate to him, after all my intense realisation on Scarborough's cliffs, because wanting to ask "Will you be my Master?" and knowing he wouldn't understand it.

I had written a few things before his first visit. I led him to my single room, and then rushed ahead of him, and drew all the curtains and switched the light off! I wanted to make it into a "dark room," a place where I could be comfortable, hidden in the darkness of God's love, a space that couldn't be violated. He objected "Mairi don't; what will people think!" But I threw myself on the floor by his knees, so that I was "at the feet of my Master", and desperately tried to explain everything I had mind-blowingly realised on the Cliffs of Scarborough about the meaning of "Master" and the meaning of "Death." But I found I couldn't, and tried to let him read the scraps of things I had written instead. He wasn't understanding, and now that he was "present" all I wanted was to sit there in my silence. He came upon a page which said something about my son, and tore it out, and commanded "Tear it up!" And I was instant obedience; as I later said to him, "not a "Yes but" in sight!" Because I was such a complete "Yes" to him, I didn't want to spoil my silence with the use of inadequate words; what I knew lay beyond the realm of words.

We had to wait in the office for a while, whilst a nurse found some information on one of his other patients. I stood next to him, just yearning in the silence. "What are we doing?" I asked. "Patience!" he replied. "But what are we doing?" I repeated. "We are just waiting," he said. A couple of days reflection on this and something dawned on me; "Patience" I always thought meant "ability to suffer"; but no, it meant "ability to wait." In the same way I had to "wait", in this limbo-land where my psyche was stuck. I discovered after a few days that I could "wait" without the sense of suffering.

So I started writing what I wanted to tell my Master, so I could keep silence when with him. "Do you see what I mean by jumping in the sea? It is a metaphor, a myth, a higher reality. All my life I have but "paddled" with my feet on occasion in this vast dark sea, but I always found it too cold and come back out again. But you know, I did it! I finally jumped in; total commitment, willing to die, to abandon everything I had known." And I wrote that I had shared in "the laughter of God," - laughter whose meaning we can't comprehend; "seen through anything but your eyes it will seem like the permanent and irrevocable hilarity of Madness."

He came again, into my "dark room." I tried to get him to read what I had written, but he wouldn't. I tried to explain my mystic understanding of Death, but found I couldn't. I tried to explain about him being my "master", but found I couldn't. I tried to explain how I just needed to be somewhere where he could have access; "I will stay where you put me." And then with a painfulness which made me blush, I said; "I will do whatever you say." He replied with a kind of impatience, "I will not tell you what to do." He questioned why I was incapable of talking and explaining things to him, and I tried to explain how I wasn't like this to everyone else; only he caught me stuck in my silence; for others could not see that part of me that was open to him. *I told him to keep secret what he saw in me, because I was stuck in a limbo-land between two doors, not able to go forward or back. The element I now lived in was one of God's love and laughter, which "sounds like madness to human ears."*

He didn't stay long, but said to me earnestly at the door "You will get well." "You mean I'll come back down to earth?" I replied. "You will" he said. He left and I stayed for a while immobilised by pain. Did he still not understand anything I was saying to him? He was wrong; didn't he understand that I would never come down to earth now because I had sacrificed the means by which I could do so, sacrificed it in order to keep contact with him? *I had told him and now wanted to scream it out to him; "the door slams shut; I turned back for* you."

I wrote again, frantically trying to express my pain with my pen, to explain how I got "locked out," how he being my Master sitting at the foot of the door, was my only contact with reality;   "I have lost all contact with the world now, with reality and human souls, except through you.   I feel a bit like Cathy in Wuthering Heights when she hopes to transcend her body and live as spirit on the heath, saying "I shall be incomparably above and beyond you all." For what I did, you

213

see, after locking myself out of the temporal world, by reaching for my bliss of an eternal heaven, was to turn back to touch you. This is what Jesus did; you deprive yourself of heaven whilst you have transcended the earth as well; *that means you are stuck, in a kind of limbo of the spirit-world, unable to go back or forward, "zilched out." It is like "being a door-stop," like "holding the door of heaven open with my left foot."*

"I have to perpetually keep the door open, unable to pass ahead myself. I can't go forward to my own bliss, but it means others can obtain bliss through me. But I have lost contact with everybody but you, because it was only you I turned back for. Jesus perhaps turned back for everyone, and everyone pursued him; I have let him off the cross as it were, letting him go free by taking his place. It's only open to you; so you are protecting me and keeping me hidden, in the same way as I now protect Jesus and keep him hidden. Jesus is behind my eyes."

Looking back, I was definitely "insane"; and dear Dr.James was the only person willing and able to listen to my madness, my only way of communication. I once said to him, as regards madness, "there is always a way back for those brave enough to take it." But this time I couldn't get out of my madness; I was stuck there.

Chapter 54
Unreality and Loss of my Son.

It was in that Summer of '92, when I was completely and mystically "mad", locked in a mental limbo-land out of touch with "reality", that Walter took the custody of my son off me through the courts; and the health-care professionals supposedly caring for my welfare, let it happen; indeed they helped it to happen by averring I was severely "mentally ill."

My purpose was still holding, as regards my wanting Gabriel to be lifted out of this situation, and away from Walter, so that he no longer be a "tug-of-love child." I still believed that he would go for adoption if I held to my principle of not fighting to keep custody. The court -case, for Walter's bid for Custody, was looming in May. Solicitors and Social workers came to see me. I begged Dr.McNeill to allow me to attend, so that I could be there on my own behalf; he refused, saying he would put a report in to say I was severely mentally ill. I told him I wasn't going to fight any more over Gabriel, and that I was remaining true to my decision of "letting go" of him, because he was being torn to bits. Dr.McNeill replied that he couldn't deal with me because I was "always changing my mind", like a typical mentally ill patient. *I replied that I wasn't changing my mind, but was holding true to my decision.* He said it was a decision I would regret.

Because my solicitor Angus Gourlay went on about "fighting for me" and I didn't want to fight, I dismissed him. He had visited and been upset by my anger at him, as I averred that he had never done any good, and never achieved anything; and I remember how, later on, I walked all the way into Kirkcraig one hot sunny morning, unbeknown to the nurses, to hand in a letter to him, saying I was dismissing his services, and no longer wanted him to act for me. So there was going to be no-one in court to act or speak on my behalf; I wanted to be there myself, but they wouldn't let me. Hence Steven Peterson the social worker brought round a woman to see me who he said would be my "curator ad leitam" and represent me. I didn't want her to represent me; I didn't like her.

My friend Maggie visited me, and said I must fight in the court to keep Gabriel, because I would regret it if I lost Custody of him to Walter. But I said to her that I wouldn't fight, convinced that Gabriel should no longer be torn to bits. *And I was completely convinced that, letting go of the Custody, I would have the Access rights, which I would use wisely. And I was completely convinced that Gabriel would soon be sent for Adoption, when it was seen that he was suffering.* My hope was that he would be seen "to fail, to suffer," and thereby be taken away from Walter. I thought how this sounded like "I hope my child will suffer because I love him," but I also thought that this sounded like the quality of God's love which allows us to suffer. And I was also completely convinced, if truth be told, that Walter would die soon. When I enunciated this to Steven Peterson he replied "But Walter might survive for years, up until Gabriel is 20." And I replied "Believe me, I know how close he is to death."

So I took this position of "I will not fight," as Arjuna says to Krishna on the battlefield in the Bhagavad Gita; I was laying down arms. There was going to be no fighting, no contest, and I was going to let Walter have Custody of Gabriel until his own death. But I believed that I would be getting "total Access." My solicitor Angus Gourlay told me that if I didn't apply through the courts for Access rights I might never see Gabriel again; but I believed that if I gave up Custody, I could expect "sensible, adult, legal arrangements to be made" for Gabriel's access to me.

So the great day at Court came, and I knew no-one was on my side there except this "Curator ad Leitam" woman who hadn't a clue about anything to do with the case, as she was only brought in at the last minute. The court was told that I was an "unfit mother" because severely mentally ill, and Dr.McNeill supported that view. *No-one spoke on my behalf. Afterwards that woman and Steven Peterson came to see me, took me into a small room, and said "we have bad news". The Custody had gone to Walter; I had finally and irrevocably lost my son. I remember sitting looking at this woman, with the thick pink lipstick and horrid coloured hair, thinking "how could it be that at the end of the day, after all my struggle, I had this unknown and unknowledgable woman to represent me, the mother, the one true loving mother!" I felt shattered and began to cry.*

Later I sobbed my heart out on the phone to Pater Leo, saying my fear was that when I ever saw Gabriel again "I shall not recognise him; that the good and loving qualities of his soul should be destroyed; and I would rather he died than that this should happen." It seemed harder to me as a loving mother to go through the pain, the anguish of fearing the qualities of his soul may be destroyed, than having him dying and going straight to God. I knew from first-hand how Walter's sort of abuse was soul-destroying; if a grown woman couldn't cope with it, how could a 5-year-old child?

Hence when Dr.James visited at the beginning of June, he found a piece of manuscript on which was written; "it would have been better if my son had died." He said "tear it up". I did so in an instant, in obedience to him, but afterwards I wrote in explanation: "It is greater grief because greater sacrifice and loss for me, giving Gabriel up into the suffering of Walter's care, than seeing him die. It is harder to have the will to let someone you love suffer, than it is to watch them die. And so my bereavement is worse than him dying."

Various social workers came to see me, and Dr.McNeill too, to talk about an "appeal," and to see if I would consistently affirm that I was letting go of Gabriel without a fight. I told them all that "because I loved him I was letting him go." When told that I must have legal representation, I coolly commented that I lived "under the law of love" which didn't assert rights, and I didn't care about man-made law. I felt really that Walter had only fought over Gabriel to get revenge on me, and now that he found I was saying "I will not fight", he might well give it up; then if Gabriel were "failing" he would go for adoption out of Walter's grasp. This is what I believed would happen.

I kept saying of Walter "I hope he dies quickly", for I believed and foresaw that he wouldn't let me see Gabriel. I believed God would take Walter's life at a time of his choosing and it "remained dark to me." *One thing I was sure of; that now I had let go of Gabriel, given him up, I wasn't going to fight over him any longer; I wasn't going to reintroduce the torment of the tug-of-love back into his life; now that he had suffered separation from his mother, it would be cruel to tug him back. "I will not tug him back."*

Then there came a mystical point when I realised I preferred to leave Gabriel in Walter's hands, rather than hoping he would go for adoption. I began to hope custody with Walter would work for Gabriel, as then he would suffer the least. *It was a point of self-immolation; "to let Gabriel suffer the least I will make myself suffer the most."* *I finally felt that I had given my son up, "yielded him up into the hands of God," and therefore he must be somehow "safe."*

Looking back, at all these mystical decisions I made and these mystical, unreal beliefs out of which I acted, which meant I lost my son: - it doesn't make sense that the psychiatric system which "locked me up" and pronounced me "insane," should then allow me to make big life-altering decisions, which in effect signed away my rights as a mother! My "life" should have been protected! I mean they take away your keys in there saying they have a duty to "protect" your property; they should surely take away your ability to ruin your own life!

Dr.McNeill made a decision of mine legally stand when I wasn't fit to make that decision of yielding up my son, with the hazy idea that he would be taken up out of the situation into adoption. I said to him angrily after realising what I'd done, "How could you let me make a decision like that, when I wasn't based in reality, so much so that you locked me up as a danger to myself?" He replied "I considered you were well able to make such a decision at the time." I retorted angrily, "Why then if you claim I was rational enough, did you keep me locked up!"

My sense of injustice and outrage lies in this; I had my child taken off me and handed over to man I hate whilst I was incapacitated in the hospital; I wasn't in the plane of reality. The courts made a decision against me when I wasn't there to defend myself; my child was taken off me when I wasn't there; when I was out of reality.

Chapter 55
The Self-Yielding Bliss.

When he uniquely mastered me and I utterly yielded, it was the greatest sweetness known in my life. On that Midsummer's Eve, I was wearing my nightdress and dressing-gown when he came to the door, and he commented, "it is naughty to be in your nightie." I was pained by his ascribing anything to me other than innocence, and felt it unfair; I'd just had a shower, wanting to be clean, fresh and beautiful, instead of hot, dirty and tired as I had been all day. I just said back, "Don't let me be naughty; I'll do whatever you say."

I took my place on the floor, next to his chair, so I was close to his knees. I said "I'm only a 19-year-old school-girl; can't you see that? I jumped into the waters of death, and have come back with a fresh new knowledge, as a vulnerable and childish 19-year-old. I have a fresh new life and a fresh new knowledge, unsullied by the tiring of experience."

"What is this knowledge?" he asked, interested. I was pained that he still did not understand that this knowledge was direct contact with the love of God, which I had given up for him. "I am so lonely; all I have is you," I replied forlornly. "Explain it to me," he urged. I replied, "In attaining this knowledge and giving it up, I have lost contact with everyone but you, so it is for you to give it to other people." "Mairi what are you asking me to do?" he asked painfully, "I am a doctor, I've to heal the sick." Pain shot through my being.

Then I tried to explain to him my knowledge of Death found on Scarborough's cliffs, and finally found the words: - "I cannot swim, therefore if I were going to jump into the eternal waters of Death, I would drown. But you can't die when you are alive. The air in your lungs brings you back up again! Like Beowulf surging upward through the mere, like a bubble coming to the surface, like Christ rising after his burial, "the only way is up." But nobody ever dies you know, because they are too scared to. They cling hold of their selfish little egos through many reincarnations; and they never find Life, eternal life, because they are afraid to die. It's so simple; it is what Jesus was saying; those who seek to keep their lives, will lose, will die; those who give up their lives, who die, shall have eternal life." He was nodding his head. *The fresh new knowledge I have is this: What awaits beyond dying? What happens when you die, yielding the self up to the eternal waters out of which you came? - Reincarnation; a sending forth into life again."*

He nodded his head in a wise and pondering fashion. At this point I tried to explain what I meant by calling him my "Master." All my life I had sought for a Master, I explained, but had missed the reality of it; a Master is the means of yielding oneself up to the Love of God. "My ability to yield myself to God is connected with you." He was looking puzzled but I pressed on. I tried to explain how the release-spring in my being which he touched, God also touched. He responded solemnly, saying it amounted to blasphemy, to equate his hand with God's. I went on, trying to explain how the "yielding" and the "mastering" were the same thing. Pressing his hand against my cheek I said, "Before I left, when you were healing me so deeply and swiftly, I said "your hand is in my being, and it is a mastering hand." He pulled back, declaring solemnly, "Mairi I cannot be your lover." Pain shot through my being; he wasn't understanding.

I was silent for a bit, seeking for a way to explain my love for him; it wasn't right for him to be my lover anyway when he had the right and power and authority of a father over me. I asked if he had seen the recent film, in which the "little mermaid" was willing to be dissolved into sea-foam out of her loving-devotion. "So am I," and I explained that I had found something very beautiful which I had written on Scarborough's cliffs; "I have only one desire, which is my heaven, one pure intent of my single loving soul,- to be so known, so mastered by you, that I am so yielded up to you that I no longer exist." He seemed moved, but intimated "it's not a pure intent." Pain shot through me again; I desired to tell him, but couldn't find the words, that my desire to be entirely yielded up to him was entirely pure; it had the same purity as my love of God.

Suddenly I was overwhelmed by a pure bliss. For he held me like a child in a father's embrace; and saying "Oh Mairi," kissed me on the forehead. It took the breath of my soul away in one long sigh of communion. My mystical self-yielding in the moment, both unto God and him, was complete, and I was enraptured by the most utter sweetness known in my life!

In the next moment, we were stood up by the door, uttering deep things. *"I want you to take all that I have and all that I am,"* I whispered. He replied with a note of distress, *"I can't Mairi, I can't."* Pained again I replied, *"If you will not take me, will you take my knowledge?" "Yes I will take your knowledge,"* he said.

The moment had a strange intensity. As he urged "I have to go," I said plaintively; "you don't know how I feel; I feel this is a precious moment which will never return or be found again." He didn't seem to understand how lonely I was; "Don't leave me alone," I whispered. I had sacrificed my contact with God for my contact with him, and wanted to say, "If you don't console me, what is there left?" His leaving of me, after such a knowing of complete bliss, made me collapse into an agony!

Everybody is looking for God, and I know how to find him. I want to tell others how to annihilate the self and get to God, without themselves going through madness, which was the way I came. They think mistakenly that they have to "mortify" and "crucify" themselves to win eternal life; but I threw my crucifix in the sea, as a false image of how you really "die." It doesn't come through an effort to die; rather it is an instantaneous and joyful self-yielding. It is He who does everything, and not us; the secret lies in allowing Him to master us.

Chapter 56
The Escape to Austria.

I returned to the hospital on the bus the next day, after that heady mixture of pain and bliss on that Midsummers Eve encounter with Dr.James. The memory of the moment gave me a continual sense of sweetness, but something dreadful was awaiting me.

In the hospital, whilst I was being happy and "high" along the corridor, Dr.Walkinshaw, who wasn't my Doctor, was trying to work in the doctor's office. Suddenly he came out angry, saying he had had enough of me; "we are going to give you an injection." It was going to be Haldol Decanoate, which was a depot injection of Haloperidol. I was alarmed; if he meant a long-term depot injection it would make me so ill, seeing Haloperidol didn't agree with me, and I would never get out of it, because they would keep renewing it, and I would be "ill", mentally dead forever! Fear coursed through the whole of me. *In the event, fear of that injection flung me all the way to Austria.*

Desperately I tried to stop it happening, saying that Dr.Walkinshaw wasn't my Psychiatrist, and so had no right to change my medication; but I was told whilst Dr.McNeill was away on holiday, he was in charge of the ward. I argued that it would make me extra sleepy or have unknown effects whilst I was away on Pass during the coming weekend. This worked; the senior nurse agreed and conceded that I should have it on Monday morning after my weekend's Pass. "But you are having it when you come back on Monday," I was told. I went off for a walk, trying to veil my intense emotion till I got out there, out where I was alone along the farm-road. *And there by a barbed-wire fence, and surrounded by sheep and cows, I yelled and screamed my passion to the skies!*

"How could you do this to me, how could you! How could this happen! Just when I thought I've found bliss, when I've got Dr.James to accept his position as my "master", everything good lying in front of me, and they are going to rob me of my mind!" It seemed to me "the greatest blow suffered in my life-time"! I yelled and kicked up the gravel with my feet in a complete anguish. I had to go! I had to go somewhere, to avoid this; I had to hide away for a month. Where could I go? "Austria"! I'd go to Austria where Pater Leo could hide me in his monastery for a month! I could think of nowhere else to go.

I was plotting and planning from then on. I took home with me from my locker everything I cared about. It was Saturday morning when I was back in KirkMichaels; I had to get money, tickets, above all a Passport. I can remember standing in the queue with all my documents for the passport, thinking "suppose someone in the queue who knows me, sees me doing this." I was so scared whilst in the travel-agents too, getting a bus-ticket from London to Munich, which was as far as I had money for. I spent Sunday packing and writing a long letter to Dr.James; I intended leaving some writings for him, and leaving him the keys to my house. The powerful stuff I had written in Scarborough I burnt on the back step, feeling it was "dangerous knowledge." Early Monday morning I went round to the surgery and insisted on going past the secretary and leaving all this precious "knowledge" on Dr.James' desk. *The irony of it is he never got it that morning, and never found it till 6 months later!*

With my luggage I got on a bus to Langport, the local station, instead of a bus to the hospital, as I was supposed to. I was very scared that someone would see me, and someone would stop me. I had decided to get the train, in order to get as far away as possible from the area, as I knew they would start looking for me as soon as I didn't turn up that morning for the injection. I wanted to get out of Scotland as soon as possible. I was scared waiting on the platform for the train, and even more scared as the train went past the hospital; I can remember looking out at the Craigdene buildings with a kind of terror. But the train passed swiftly on, and it wasn't long before we got to London. My fear abated a bit there, because I thought I wasn't likely to see a Craigdene nurse milling round London.

The problem now was the hot, dusty and noisy traffic; I didn't like it. Whilst asking the way to the Victoria bus-station I found a young girl who said she was herself going there, and would go with me on the bus. So there I found myself in the midst of a summer-heat-wave capital city, on the run from the law; I flinched every time I caught sight of a policeman. I had a long wait in the Victoria bus-station, but eventually I was on my way to the Dover Ferry. I was scared going through the passport control, as I thought I might be officially "wanted". But that was OK, and I felt a great sense of relief when the boat set off and I was officially "out of the country." I remember hanging over the edge of the boat, watching the moon reflected in the inky waters, thinking how I would not dare ever come back!

It seemed a long way on the coach to Munich, and I felt grubby and sleepy when we arrived there. We stopped outside Munich Railway station; so now what was I going to do? I decided that my best bet was to spend the rest of my money on getting to Pater Leo's monastery by train, as it didn't matter to me that I would have no money left for coming back. So I went into the station and got a ticket to the nearest station to St.Peterskirche, via Salzburg; and then I got on the next train to Salzburg, which happened to be the last train out of the station. So what happened? The train pulled into Salzburg station at about one o'clock in the morning, and there were no other trains out until about 7 that morning. I did not like the thought of being stuck in Salzburg railway station overnight. *I suffered there one of the worst and most frightening experiences of my life!*

What happened was this: - The station was dreadfully deserted, with no trains, and no waiting rooms and nothing open, but with lots of drug-pushers and users in shady corners. I was scared. There where lots of unsavoury characters around, fighting with knives, squabbling. It was becoming very cold. I tried to sit on a bench, but these frightening characters kept sitting on the other end, ranting, swinging bottles of alcohol and blowing cigarette smoke in my face. I was frightened, cold, miserable; I thought that if I went out into Salzburg on my own, it was likely to be worse and I would be in danger of being found by the police. And I desperately needed sleep; but how could I sleep there, with all these dangerous people about! There was one guy looking at me nearby who seemed quite nice, so I went up to him and asked "Do you know of anywhere to go, that is more warm and more safe, where it is possible to sleep?" We talked for a bit, before he said he would take me to his flat in his car with four of his friends. I was hesitant, but I was at an extreme point of need, so I went with them.

What followed was ghastly and very dangerous. They took me to a place which was more like a clothes shop, and there they lit candles and started drug-taking and drinking. They had locked the door, and I felt trapped. I bore it bravely for a bit, then asked if there was somewhere I could sleep. This guy took me to a small room, with more clothes on the floor, and promptly jumped on top of me, and tried to have sex with me. I can remember there was a knife involved; he had a knife in his hand, and I was very scared. *I had round my waist the golden silk rope used for a belt, which I had worn with a promise that I had One Love, and would never let anyone or anything else "master me." I now clung to this belt round my waist, and enormous energy surged up in me, as I screamed, in German, "Let me go!"* He tumbled off me, and I went in to the others and bravely shouted, "I am going now, unlock the door!"

And so I found myself in the middle of Salzburg in the middle of the night, not knowing where I was, and not knowing the way back to the train-station, and feeling the need to keep out of the way of the police. And so I was glad when one guy followed me out, saying "I'll show you the way back to the station if you like." I agreed to this, and we walked a long way till we came to some dormant trains, which he said would move in the morning. We climbed in; I just wanted to sleep! I tried to get him to go, but he wouldn't. So I was in another pickle. I let him kiss and caress my breasts, thinking that if I thus humoured him, I would get away with it lightly, though his beard made me sore. But the morning eventually came, and I left him there and sneaked out of that railway carriage, and soon got back on a train heading the right direction. I felt really rotten, really "dirtied." I also felt glad that I was still alive; as I felt the events of that night had been very dangerous.

I reached a place by train about five miles from Pater Leo's monastery; from there I hitched a lift in a car. When we finally got to St.Peterskirche the kind lady said she knew someone whose house I could stay at for a while, because Pater Leo was not there; he had never receive the postcard I had sent and was away on business. The first thing I did in this lady's house was to have a shower, to wash off the dirt and unpleasantness of the journey, telling myself that the experience was behind me. But Pater Leo was nowhere to be found for a few days; when he did arrive back, he transferred me to a room in the monastery, next to the cook.

And so I put behind me the horrible experience of that journey, that "escape" from Craigdene and from the horrors of psychiatric drugs. And "freedom from" became "freedom to," as I became happy, creative, blissful in that Austrian paradise where true "adventure" began.

Chapter 57
The Austrian Adventure.

The first thing I did on arrival in Austria was to sit on a bench, halfway up the hill behind the monastery, and just sit, longing and yearning for my "Master," Dr.James, who was far away across the mountains and across the sea. It was a kind of terrible homesickness. And then I spent the whole of my time there writing an endless letter to him, trying to explain how he was my "Master" and must take on the task.

Pater Leo understood that I must stay there for at least a month, to allow my section to lapse, and employed me in the kitchen, helping the cook. I spent endless hours, filling up the dish-washer and polishing the glasses which came out of it. I walked around the hills and forests, feeling constantly very tired and out of breath, because of the altitude. On my second day there Pater Leo took me with him up a mountain, to say Mass on the top; he just went straight up, through all the thorns and barbed wire fences, and he climbed so fast that I couldn't keep up with him and it became painful for me to breathe. He kept saying "I know the way," and "you haven't any faith." "I haven't any faith that there is a path up this mountain," I replied. I never climbed a mountain with him again after that.

I had asked him to send a particular book to me, getting it from my house, and finally it arrived, and this was the book which saved my soul in Austria, because I turned then away from my unendurable aspiring yearning, towards the enormous and joyous creativity of writing, of finishing this book. It was called "The Book of the Beloved," and based on a revelation of God's love, of "the Star-love," I had when a child.

Once I started on this I was absorbed by the intense creativity and hard work; I was working all the hours God sends, either on my book or in the kitchen, with only short snatches inbetween, of visiting my favourite place in the forest by the fountain, or going out at night to see the magnificent starry skies. And suddenly that place, that limbo-land of Austria, like "Aslan's country", was no longer a refuge, a "freedom from" the mind-robbing power of a psychiatric system, it was a "freedom to" complete a God-given task, a sublime fusion of my understanding of my entire life, and of sublime things for others to know. *I wrote there of "the Way to Bliss"; and what drove and fuelled my knowledge of "Bliss," of perfect "self-yielding to the Star-love," was my memory of that one time when I had "touched the pulse-point" which was my direct contact with God, the greatest sweetness of my life. I wrote to Dr.James that I knew of it by remembering being in his arms.*

I had a couple of very romantic experiences. There was another dance one night in a tent several miles away from the monastery, and I went there with this young coloured man, who was a worker in the monastery who depended upon me to get him back in the door as I had the only key. I enjoyed the dance, sensing it was a "sharing in the one life," but when we started back along the long road in the utter darkness, this man started getting sexual with me, and tried to attack me. So I went back, and asked a nice man whom I had danced with, for some help, and he gave me a lift back; and we stood there on the bridge over the stream talking earnestly about our life-situations. He was astonished when I told him how the law had taken my child off me, and he told his equally sad tale; we agreed how awful it was to have a destructive and unloving relationship imposed upon you by law. The purling water, the moon, and the wide surrounding darkness, and our earnest conversation, made it strangely romantic.

A few days later I met this Johan again whilst walking through the woods, and he was driving up the mountain to feed his cows. And we went up to the mountain-top together in his car to see the sunset. I had no fear of him, because I always believe that adventures with strangers are "God coming towards us," and I could see he was an earnest, simple, honourable man. Sunset on that mountain-top was one of the most magnificent moments of my life. We could see far off to the North the Niedertauern, a magnificent range of high mountains, jagged and covered in snow; the hills and forests around stretched endlessly and were darkening, as the orange sunset-glow and pink-tinged clouds gave way to the first stars in the night's dark mantle, and down below, far below, the monastery and village nestled, and clustered itself around its little bright lights.

"You can sense what eternity is up here, can't you?" I said to Johan. Everything seemed set in the context of eternity, and for the first time I grasped and understood the Anglo-Saxon world-view; the intensity and beauty of that mythology which sees the dark unknown eternity filled with giants and dragons, pressing in upon the small habitations of men. It is of course so different from the modern world-view which is arrogant, and I explained it all to Johan, saying that "the outer space, the eternal darkness which rings us round in its gigantic nature, which dwarfs us, is where God reigns." I then explained to him with free-flowing words, as the stars came out, my concept of the "Star-love." I explained why I chose that word for God, and in explaining to him, how the love which moves the stars is always there, how it embraces and encircles us, how it shines in the mystery if the darkness, I understood the concept myself. This earnest man was overcome, saying that he had never met such an "intensely spiritual woman," and that intensity shone from me, and that he would never in his life forget the experience we were then sharing.

Pater Leo at this stage began to tell me that I must go home when the month was up. And I wouldn't go. He was a man used to obedience, being an Abbot, but I wouldn't be obedient. Initially I had been too scared to go back. The coloured man I've spoke of, who was a political refugee, told me when I first arrived, that I could not possibly ever go back to Scotland; he said I should stay in Austria by getting married and starting a new life. I had said No to this, because I felt dedicated to the one end, "single-minded in intent." And this "one end," this one task, was to write what I knew of the Star-love; I knew that I was there in Austria "to take up my connection with my knowledge," and I wrote endlessly to Dr.James about it. He had told me how the police were looking for me in Scotland. Now I knew that I had to finish my book before going home, though Pater Leo didn't understand this, because I knew that once home I would be too paralysed by fear to do creative writing. *It was then and there that I had the mastery of the whole thing, that I comprehended this "Bliss" which was direct contact with the Star-love, so I had to complete it.*

And so I started seeking for somewhere else to stay, praying that God should find me somewhere so I could finish the book "single-minded in intent." I only needed a further ten days grace. Finally I found a farmhouse halfway up the hill, belonging to the Kaufman family, with whom I had stayed before once, decades ago; they said I could "help to look after the cows," especially if there were any births of calves in the middle of the night. I was a bit dubious about this; in fact I did on one occasion help to pull a calf out of its mother with ropes attached to its hind legs. I liked it when I move to that farmhouse, because I could look out on a beautiful farmhouse scene with farmhouse noises, instead of being disturbed by the noise of the roadworks outside the monastery window. I worked frantically and harder than ever. I lived in an idyllic place, an idyllic landscape, in perfect summer sunshine, yet all I did was shut myself inside writing about ten hours of the day. *I was seized by the fulfillment of my creativity, writing a book about how to win eternal Bliss, trying to understand what that Bliss was, and charged with my memory of Bliss; I felt I was "ringed round by Bliss."*

What about Gabriel, and where did he figure in all this? Well Dr.James had been saying that I must "fight for him" on getting back, but I replied that I was no longer going to fight with Walter over Gabriel; I wasn't going to fight to get him back, because it seemed as though the only way it could have ended was to have "the connection cut." I blamed "the System" for it; by insisting on "father's rights" they had destroyed the relationship with the mother, and this was in the equation from the beginning. I felt I was doing what God wanted me to do; "I had taken him up as a baby to love because I believed that was what God wanted me to do; and out of the same love I lay him down, because I believe that is what God wants me to do." I felt an awful anguish about his feet, and how Walter would do them damage by not getting proper fitting shoes. I had to somehow cease to care about him, because "I can't afford to care about his feet," or his whole being which would be damaged by Walter's meanness. *I felt how, if he ever asked me, I would say to Gabriel "I didn't abandon you; you were torn from me, so out of my love, I let you go."*

I felt really that I didn't need a relationship with him any more, from my side, "so completely have I taken to myself the immolation of my motherhood." But on the other hand I wanted him to have Access to me, because I wanted and desired to "be there for him." Hence, a few days before I was due to leave, when I received a letter from the court, who had presumably got a note of Pater Leo's address through Walter, I was galvanised into action. It said that if I were not present or represented on the 13th of August "the action would proceed against me in my absence." I intended to be there! And also, seeing it was now known that I was at Pater Leo's monastery, it could be dangerous for him, as he was breaking Austrian laws by keeping me there. And so I knew I had to leave.

First came the adventure of that electrical storm. I had gone down to the village in the gathering gloom, and it started to pour down, and then came frightening lightening and thunder. I went to shelter at the house of a lady I knew, but I knew I had to be back at the farmhouse before the time they would go to bed, as I had no key, so I set off again with the umbrella that the lady's daughter gave me. This teenage girl had been telling me frightening tales of how you can die of a lightening-strike if it hits the ground somewhere near you, and how lots of people yearly die of lightening strikes in Austria, several from that very village. That walk up the hill was terrifying, because I realised half-way up that this umbrella had a metal spike, so it would draw lightening-strikes. The rain was pouring like sheets, and the storm got worse, until forked lightening was striking the hillside in front of me, with the unbelievable crashing of thunder. I was so scared!

When I got back the farmer told me I was a complete idiot for walking outside at all, let alone with a metal-spiked umbrella, during such a kind of storm. He explained to me that you must stay indoors with the windows shut; you have to shut the windows, because other wise, if lightening strikes the house, the electricity leaps inside in the form of a lightening-ball and kills you. He impressed upon me how dangerous was what I'd just done, telling tales of people he knew struck down, and I went to bed really frightened.

Finally the day, the moment came, when I finished my book, concluding with the words: - "And she was brave enough to take the Star-book and go, knowing that the Star-love and his bliss would go with her." I could see how the book itself was my knowledge of the bliss, and I could carry it with me under my arm! The first thing I did was to fling my arms wide open at the window, and cry out the words from an old Hindu text,-"Adoration unto thee, a thousand adorations, and again and again unto thee be adoration!" I knew that the ecstasy achieved in that moment of fulfilled creativity would not last, so I hurried down the hillside to the Mass in the small church, without trying to make it last.

That evening I lay in the meadow, between the sunset and the first stars appearing, realising I had written a book about how to win eternal Bliss. I said to myself, "this is the closest thing to Paradise I have ever known." I would be returning from Paradise; "my time in Austria will live in me as a delight forever!"

On the next day, my last day, I intended climbing that mountain-top! Rising through 7,000 feet, it was hard to climb! I was so breathless and the sun was so impossibly hot! I was scrambling up rocky paths and through endless forest, and so aware of the solitariness of my consciousness. I felt how I really wasn't fit enough for it. Two-thirds of the way up I had to phone Pater Leo from an inn, to ask him to tell Frau Kaufman that I was going to be very late back, as I was so struggling to get up there. I felt that if I ever got up there, I'd stay there forever! When nearing the top I felt how I had reached my goal in every way; in what I had written, created, understood, achieved, and it seemed so symbolic that after I'd reached my goal, I must then go back down the mountain into the world of men. Several intense experiences awaited me on that mountain-top.

I approached a wooden cross near the summit, with the words "in this sign you will arise," and I was overwhelmed in realising it was the same cross I'd found there decades earlier in the company of Pater Leo; "this is the cross that is actually in my book!" And I threw my arms around it in a veritable ecstasy! And then, I was lying on the grass in front of a magnificent panorama of mountains, when a cow came up to me and started nudging me; I kept saying "go away," but then imagine my shock on realising it was a bull! A bit frightened that I was going to be pushed over the edge by this bull, I moved away to the cairn at the very top, and whilst standing there a man came along and asked me out of the blue, in German, "Are you the Scottish woman who is a writing a book about the love of God?" And I was astonished, for how could he possibly know that! He explained that he had momentarily met me when I had first arrived, and it had stuck in his mind that I had said I had no interest in men, and I was writing a book about God's love; and he said that everybody in the village and neighbourhood had been talking about me. I was astonished that I had won such local "fame."

I stayed up there on that mountain-top for five hours. Pater Leo had told me "Don't stay up there for long" and I had no comprehension of why he should say this to me. However I soon found out why, later that day. My face and shoulders were so incredibly burnt that they were painful; one is not supposed to stay long on a high mountain where the sun's rays are so strong! But I stayed there reflecting, mulling things over, and I developed a marvellous sense of choice and freedom. When a great jet came high over head, leaving its trail, it increased this sense of freedom, of choice to do what I wanted and go where I wanted. And I shouted into the wide sky; "it is decided; I am not going to go back to stay and live in KirkMichaels." *Then the time came to say goodbye to my bliss amongst the Austrian mountains, and I prayed fervently by the cross; that I should keep this knowledge of Bliss within me, that I should kept true to God and true to my task, "keep me true to you and keep me like a child." And so I set off homewards, down that mountain, knowing that I carried Bliss with me.*

And I had a terrible time being chased by a bull, most of the way down that mountain. It really frightened me, especially as sometimes there were some very steep drops. Finally it stood in my path, and was ready to charge at me. I gazed at it straight in the eyes, commanding in German "Go away!" And it meekly turned around and did go away!

It was very sore taking a rucksack on my shoulder when I caught the train the next morning, because the sunburn was so painful. *And the last thing I remember was that Pater Leo, perhaps realising how scared*

I was at going back, gave me a card which said, "You will walk through fire and it shall not harm you."

232

Chapter 58
The Mad Knowledge.

On that weekend before had I left I had written a long letter to Dr.James, saying I had to go, "and I can't know that I shall ever find my way back to you." I intended leaving this letter together with my keys and a lot of my writings. "Please keep all my writings and all my knowledge safe. You said that you would take my knowledge, and I hold you to that. I would have sacrificed my life, to save this knowledge, so you must save it." I urged him to tell people that it is only by truly dying in the arms of God, yielding the self up into the eternal waters, that they can truly live and have eternal life. "Impart to others the knowledge I leave you, because it is life-giving; if they understand what is meant by "dying into the love of God," then they shall not die." "I leave for Austria, above all conscious of the purity of my yearning toward you. I don't know when I shall ever see you again. When I encounter you again, I trust you to recognise me, and if we are as angels, I trust our bodies will melt into each other. I will live in the hope of seeing you again, of somehow making my way back to you. For the earth is round, so I have hopes of seeing you again on the other side of it. My love of you and love of God are inseparable; that means my devotion to you will last forever."

The first thing I did on arrival in Austria was to sit on a bench, halfway up the hill behind the monastery, and just sit, longing and yearning for my "Master," who was far away across the mountains and across the sea. It was a kind of terrible homesickness. *And I wrote a letter to him, with a powerful and sad sense of yearning; "I have this longing for you which never goes away; my self-yielding to you is so fastened to the core of my being that I can't stop this perpetual yearning toward you; it won't let me go; it is fastened to the core of my being. Your mastering hand is needed by my whole being; don't ever take your mastering hand away from me."*

When I went to a dance, that first week in the market-square, I was overcome by a great sense of sadness and loneliness. "I have lost my son , I have lost everything, " I said to myself, "What on earth am I doing in Austria!" I felt I'd left everything behind me, and whilst everyone else was laughing and dancing, I felt a bottomless, hopeless yearning that was like despair. I poured out endless strong feelings to explain this yearning in my writings to Dr.James, saying he should "never take his mastering hand away from me," explaining how I had "given up bliss for him," stressing that I was "perfect self-yielding to him." *I wrote, "you have great power on the one hand to make me whole and happy and loved, in a way which is needed for the creating of my being, or on the other hand to destroy my wholeness and happiness in a way which would make me despair." I said that if he didn't "take me up with a mastering hand," in the way I was asking, "then I may as well bury myself in oblivion and despair forever! You are the reason for my being alive!"*

I spent my time lying on my bed or walking through the forest thinking perpetually of him, and of that point of self-yielding to him which was such sweet bliss. I realised that I had an enormous task trying to convince him to be my "Master" in the way I meant it; I spent the whole of the rest of my time in Austria in effect, besides working in the kitchen and writing the "Book of the Beloved," trying to convince him and persuade him of what I meant in an endless and perpetual fashion. I worked on the things which were his frequently expressed reservations, such as "I cannot be your lover." "It strikes me that asking you to be my Master, and asking you to be my Lover are two quite separate things; I am asking the one of you and not the other." I explained that my feeling for him was "pure," because it got a hold of my being when he wasn't physically present, and it was "made in heaven" because it was created at some eternal point where my soul met God. *I was trying to explain that he "mastered" me at the same point where I yielded myself to God; "my yearning for you is something like trying to be one with God; my self-yielding to you is that point."*

He had said to me about giving up the bliss of God's love for him on those Scarborough cliffs; "the idea that you gave up bliss for me I find totally unacceptable." So I tried to explain, tried to win him round to understanding it; "I somehow let go, and came through death back into resurrection life, and gave up the ability to remain in the loving arms of God, through wanting you to love me, know me, master me, through my not wanting to let go of you. I let go of God because I didn't want to let go of you." Over and over again I tried to explain to his understanding in a way he could accept, the explosive event for me on Scarborough's cliffs. And the explanation went on and on; - - about "being left suspended in a Void," about "being alive because I wouldn't let go of you," about "giving up my Nirvana for you," about "the eternal quality of that love."

Then as I started earnestly to write my book and became totally absorbed in it, I saw that I was writing about that "pulse-point" of touching and self-yielding to God out of my memory of self-yielding to him. "You touch me at the same point where God touches me; and it is like a spring; I now have my finger on the pulse-point of my being. All my life I have jealously guarded this "pulse-point" from being known by anybody else." By recalling that memory of self-yielding to him, I was writing of mystical Bliss! "I have never been a perfect Yes to anybody but you, and being yielded up to you is a sweetness I have never before experienced; it is the closest I have ever come to the bliss of Oneness with God, to that eternal sweetness." The book seemed highly-charged sexual stuff, but it wasn't, it was mystical; I was worried it would seem to him that it seethed with sexuality; he had once said that St.Theresa's mysticism was confused by her with sexual climax. So I tried to explain, *"Sexuality is a quality of soul with which God created us, by which we can know him; sexuality lies with spirituality at the core of our being."*

I was beginning to see my whole life in terms of this book, this "One Book," which I was writing about my "knowledge" of God, of "touching the pulse-point" which is self-yielding to God. And my whole life made sense; I had a marvellous clear vision of the whole of it, every bit making sense. I realised, I knew, that I was "mad," barking-mad; "out of this world." It was as if I lived for a while in a limbo-land, staying in ecstasy, not coming back down to earth. I realised how I always knew the best in my madness, for I touched God's love; my knowledge of God's love I had attained through madness, but I didn't want others to have to tread the same path; I saw my task as showing others the way to Bliss, and that's why I was writing the book, so "single-minded in intent."

Sometimes my whole being was overtaken by an intensity of yearning; I used to sit on benches at dusk, watching the moon and the first stars appearing, thinking how my Master, far away beyond mountains and sea, was yet "under the same moon." I yearned for a deep union with him and God simultaneously, a union eternal in its nature.

I wrote to him a lot about "dying," about yielding up the self; and how with real "knowledge" the soul which goes round the cycles of existence, can opt out and find union with God at the centre of the circle; "understanding how to die and dying are one and the same thing, one complete act." I wrote, "If you ask whether I am saying that I have a special knowledge which can save souls, and bring them to the consummation in God's love which is eternal life, I would unashamedly answer Yes. To attempt to give away such knowledge is an unenviable task." I explained how I wanted him to share in this task; "this is because you must stay at the door listening to me."

Then I explained about the "Door." "I travelled repeatedly into the Void, where madness is possible, in order to find that door and open it. That is why I've said so often in supposed madness "I know the Way; I know where the Door is." That is the door behind which Jesus was shut; I went through, and took his place, setting him free, and now I'm stuck. And now you take my place; you sit at the door keeping it open for me; it is only through you that I have contact with the earth. I cannot ever really and completely "come back." I am stuck somewhere as I've said, having let go of heaven on the one hand, and never fully able to get my feet on the earth on the other hand. I need you to be there, because it is you who fastens me to the earth."

I realised during an electrical storm that the image I had was that of a lightening-conductor. "Through you the energy of this knowledge can conduct itself to earth; I want you take it from me so as to render it safe. It is you who fasten me to earthly reality; that is why you are my Master; because you can take the knowledge which I conduct; it is you who have mastery over me; I am like Ariel in Shakespeare's Tempest; and you are like Prospero, because you are fastened to the earth and I am not; my only purpose is to wait upon you." I told him that my only purpose was to transmit to him the knowledge I was possessed of; I was like a "spirit" or ghost who had passed beyond, detained for a while.

And thus I spun a whole "philosophy" around my condition, around my madness and my need for a Master. It was totally mad. And I knew I was mad; I wrote begging him not on any account to show what I wrote to anybody else, because I would be in danger of getting locked up as permanently and irretrievably "insane." "Please don't show these writings to a psychiatrist! I was aware of this fact; if it were known that I was still talking about "holding open one-way-opening doors in the Void," I would be considered still mad!

"I would be judged as permanently and completely mad, by what I write now. You see you don't have to do anything to be certifiable, you only have to "think something" certifiable. And to think "I know what Jesus knew" is an extremely certifiable thing to think! The reason I keep being locked away basically, is because it is perceived that I claim to have some special knowledge. It is thought that I think "I am Jesus" or "I am the Virgin Mary" because of the way I talk. But all I do generally, to make people think I am getting better, is to learn to keep silence. Then when I no longer speak of such things, people say "look, we have made her better"! But all that has happened really is that this

*knowledge is plunged deep down into me, so that in daily life I too have
lost touch with it.*
*But I'm not losing touch with it this time, that is the point! What I am
saying is that this time I am not letting go of the knowledge that I have
always caught glimpses of in madness; if this is known I shall be
considered "permanently mad"!*

I tried to bind him to me, by an endless explanation of that "nuclear
event" which happened in Scarborough. I said it was like a nuclear
bomb in that a large amount of energy came out of the annihilation of a
small amount of matter; what was annihilated was my connection with
earthly reality; "what got burnt-out was me." I explained how I went off
to Scarborough having found "the secret of dying," from being
mastered by him. "I needed your attentive gaze; I needed someone to
know me and gaze into me. You have always compelled me to
obedience, and had this mastery over me; you had perfect compelling
knowledge of my soul's centre." In Scarborough I "momentarily died,
but not completely; I died so quick that my body didn't have the time to
follow; so I came back, reincarnated into a body which had not died.
And now I can't properly get back down to earth; my being is
attenuated, stretched as if buttered too thinly; my love of you upholds
me in existence."

I tried to explain to myself what this "knowledge" was that I possessed;
"nothing on earth shall ever separate me from my knowledge," I had
said above the dark inky waters of the ferry. I appealed "Don't leave
me alone in this Void forever; for I am possessed of a knowledge which
makes me alone." I knew what Jesus knew; "I know where the Door is
and I hold it open." My knowledge was the secret of "dying", the secret
of yielding up the soul's existence, the secret of "blowing out the
candle." Extinguishing one's own light of life, "letting it go out, without
putting it out," means perfect self-yielding. It was he who had thrown
me open to God in this way; "it was through you; you were the key
which sprung the lock, throwing me wide open to the love of God."

*In madness you annihilate the self and find a Void. What do I think in
my sanity of what I write in madness?- It attracts me as sublime,
containing a knowledge I now lack. "You seek and seek, and when you
find the centre of the self - there is nothing there!" This is what my
madnesses were; a greater knowledge, a touching of the centre of the
self which is a Void; and when trying to find God in that Void, I lost
contact with reality. People kept saying the knowledge I thought I had
was "illness", but that is nonsense; "my madness only rode on the back*

of my enlightenments." First I had knowledge, and then my selfhood was lost in a Void. Madness is what is left after you annihilate the self.

Childishness then dawned on me, as I tried to explain that the feeling I had for him was essentially childish. I wanted him to be my Master in the same way my Grandad had been; "it is because I am returning to being a child that I need a Master," for it was only as a child that I had "direct touch with the love of God." I explained how I had this bliss when a child, but the world ensnared me and it was lost to me; but now I had been baptized again into a fresh eternal youth. I explained it wasn't human love between us because it was essentially one-sided; he remained a mystery to me whilst having the key to my self-yielding; it was really like the childish obedience I owed to my Grandad. "It is childish obedience I offer you; I'm asking you to take responsibility for the key you hold; I adore you childishly, in the same way as I owe God my childish love." *In Austria I had become completely childish; when I came out through the customs in Salzburg, I knew I looked and felt a complete child!*

As my days there were coming to an end, I became very afraid at the thought of going back. I had existed there in the innocence of my childhood, and had appealed to this man who meant so much to me, in a completely "mad" and childish way. I realised returning would be one great act of faith in him, because I feared that if he revealed to others the "mad" way I was thinking, I would be locked up as irretrievably insane. I had discovered in Austria that I hadn't given up my "knowledge of bliss," but was living in direct contact with the love of God; my blessed consciousness, my childish consciousness, wasn't failing me. So I was fearful of going back, of being robbed of it by the drugs of the psychiatric system; "I am fearful of everyone and everything, including you." And I knew I was going back "as a child" and she wouldn't have the wits or the understanding to cope with the real world. But I wrote that I would come back trusting him utterly, "with a blind childish trust." I said he would have to say that I was "a spirit-child, come from the mountains, who has happened to attach herself to me." For being a spirit-child attached to him, was my only purpose.

Painfully, laboriously, I carried all this mystical knowledge back with me, in an old rucksack on sore and sunburnt shoulders, from the Austrian-Benedictine-mountain-tops, to a sad sick place by the sea, where I was raped in my soul, and robbed of my Bliss.

Chapter 59
The Mystical Secret of Dying.

Our life really is a desire to be One with God; this is what my "Book of the Beloved" is about; she goes "into the dark Void" where we meet the Star-love, but she cannot comprehend why it is dark or why she is not loved, what she suffers or why she cannot attain what she seeks. But with a kind of "graciousness" the Star-love meets her in that darkness; and at the end of every story she attains the bliss of being "One with the Star-love." It is an explanation of what we are here for, the desire which keeps us alive.

To die only has one meaning; the complete yielding up of the self. And understanding how to die and dying are one and the same thing; it is one complete act.

People are afraid to die; they cling on to their own little self-centred lives, and think that the meaning of "eternal life" is that little life going on forever. They are afraid to die, afraid to yield themselves up to God's love. For this reason they go round in the cycles of existence endlessly bound to their own self! And so they can never reach Heaven, bound up in the illusion of the world of "Samsara." The Christian world-view, that the soul travels in a straight line, and after death achieves heaven or hell, is nonsense. The truth is that the soul is unable to understand what "dying" is; until finally, being enlightened and really "yielding itself up," it opts out of the cycles and reaches the middle-point, which is union with God. *And the only way to get to God lies in knowing how to "die."*

And real "Death", the charnel -house extinction, the ending up of the soul in the grave where there is no life, is due to this lack of "knowledge" about God's love, and how to yield to it. In this way souls are either heading toward heaven, or heading toward hell; hell being of course the everlasting separation from the knowledge of God's love.

There is a Zen story of how a nun achieved enlightenment; for decades she strove for it, and daily carried a pail of water back from the well. Then one night the bottom suddenly fell out of it, and she instantly reached her goal; "no more water in the pail, no more moon in the water!" *She suddenly understood, you see, that the struggle and the effort and the holding of the self, could be annihilated in one single sublime act of self-yielding. Now that I have written "the Book of the Beloved" I can carry the secret of this self-yielding under my arm!*

239

Our struggle is to keep our own light of life burning. God does not take that light from us; that is not what death is. He doesn't take it from us; we have to give it up ourselves; we don't have to wait upon God to die; first we have to die, to give up our own light of life, and afterwards we meet him in the dark Void; we have to "go out to meet him." *I have discovered the secret of "letting the light go out."*

The struggle within ourselves which keeps us alive, is, on the one hand trying to keep the flame burning because we are afraid of death, and on the other hand our longing for the light to go out, because we guess that once this light goes out, we will find "eternal" life and light. It is the struggle that keeps the candle-flame burning. But I have discovered the secret of ceasing the struggle. "The light you can put out is not the eternal light." People are idiots when they think that "eternal life/ eternal light" is simply the littleness of their own "light of life" going on forever. That candle-flame has first to be put out before we can experience "the eternal". It is like finding a way to jump from the circumference of the cycles of existence into the centre; *and I have discovered that secret.*

What strikes me is the great difference in the quality between human love and the Star-love. *When men achieve the self-yielding of the soul in sexual union, when they attain that "mastery," they say "I love you less after the event," or "I don't want to love you any more; I got what I wanted, I achieved the end of my desire, - that was it, - I've finished with you now." But the Star-love, when He loves and achieves the mastery of the soul in its dying, its self-yielding, He says "I will take you up with an everlasting love, I will love you forever; never shall my love wane or let you go, after this intensity of the moment; and I shall be forever with you, and close to you, and loving you."*

There is another great difference between human love and the Star-love. *Men's love always wants to overcome the centre of the will, to compel. "I love you" is generally a euphemism for "I want to overcome you when I want to overcome you." It seems to me that is why men get married; so at any time they can compel and overcome the will. The Star-love is essentially different in quality, saying "I want you to love me, I want you to respond to my love; I wait upon you, upon your understanding and self-yielding."*

And so the "Mastery" of the Star-love is essentially different from the mastering of human love. *Men's love masters by overcoming the centre of the will so that the yielding is essentially unwilling; the Star-*

love masters us by touching the springs of the will and the love that is in our souls, so that we yield to him a "perfect Yes." The Star-love cannot "rape" as human love can. What the Star-love demands is: "I want you to love me back with the eternal love I have put within you, so that we can be One." - - Men's love compels the will, and the Star-love releases the springs of the will. So men's love enslaves, whilst the Star-love liberates.

I see another way that human love is different from the Star-love: - *Men's love can always reach a point where it stops; "you have disobeyed me, offended me; that's it, I don't love you any more." But the Star-love never reaches such a point. And it is not a point in time, but a point in quality. The Star-love is gracious and compassionate and tender; he "bends" toward the soul with such graciousness!*

Chapter 60
A Manic Return from Austria.

I did indeed on my return feel like "a spirit-child come from the mountains, straight from God"! The journey was horrible, for I had to carry the full weight of my "knowledge," of all my writing in a rucksack which chafed sore and sunburnt shoulders, and I suffered from the horrid pain of an ear-infection. I had to walk for miles it seemed with my luggage between trains and ferries, and I was stopped and searched for drugs on my way through the Dover customs.

It seemed as if "shades of the prison-house" were closing around me, the closer I got to KirkMichaels. I noticed how through the Austrian mountains when the train stopped, everybody piled out and everybody piled in, and everybody talked happily and gazed out of the window. Once I'd reached London, everybody queued, even queuing before going on to the platform, and everybody stuffed their heads in newspapers in a taciturn manner. I couldn't stand the sense of claustrophobia I was getting, and determined that I wouldn't stay in KirkMichaels, as I had said to myself on that mountain-top, but would go off somewhere like Ireland. I was only really returning to KirkMichaels, in order to make my bid for Access to my son in the court, which, as I had been advised by that letter to the monastery, was the following day.

Finally I arrived, at about midnight, and went straight by taxi to Dr.James' house. He answered "Who is it?" - "It's me" I replied, sure that he would recognize my voice. I was full of trepidation as this was the man I counted as my "Master", having written endlessly to him from Austria. When he opened the door and handed me the keys he told me to go straight home, and he would come round the next day. Once home, I heated water for a bath, finally got to bed, but couldn't sleep at all because of my painful ears. He came knocking on my door at 12 noon, and shouted at me, "What are you doing still in bed, at this time! Come on get up, you only have 4 hours till that court hearing!" "Please don't be angry with me; I can't bear it," I replied. He stood in the doorway and said "I am not angry with you, I am just raising my voice!"

I knew I had to get to court on time, and my phone had been cut off, so I went to the Baptist church and made calls from there to see if anybody might take me and give me some support. Finally Hugh Yates agreed to take me in his car to the Kirkcraig Sheriff court, which was about ten miles away. I had written what I had wanted to say, and then learnt it off by heart. So when it came to the point where the court was

242

asked if anyone was there on my behalf, I bravely stood up, went to the witness-box, and recited this speech I had learnt.

It went like this: *"I have travelled, with all the haste possible from Austria, from a 7,000 foot high mountain-top, at considerable personal cost to myself, both financially and in terms of physical pain, to assert, that I love my son and I am his mother."* - There were cries of astonishment from the court, but the judge said "let her speak." I continued -*"To assert, that I love him too much to tug him to bits, that in my true mother's love, it not being possessive, I love him enough to let go of him. Despite that, to assert, that my son needs me and needs access to me; and above all to assert, my desire and willingness to be there for him. I need not have come back, but I have come back to be here, and to assert these things."*

There was a hulaballu in the court. Walter's solicitor, a female, pointed her finger at me shrieking "She is mentally ill, she is mentally ill!" The judge was saying he hadn't expected me to be represented in the court, as I no longer had a solicitor. The female solicitor was meanwhile arguing "I move that she have a curator ad leitem, because she is not fit to speak herself in the court because she is mentally ill!" I was overcome, I hadn't come all the way back from Austria to be accused of being "mentally ill" like this!

Finally the judge gave his decision; "You are obliged by law to stay in your abode of 109 Dumchapel Drive, until social work reports have been made into you mental condition, and the whole situation." I almost visibly collapsed in the dock; there was no way I could abide living in KirkMichaels for a month, to be investigated; I wanted fresh air and freedom; I planned to go to Ireland; now I was condemned to something as bad as a prison! When we were driving back to KirkMichaels Hugh Yates commented "we won." *"How do you work that out?"* I replied, *"I lost, I completely lost."*

Dr.James came that night; I tried to express to him the whole thing that I had comprehended and written of in Austria, by reading out snippets back and forth in my letters, trying to keep my silence toward him, trying to establish this "spirit-child and Master" relationship. But it didn't work; he saw me as distraught. *I told him why I felt distraught; after all the fresh air and freedom I knew in Austria, after all those walks through woods and mountains, when I was solitary, and not another consciousness for miles and miles around, now I was so crushed and rendered claustrophobic with these thousands of consciousnesses, of minds, pressed into a small space; I couldn't stand it!*

243

That night he said to me "I want you to take some tablets"; I replied "I'll do anything you say," and without enquiring what they were, let his hand slip them down my throat! I was trusting "his mastering hand." When I woke in the morning I felt so very ill. I couldn't breathe or speak, my tongue wouldn't work; I recognized all the ghastly signs of Largactil. But he never gave me the antidote, the Procyclidine, which releases the side-effects. I was scared of remaining in the house in that condition, in case someone official came to the door; I would seem mentally ill. So I went out, at 6 in the morning, thinking I would try and get out and away from all these oppressive consciousnesses. I headed for the long solitary stretch of the West sands. I can remember pinching a bottle of milk from outside a hotel on my way. I can remember being disgusted with the mud and effluence on the beach, comparing it with the pristine cleanliness of Austria.

I can remember how I had also become disgusted with the water, refusing to drink any, as it came though pipes in a district of low-lying manured farms; Pater Leo used to say that it was only and always safe to drink the water that flowed down from mountains. I can remember how I was also obsessed with milk, and drunk milk instead of water all the time; I felt milk was precious and pure, for in the farm where I stayed the milk from the cows was considered too valuable to drink; they had to sell it in order to buy all other commodities. *Hence my manic obsession with water and milk; it wasn't "mad," for it made sense to me.*

Dr.James came back that night. "Where've you been? I've been looking for you," he said crossly, "And what was I to think with all the ID cards and money torn up at the door?" "You gave me poison!" I said with some sting. "It wasn't poison, it was Largactil" he said defensively. "I had to go out to get milk," I said. "I've brought you milk and yoghurt, and left it in the fridge; didn't you even look!" he said crossly.

Then we calmed down a bit. I told him I'd found a way to cope with all these minds around me all the time. I showed him a quote from "the Prophet"; "Build of your imaginings a bower in the wilderness before you build a house within the city walls." I said my plan was basically to stay out there, in one of the shelters, way out on the West Sands, and I would leave number-messages by Henry's door to say when I was out there. He didn't like the idea; "Don't you realize all the drug-pushing and using that goes on out there late at night?" I was adamant that I was going to spend as long as possible out there, in order to get myself a sense of freedom again, and to save my sanity.

The next day I again walked out along the West Sands, and walked bare-footed, as I was becoming obsessed by the Austrian hiking-boots which Pater Leo had bought for me; I felt they should be saved for mountain-climbing, and as they came from a pure place they shouldn't be worn with socks. Accordingly my feet were getting sore, so I walked bare-foot as far as the Holy Martyrs church in the centre of town, where I got my self inside the railings, and sat there cross-legged singing religious songs. I can remember feeling like "a Spirit-child from the mountains," having nothing to do with the abodes of men. I felt that being inside the church railings was a "safe" place. I partly needed to be safe from the police, because they had been hassling me; even the visiting priest from the local catholic church had told me to "move on" and not stay praying in his church; I must have looked a suspicious character carrying everywhere with me an old rucksack, which was full of my precious "knowledge."

When I was inside these church-railings many people stopped and talked to me. I can remember an old friend called Nicola leading me out of there for a bit, but I got a sense of evil and danger, so I went back, feeling safe inside those church-railings. It was as if I were claiming "sanctuary" where human law couldn't touch me. But I was aware that my "Master" didn't know where I was, so talking to man who was enchanted by me, I gave him my watch, telling to go give it to Dr.James asking him to come for me. All day I stayed there, and he never turned up, so I set off to his house, going bare-footed all the way, walking straight across the main road "like a bull." I later said "I walked straight across the main road like a bull, and all the cars stopped for me." Dr.James replied "I bet they did!"

When I got to his house he was still away working, and for some strange reason his wife and daughters agreed to give me a bath when I asked for one. And when he came home he handed me my watch saying crossly "What are you doing here? A man came and told me you were waiting for me in the town church; here's your watch!" And I flung it at his head with a great violence. It missed his head and hit the window; he picked it up saying "it's broken." *Looking back I think he was at a loss how to deal with me; he could see I was becoming manic, and really couldn't cope with it.*

He gave me something to eat, letting me share pizza with the family, then told me to "Go home". I can remember feeling that this was an incredibly cruel thing to say, as I felt my "home" was that mountain-top I had come from, and I only felt imprisoned and in danger in 109

245

Drumchapel Drive. But I left, and on my way, seeing milk on a friend's door-step, rang at the door to ask if I could have it; I was obsessed with milk. My friend Elizabeth invited me in, and I took off my Austrian boots at the door. She foolishly gave me a cup of tea, which was stupid, because being manic I tried to pour it all down my throat at once and scalded myself. She meanwhile had phoned the doctor, as she could see I wasn't in my right mind. When Dr.Miller's car arrived, I yelled at her that she had "betrayed me", but the doctor simply gave me a lift back to my own house, which I was very glad about. But I felt I couldn't stay there, so I went back to Dr.James' house.

He yelled at me this time, "Go back home; go back to your own house and stay there!" I felt I couldn't ; how could he not understand that "home" for me was that Austrian mountain-top? So, though I was shut out, I stayed on his lawn, and sung with my loudest voice the "Salve Regina" in Latin. But he wouldn't open the door, and I remained in his garden, till a teenager, his son, saw me there on coming home. "What are you doing here?" he asked me, where I sat cross-legged and bare-footed on the grass. I held his head caressingly in my hands and said "You are beautiful; are you a boy or a girl?"

Seeing I felt I had nowhere to go, I decided to set off walking with my sore feet in my sore-creating hiking boots into the night, because it was a beautiful starry and moonlit night. I ended up walking all night, arriving in Kirkcraig, ten miles away, in the early morning. I remember I walked through Cameron Park in the lovely sweet moonlight, pondering over and over why I couldn't make a "Spirit-child to Master" relationship with Dr.James; it had all gone wrong, and I wished I had never come back from Austria. And slowly it dawned on me that really the relationship was "child-Father"; and it dawned on me, he was like a Father to me, if only he could accept it like that. Then I walked on the country roads for miles and miles, feeling that this was my task, to walk around converting people, without an abode of my own. I can remember how a man who was repairing something leafed out of the darkness, and he was fascinated as I told him I was walking homeless over the face of the earth, sent on a mission by my "Master."

In the early morning, about 6 am, I got into Kirkcraig, and I saw a man by a van loading bread from a Bakery. I said to him "Do you happen to know anyone who would be going to KirkMichaels?" My great urge was to get back to my "Master" to tell him what I had discovered. "I'm going to KirkMichaels; hop in!" he said. On the trip I told him that I was Dr.James' "long-lost daughter" which he never knew he had; he promised he would phone this fact through to him after he had set me down from the van. It was now raining; and I got the urge to get really wet, before seeing Dr.James, so I found an over-flowing water-drain and stood beneath it, till I was drenched. I then made straight for the surgery, which was just opening, and insisted on waiting in Dr.James' room till he should come in to work. There I sat on the floor, cold with bare sore feet, absolutely drenched, yet passionate and intense.

So Dr.James eventually came in and there was this absolutely passionate, crying, cold, wet young woman sitting at his feet, clasping his knees, yelling "you are my Father! I have found it out in the night, I got proof of it; you are my Father!" He mulled it over in his calm deep considering mind, and said "Yes a man phoned me to say that my long-lost daughter was coming! I suppose it is just possible, seeing I am 13 years older than you, if I had an early start!" Then "Come with me," he said earnestly, "I'm going to take you back home in my car; I don't want people seeing you barefoot along the street in this condition!"

Thus I ended up at home again. That night wanting milk, seeing I wouldn't drink any water in any form, I went to a neighbour's house, and asked if they could give me some milk. I said "I have a baby, I have a baby to feed, and need milk." So they gave me milk, at the same time as phoning the doctor, as it must have seemed strange; I told them to contact Dr.James about it. Shortly after, he came round when I was washing my feet in milk, - it made sense to me as my feet were incredibly sore, and I felt that milk was kinder than water. He was busy telling me I was getting dangerously close to being hospitalized, when the "Craigdene squad" burst in the door. "Oh No, I left the door open," bewailed Dr.James, and from then on it was out of his hands. Looking back, I'm convinced it wasn't he who had called for the Craigdene nurses; he had been doing his very best.

So I ended up back in Craigdene, back in the lock-up Ward, after my 2 months of glorious and blissful freedom in Austria! And so I learnt that the words of Pater Leo didn't come true; "You will walk through fire and it shall not harm you." For I was very harmed. The first thing they did was to give me the long-term injection of Haldol Decanoate which I had so fled from. For the ensuing months it made me soul-dead, unfeeling and stiff in my mind, body, and soul, until such a "living-death" drove me to commit suicide by jumping off the pier into the dark cold waters of a November night! *The irony of it was, that after being given the impetus of going all the way to Austria, by fear of that injection, that very same thing was waiting for me; it met me on my coming back!*

Chapter 61
Suicide.

Somebody told me that I had "attempted to commit suicide," but "failed". Nothing could be further from the truth! I *did* commit suicide, in that I committed the irrevocable act of suicide, in jumping off the pier. And I didn't *fail*; rather I transcended myself; I transcended my desire to commit suicide, in that I took hold of even more courage, to face life.

It was a dark cold November night, 11 o'clock at night, when no-one else was around. The pier of KirkMichaels looked a cold and forbidding place. I had been there earlier in the day, but there were some odd people about, who I thought might rescue me. *And I didn't want to be rescued; I intended to die! Why did I want to die? Because I despaired.*

It was 1992, and I had just spent another 4 months incarcerated in Craigdene hospital; I wasn't at all ill for 3 of those months, having quickly come down from a "manic" condition, but still Dr. McNeill wouldn't let me out, and I felt I'd been imprisoned for ages. I had not seen my son for ages, and felt I was never going to get the chance of seeing him again; I had irrevocably lost Custody of him; I was a grieving mother. And then, before allowing me out on "trial leave" the regime of Craigdene had forced me to embark on a "depot injection"(i.e. a slow-release deep-muscular injection that is repeated every week or so).- They were the bane of my life, these injections, because it meant you were forced to have mind-sickening chemicals in your brain, which would take ages to wear off. It was "Haldol Decanoate," and I had a very bad reaction to it. *They forcibly injected me with this, and I realised with horror that before it wore out of my system they were going to give me another one; i.e. I would be forced to be on this for the rest of my life.*

It made me really ill, - I had felt alright before they gave me it. I couldn't do anything, I just couldn't cope; I couldn't do a simple thing like brush my teeth; I was all stiff, - even my eyes were stiff. I couldn't think, I couldn't feel; I was like a zombie. *And I was going to be like this ever after?! - I despaired. For the first and only time in my entire life I completely despaired. I decided that I couldn't tolerate being dead in my mind like this, - I preferred to be all dead.* I couldn't tolerate being physically alive but mentally dead. This is what I told Dr Hughes when they had pulled me out of the water, when he came to the hospital, where they had wrapped me up with tin foil like a turkey, to increase my temperature. "I can't bear to be dead in my mind like this, I'd rather be all dead," I said to him.

It took a great deal of courage to jump off that pier; it took "guts". I went back there, late at night, intent on my purpose, and before I set off I posted a letter which was a suicide note to Dr.James, thinking "Right, now I've got to go through with it." This suicide note ended; "And may the Lord have mercy on my soul," because somehow I felt I was guilty of a great sin in trying to end my own life.(I have still felt this, years later, and sought absolution from a priest for my "sin".) I couldn't do it for ages! I couldn't swim, so I thought I'd drown quickly, but I just couldn't bring myself to jump off the end of that pier! It was all dark and cold, at 11 0' clock, and there was nobody anywhere around. I thought it was a sure way of killing myself; I didn't choose an easier way like an overdose, because of the risk of failing in the attempt; this had to be it! - *an irrevocable act, the taking of my own life!*

People make the effort to live, to stay out of Death, because they are afraid. It is only by truly dying in the arms of God, yielding the self up into the eternal waters, that they can truly live and have eternal life.

Finally the only way I could jump was to take a run at it; I ran half-way along the pier and threw myself off. *I seemed to fall down and down for ages; it was like "Alice in Wonderland" when she falls; it seemed to take ages before I hit the water. Then a cold splash, and it hit up through my nose and took my breath away. I floated back up to the surface, almost surprised that I wasn't dead. It was so cold!* I thought "How long is it going to take before I die?" I put my head down and breathed in the water on purpose, thinking that it would fill my lungs and sink me. Time passed. I became so so cold! I kept saying to myself "I want to die, I want to die." Time passed. I had a heavy voluminous anorak on, and the brand new boots my Mum had bought for me; I thought these would drag me down, but still I floated. I became so cold that I thought I was going to die of it. It was only later Dr.James said to me *"You don't die of drowning, you die of cold!"*

Finally, in what I thought would be my last conscious act, as I tried to "surrender myself" body and soul, I said; *"When I open my eyes, I want to see the face of God."*
And I opened my eyes. Now I thought I had been floating face down in the water, in that I felt the warm ring around my face, but my skin must have become colder than the water, because in actual fact I

was the other way up. So I opened my eyes. And what I saw astonished me. I saw the pier some distance away, and on the end of it, two figures looking down at me! It took me some time to orientate myself to realise what I was seeing. They were two children. What I suddenly felt was that God didn't want me to die after all; He was rescuing me. *Suddenly a hope surged within me; I wanted to fight for life. I had the image of myself, cold and wet and dead, found on a sea-shore; I suddenly felt life was worth fighting for, no matter what suffering it entailed. I suddenly wanted to live!*

I don't think the children would have seen me, as I was some distance out from the pier, if I had not waved and shouted. I waved and shouted with every ounce of me, even though I felt my life slipping away. "Help, help! Can you see me? Help, help! I want to live! *I don't want to die, I want to live! I have a son , I want to live!*" Afterwards I always thought it strange, how I cited the fact that I had a son, as reason to want to live! But I suppose in the back of my mind, I had thought what it would do to him if his mother's dead and bloated body were found, and I saw that, even though I couldn't see him and had veritably "lost" him, yet having a son should give me hope and courage to live. So that's what I shouted.

And to my horror, one of the children disappeared for a bit, for what seemed a long while! She had apparently gone to get a life-ring to throw to me. But I rather thought they hadn't heard me, and I lost the energy to shout to the small boy who was left there. So as I drifted, so cold in the sea, I felt that I was going to die after all. *This seemed to last for ages, floating, so cold, so hopeless!*

But then the girl came back and threw this ring to me. It was still some way away, and I struggled and struggled to get to it; I fought through the water, hellishly, to get to that ring, that promise of life which I saw in the water. I thought "I will live, I want to live." I didn't think I'd make it, but I did, and the girl and her mother pulled me in, till I was standing dripping wet on the pier. I was still so so cold! I was suffering from hypothermia, and they wrapped me up in something like tin-foil once I got to the hospital, in order to raise my body-temperature. Then the nurses from Craigdene came to fetch me. I was horrified, to realise I was being put back in Craigdene, but then again, I was only too glad and thankful, to be alive!

Chapter 62
Bravery.

I was glad I'd tried suicide that November night, because as a gesture of protest it was invaluable. Dr.McNeill took note that I was "suicidal" on that Haldol Decanoate injection, and mercifully he stopped it. I rapidly got better once it was stopped, *and I thought it strange that I was "returned to life because I tried to die."*

There were a couple of other things which had urged me to that suicidal act of jumping off the pier, two things which aggravated that sense of complete despair. Firstly Dr.James had been to my house, saying he could not ever come round to see me again; and secondly Walter had said he wouldn't allow me decent Access-rights to Gabriel. And without Dr.James and Gabriel in my life, I seemed to have nothing to live for.

We had a social work meeting with Walter, trying to establish some kind of Access visits for me and Gabriel; and Walter had made out that Gabriel had been fine until he was upset by seeing his mummy again, and he said I had problems he didn't want his son to know about. I had replied angrily "I could have said that to you, that his existence was happy before you came along." He said he didn't want anything more to do with me because he had "found another woman"; he would allow no more than my seeing my son two hours per week, supervised. I thought he was a "piece of slime"; he used my illness against me every step of the way!

Walter used the opportunity of my illness to steal my son away from me.

And so I found myself picking up the pieces in December again, once I was back out of hospital. *I had a feeling of how "brave" I was; "brave in faring forward into life, brave in picking up the pieces."* There were a lot of things to try and mend this time; loss of a crucifix, a son, a novel. But I had a deep acceptance of things; "things get smashed, but you have to pick up the pieces and walk on." I was proud of my madness and the creativity that went with it, proud of how brave I was in facing it. I thought I'd try and build a new life.

But I had no support! There was no "support system" given me, now that I was on my own without a child! And without this precious child, the direction of my life lay downhill. I was sadly rejected by all my friends, largely I think because they were afraid of my illness; these mothers with young children who had befriended me when I had Gabriel, dropped me like a red hot brick when I was without him. I felt lonely and unloved. I got no help from my parents, who refused to let me go home for Xmas; they treated my illness as though it were some deadly disease. I felt so alone, in that everybody else seemed to have children and family around them; "everyone seems to have a rich emotional life but me!"

When I blew out the candles on my birthday, my wish was that I could somehow get Gabriel back. I felt that the two hours a week, supervised by a social worker, was nothing. I couldn't tolerate the feeling I had about him, and the raw-nerved loneliness it caused me. Walter had stolen him from me, and I wanted him back! But I knew as I said it that I would never get him back. That cold pain was due to the fact that I felt I wasn't his mother any longer. I needed a child to care for; to look after, dress, feed, cuddle, hug and be close to; I was screaming in my motherhood. I was so lonely now that I'd lost Gabriel; I felt he might as well be "dead to me." *I knew I had irrevocably lost my son.* "Because my illness counts against me, I'll never get Custody back!"

I felt so lonely and unloved, especially with Christmas approaching. "Nobody really is a friend to me, nobody wants to spend time with me." It felt particularly sore because nobody had invited me to Xmas dinner; I had no feelings of being accepted, wanted, loved. The way people treated me made me feel; "I am one of the unwanted, one of those you have to show charity towards; I am one of the dispossessed."

It is those who are dispossessed of their children, who are really poor.

I began to wish I could have another child! And I began to wish I had a boy-friend. When Dr.James came to visit, I told him how I wanted another child. It was partly because no-one would have me because of my illness and no-one would employ me. Having a baby would be a way of getting my own back on the world, as it was a thing no-one could stop me from doing. I knew this was bravado, and not the best reason for wanting a child; I felt like this because the world wouldn't allow me to fulfil myself, wouldn't allow me to achieve anything, or give me the opportunity to use my gifts and talents. And the one thing I could do, was to be a good mother.

Dr.McNeill didn't help by rubbishing me! I asked why, after labelling me at the time as mentally ill, did he then accept what I said? He said back very unkindly, "you are always changing your mind. - I must have known 20 different Mairis.- You do strange unaccountable things. - It

252

was your fault for going off to Austria .- You are lucky we let you keep him for the first 5 years." He was a swine for the way he rubbished me! What kind of "support" was he?!

And then Matty arrived in his car one night, like a charging knight in shining armour! He said he wanted a baby too; "I want a baby and you want a baby, there is nothing to stop us." However I wouldn't let him make love to me; I was charged with the moral awareness that in love-making you have to say "a perfect Yes." So I told him that I wanted to wait a while to make sure of him, because I wanted us to be committed to each other before having a child. But at least he made me feel wanted.

But that Xmas Eve Dr.James invited me to Christmas dinner, with his family at his house, and I had an intensity of feeling toward him which was like pain, and I realized it was him I was "saying a perfect Yes to," and not Matty. In comparison having given Matty dinner on Xmas day, I felt he didn't have a mind that met mine; "it would be immoral to make love to him, as it's not him I'm a perfect Yes to, not him I'm in love with." It seemed to me that day that the love which makes you happy is of the mind, and nothing to do with sex and food.

After that realisation, my relationship with Matty began to go downhill. There was no rapport between us, when I compared him to Dr.James, and I was thinking about Dr.James all the time; just talking with him was "mind-blowing, and sent me full of stars." Matty did his best to get a committed relationship with me, and I could see that he had good qualities, but I just couldn't love him back when Dr.James was absorbing all my affections and intense feelings. And so a short while later I told Matty he would have to leave me alone, because I was "in love with somebody else"!

As for my son, I realised "I've scrapped him"; (Dr.James always used to joke that when babies grow to school-age, you should "scrap them" and start again!) I mean, I realised I had to come to terms with my loss of him, and the fact that they would never give him back to me; the only thing to do was to have another one. I wanted to be free from him because he bound me to the murkiness of my past; but on the other hand, I realised I couldn't reject him and had to go on loving him; *I had to "take on the pain," because to escape pain is to escape life.*

That New Year's Eve was a memorable experience for me. My intense feelings were set in motion by a minibus driver, who said to me "Where is your boy?" When I told him I'd lost him to the father, he responded

253

with sympathy "that's bad, that's terrible; it wasn't fair when you had done all the dirty work, all the nappies and things!" He asked me "Why did you leave the father? Did he beat you up?" I replied "He never beat me up physically, but he did emotionally, which is worse." And so I arrived in town with the vivid memories of how I let myself be used and abused by Walter, memories of the tarnishing of my pure soul. *And as I walked in dark and lonely places overlooking the sea, my thoughts were: "I don't want to be bound by this dark and murky past; I want a fresh start without that murkiness of Walter and what he did to me; I want to build a fresh new life."*

My suffering was that of a dark and lonely soul, who had heavily lost my only son, reaching out for a meeting of minds to the one person who made me feel loved and accepted. And that was the feeling, on that New Year's Eve of '93, which catapulted me into seeing my love of Dr.James as a star in the darkness, enabling me to be pure. "My love of him will give me wings, will be like a star to me."

Chapter 63
The Lone Star.

It was partly due to the crumbling of my friendship with Dr.James that I attempted that dreadful suicide, jumping off the pier on that cold November night. For I had come back from Austria full of this concept that he was my Master, and he hadn't at all understood it. I had only had a short time to explain it to him before I went manic and got put back in hospital, and then when I was doped up the whole thing was lost to me. There was an occasion when he visited me when I was out on Pass; he asked "How many men have you seduced Mairi?" and I replied "None." But he doubted my intention, seemed convinced I was dangerous to him, and suddenly he was out of there, declaring, "I can never come back; not after this!"

And so it was important to me, when trying to get my life back together, to go round to his surgery to try and appeal to him to visit me again. He said that 99% of doctors would have nothing more to do with me, and he seemed to blame me in some way; I appealed to him "Because our relationship has to be asexual, it doesn't mean you can't relate to me; can't we be friends?" Suddenly and unexpectedly he consented to come; I couldn't understand why he had changed his mind; but I felt an enormous sense of God's grace, and was so grateful.

And so he appeared to visit me when I was discharged at the beginning of December. I told him "I find the purity and intensity of what I felt toward you in Austria very beautiful," but he seemed embarrassed by the subject. So I talked a bit of my suicide attempt, and he said "Don't do it again." The important thing was, after saying he could never come back, he had come back, and "there's hope in that!"

When he came again a couple of weeks later, I unburdened my heart to him, saying how horrid it was to have my son stolen away from me, and how I had my heart set on having another child. I said even if I were to become ill again, it wouldn't prevent me from employing my talents in child-care. We stood earnestly talking by the door, leaning against the wall. I said "I'm lonely." "I bet you are!" he sympathized. "I don't feel as though I am a mother anymore" I complained. He said I had to be careful not to get pregnant. But I explained earnestly that I wanted a child, because it was a way of achieving something; it was a matter of using my gifts and talents; the world denied me fulfillment because of my illness; I wanted to achieve what I could by being a mother of a child. He took me by the wrist and said earnestly, full of care and concern, that I had to be careful if I were trying to find a "Mr.Stud." I blushed, and was made glad by the sense of chemistry and magnetism there was between us. I was thrilled that the day had re-initiated some kind of closeness between us; it put hope in my life.

The day before Xmas Eve he unexpectedly called round to invite me to Xmas dinner, interrupted me whilst I was typing, saying "I only have 23 seconds." First he pointed out that his family have Xmas dinner on Xmas Eve, as is the foreign custom, then he asked if I would eat turkey, being a vegetarian. I was rather scared and thrilled at the same time, but of course replied; "Yes, I would love to; it's very kind of you to invite me." Standing by the door in the dark with him I said "I have something to tell you." It was all about meeting Matty and "the perfect Yes;" but I couldn't express it and was all tongue-tied. What I said plaintively was "Will I have chance to talk with you tomorrow?" He said Yes, and the whole family would be there; I meant to ask if I could speak with him in private; I always seemed to miss my cues when talking with him. But I was all tongue-tied, as he swiftly left. I was so surprised by this event, so amazed and thrilled, that I was for a while paralysed by emotion, repeating "I just can't believe it!" I felt I couldn't understand the half of what came from him; but the important thing was that it made me feel loved and accepted.

At last the Xmas Eve dinner arrived. The intensity of my feeling toward him in the intervening hours was like pain; I so much wanted to confide to him the fact that I had never been "a perfect Yes" to anybody but him. I had never before related to him socially like that, seeing him eating and drinking, laughing and talking, taking issue with him, arguing about historical and biblical things. I was wanting all evening to tell him about Matty and "the perfect Yes," but the opportunity didn't arise until the very last minute when his girls left and his wife offered me a lift to the church. I seized the opportunity, telling him in a rushed manner how Matty had arrived like a knight on a charger, and how he wanted to give me the baby I desired, how when he wanted to make love moral awareness rushed into me, because I couldn't say a "perfect Yes" to him. He listened with attention. I got my coat and, as I picked up my presents, with him in front me, I thought "it's now or never" and steeled myself to speak the words;
"I can't say a perfect Yes to him, as I've said to you." It was my way of saying "I love you." As he ushered me out in the darkness of the

vestibule, we said formally to each other "thankyou for coming" and "thankyou for having me." But I stood there next to him in the darkness, thinking only "I wish he would kiss me!" He urged "Go, just go." During that Xmas Eve Mass I knew I had found my own "source of pure joy;" I was in a veritable ecstasy!

I was with Matty that Xmas day, but found he meant nothing to me, compared with my intensity with Dr.James the night before; *it had been an experience purely of the mind, but it effected perfect radiant happiness in me!* And so I discovered that true sexuality is exuded from the mind, from words; he had a mind that met mine. And so, right there, I missed the chance of a family life and children with the man who could offer it, by chasing a "marriage of minds" with my doctor, who could really offer me nothing. And it was indeed a bliss "in the mind"; I did not need the relationship to become physical and sexual. I knew from then on that I would have to let go of Matty because I was in love with Dr.James; my intensity of feeling for the one prevented my relating to the other; for I realised I didn't love Matty, by the measure of that other love.

Dr.James put moral awareness into me by virtue of making me aware of what a "perfect Yes" was. *And I found in the coming days that this "moral awareness" of this "perfect Yes" restored me and healed me at my soul's core, for it was "pure."* I discovered there was still "something pure in me," so I no longer felt besmirched by my experience of the world. I discovered that having love in the core of me had purified me. And it was kept pure by him. I wanted to say to him *"What is pure in me is my love of you."*

On New Year's Eve, because he didn't come round for me to tell him this, I was bold enough to go to his surgery. I tried to explain to him as briefly as possible how I was made happy on Xmas morning, and I had discovered there was "still something pure" in me. But we said a few words misunderstandingly about pregnancy, love-making and my loss of virginity, which caused me embarrassment. I remembered how he knew about all my sexual misdemeanors, and had the sense of how intimately he knew me, and tried to make a joke about colouring my hair - "Look, no grey hairs!" But I could have kicked myself afterwards, in realising that the one thing I really wanted to tell him I had failed to tell; that this "pure moral awareness" had its source in him!

Later in the darkness of that New Year's Eve, all I could do was stand dark and lonely by the Martyr's monument, overlooking the moody

257

and tumultous Northern Sea, seeking answers. And I saw, gazing at stars, out of the lostness of my dark and lonely soul, *that my love of Dr.James was like a star, a lone star, in the darkness. It was a means of my making a fresh start, without the murkiness of my past; something which could make and keep me pure. I saw that my love of him could carry me on wings! And so it did! As I started jogging and praying in the New Year, I had the sense of the world of nature belonging to me, the sense of a fresh power to create my life; and I was soon taken up by the sense of a joyous and soul-creating love-affair, which made '93 the best and happiest year of my life!*

Chapter 64
Love's Rapture.

In the month of January I felt beautiful, because I was genuinely "in love," bursting with it, and full of its gladness! On the night of Tuesday the 5th something very deep happened between us, which changed things forever; in that I recognized my physical yearning was slipping from the heights of this "platonic love-affair of the mind"!

What happened that night was, that after talking long and deep, and taking off like an aeroplane into new and deeper realms of communion, we were left standing facing each other on the hearth-rug. I said earnestly "you are my vision; my love of you is a star to me; you are a brightness in my life;" and he listened and smiled. I talked of that "little mermaid" intensity of devotion I felt on Scarborough's cliffs, *then put his hand on my neck, saying "Just touch me and I dissolve." My whole being was electric to the touch, as I stood in front of him trembling with intensity; as if the whole of me through every pore were crying out to him, needing him. I just wanted him so badly to caress my hair and to kiss me! There was nothing in my life to match the trembling sensitivity of that moment! But he wouldn't!*

After this event we both felt differently; on the one hand it put in me an enormous new sense of tenderness and care; on the other hand I felt it a "lapse in moral awareness." I was full of solicitude for him, in that I knew he was feeling bad; I knew he found me overwhelming. I wanted to get across to him the message that it wasn't so bad, and I would try not let it happen again. I saw the event as a "lapse" or "a dip into the physical" from the pure platonic heights of our friendship; and the trouble was, it added a new complexity into our feelings for each other.

But "Love" isn't safe! You aren't "safe" when you love, because it throws you open to God and "How can you ever be safe from God?!" ("God isn't safe you know!")

So I was round at his surgery on Thursday morning with a letter, wanting to urge him not to let it make any difference to our friendship. When I asked if I could see him at first he said "I'm too busy;" but then he called from his room "Mairi come here," and I was instantaneously there! He read the letter which made reassuring points; that he could trust me, that I felt beautiful, that I honoured and adored him as much as ever. I must have said the right things because he smiled benignly; "I'll put this on the wall and frame it." "Are you feeling bad?" I asked, "my concern is for the way you are feeling." Then I said what I intended; "I care for you too much to want to hurt you." I continued, "It really isn't so bad; it makes no difference to my feeling for you; you can trust me not to let it happen again." He was still smiling benignly, so I continued; "I mean it when I said I'd rather have you as a friend than a lover; I don't think you understand the theology of the perfect Yes." He touched my wrist for a moment, whilst I was saying "I feel nicer toward you than I did before," and I felt it a blessed sign of his acceptance.

I lived in a complete bliss for a while; the thought of him made me ecstatic; I related to him all the time through every pore of my being. I had a powerful dream about his hands; "I would kiss your hands; they are the kindest, most loving, most healing hands that I know." My daily life became a veritable constant ecstasy; I wanted to say to him "you have the same effect upon me as the Eternal You; I speak the same Yes to you that I speak to God." The echo came from Austria, "you touch in me the same pulse-point where God touches me." *As for the morality of what was happening? Well I was too busy being mystically entranced by the whole thing, to be aware of the real morality. I wrote, "the point is, I encounter the Eternal You through him, I love him with all my soul, he is my You."*

On the next Tuesday night, my journal was the issue. He had said to me on leaving his surgery "Do me a favour and don't write about me in your journal." But that day he discovered what I had written, and made me reveal it, and made me tear out pages of it. At first he forcibly insisted "Show me your journal Mairi," and I wouldn't! My journal was just too private and intense for me to let him read it; he was asking the impossible of me, and I wouldn't submit to it. But I couldn't bear him to angrily walk out saying, "Now I see how things are between us; you are not being fair to me." So I submitted to reading it out, though feeling he wasn't "kind." I blushingly did so; it was "awe-full," it prized apart the fibres of my nature. Such pain and bliss together I found unbearable; nobody on earth could have made me do that; I completely submitted to his "mastering" of me at my soul's centre!

The next day I was back at the surgery, saying that all that mattered to me was that he "threw me open to God." I was hurt when he said back, -"Liar!" I said I spent too much time trying to be honest before God to be a liar, and "I purely wanted a soul to relate to my soul, and I wanted your soul because I loved you." He replied "I haven't got a soul; I lost it a long time ago." I went away feeling I couldn't bear to let him think of me as a liar, when I had been so pure toward him. The echo came from Austria; "my love of you is as pure as my love of God."

So there lay the problem which we fought with; - that our spiritual and intense friendship had on my side slipped a little into the physical plane; I was constantly yearning to have my hair caressed. But we established things quickly on the platonic plane; for most important to me was my soul-friendship with him, in his role as my mystical "Master." This was what I needed most, as I would have been lost in a Void without him!

The result of being "in love"on my whole being was like a fairy's magic wand; it transformed me; life shone in me, flowed to my fingertips, and shot through to the very tips of my hair! I felt for this first time in my life genuinely and completely wrapped-around "in love," and it was a kind of pure rapture which was new to me. I kept thinking "my intention toward you has always been pure; when I think of you, I think not of you, but of the fragrance of your power over me." The whole of the air seemed to sing and waft with fine fragrance.

I explained to him when he next came that I wasn't a "liar" and had a "pure intention," though he questioned whether I had sexual yearnings toward him. I admitted that when close to him it felt "like an electrical charge all over my body." He read my journals again, and I said "forgive the foolishness of my writings!" I explained that I never wanted him to stop coming to see me; I yearned for him to fondle my hair, but what I felt toward him was just "pure, simple, complete love."

Then I had the idea that I could write to him as the "You" of my journal, because it was the best love of my heart that I could offer; this idea streamed into me with the rays of God's grace. He was pleased about this, the next time he came, but said he felt things had been spoilt between us, because "you look on me differently than you used to." I said on the contrary he "put me in touch with the life at the centre of myself.," and I adored him "in the purity of God." He said suddenly "you have nothing to lose, and that makes all the difference." I replied with all earnestness, "I have my integrity with God to lose, I have my soul to lose!" I reminded him of how he had said that Midsummer Eve "I will take your knowledge," and went on about him being my "Master." I appealed at the door that he should continue to look at me "as a child, a daughter, that God has given to you!"

I was gloriously happy for a while; that momentary "dip into the physical realm" had made no difference in the platonic realm where I truly loved him; in fact it augmented my feelings and gave me wings. "I adore you" meant to me "I continuously hold you up in the brightness of God's presence, in the radiance of the love of God." My love of him threw me open to that brightness. I had wanted something pure and bright in my heart, and my love of him was "that pure bright thing." He had encouraged me to start creative writing, and I was jogging, and my life was full of bright moments and perceptions; I lived in a world where I could "turn a stone and start a wing,"- an existence enveloped by angels!

The evenings we spent together at the beginning of '93 were sheer mystical bliss, with the friendship on a beautiful platonic plane. When he pronounced "I think we can carry on as friends," it was bliss to my ears. I used to sit happily at his feet, reading to him my stories, feeling he knew the springs and sources of my being. He filled up my need! When I told him "you fill up my senses, and my need to relate; you make me replete with the brightness that comes from God," he replied with humility, "all I have been is a catalyst." But I told him how he "filled me up with God's wind and sunlight." It was the most blissful period of my entire life!

Chapter 65
Love's Penance.

My bliss was spoilt on the Eve of Ash Wednesday, when the intensity of our platonic friendship slipped into my own feelings of physical yearning again. It was a happening which left me feeling tragic and complex, because I knew it was entirely my own fault. *After that I had a new and complex sense of sin and sorrow; it put a new awareness of "ashes" into me, and of the earthy nature of all love and life.*

I set off walking in the dark to the church for the Ash Wednesday Mass, heavy with thoughts, and in that dark walk my understanding came together. This was "wrong," not in terms of some morality applied, but wrong from the inside, from the nature of the relationship. It flooded into my memory, how the last thing I wrote before returning from Austria was, - "my only purpose is to be a spirit-child attached to you;" and how I had thrown myself at his feet that morning, wet and barefoot whilst manic, yelling "you are my father!" I felt this gave me new strength to say No. "You are my father in some sense; and I, as a good daughter, should be doing the controlling." I felt I had got it then! I could handle it now!

This revelatory understanding that I gained seemed confirmed by my receiving of the ashes. As I was touched and marked by the ashes on the forehead, I felt that God touched me there. I had gone forward with the sense of "mea culpa," as fault and blame was mine, but I felt struck with a sense of conviction, and God's knowledge of me. Those ashes were a meeting with my Maker!

The next day I was feeling very bad, as if seeing clearly that I had "committed a very great sin." I felt a great need to unburden myself of this sin by going to confession; it was like King Midas in the Greek myth wanting to whisper into the reeds his secret of "Midas has asses ears." So I travelled to Kirkcraig on buses, which was a physically miserable experience, to make confession to the Catholic priest there; I saw how long and deeply I had sinned; my phrase of "I'll do whatever you say" meant a daughter's obedience and not accessibility. It left me with a sense of grace, but also a sense of needing to do "penance"; I suddenly realised that penance was to express sorrow. My desire to do penance was boundless and I imposed them upon myself; I would eat nothing but bread and barleycup for days, show him my offending journal, and spend an hour in church every day of Lent, with only the bible to read.

I wrote him a letter, and delivered it as if freshly and immediately written in blood; "I'm sorry; I have wronged you; I am to blame and not you; when you next come you will find me with an answer in my understanding, but very penitent; sackcloth and ashes wouldn't suffice!" And when he came and I expressed to him my sense of sin and sorrow; he said he'd forgiven me; "I was to blame" I said. And so we were wrapped round in a marvellous sense of forgiveness. And so we had a fresh new start; forgiveness like that could wipe out the past!

In the coming days of my bible-reading in the church, which was my "penance," the meaning of "God's law" grew upon me, and I felt frightened by the power and the fatherhood of God. I felt I had drawn a law in the ground of my being, and I felt Dr.James similarly "frightened" me now, as God's law and God's fatherhood.

When he next came to see me, on the 2nd of March, my self-yielding to him, though purely a soul-thing and not physical, "exceeded the bounds of the known universe!"
I ended up saying Yes to him more utterly than ever before. This was because he had said "Do you remember the anger you threw at me that day in that hospital?" and he meant that occasion in the "dark room". "Do you remember, do you remember?" he repeated, whilst I said "Yes,Yes." The memory was making me go dizzy into a mystical bliss. I said "you frighten me," and when asked why, I said "because of the force there is in you." I meant the power he had to make me yield, for the week earlier I had handed over to him my journal; "If ever I don't do as you say, remind me of the moment I gave you that manuscript, what sorrow I felt toward you." He marvelled at this sense of my utter yielding obedience. But he commented "how long will it last?" And I replied "it will last forever."

That night I was too happy to sleep, and when the milkman came in the morning I lay curled up with a great understanding flooding into me. I felt as if lying still like a child in God's hands, whilst a formless understanding flooded into me, deeper than the realm of words. I realised what went wrong between us on my return from Austria; I couldn't put him in touch with the pulse-point where he mastered me! I had lost touch with that pulse-point in leaving Austria, and needed him to put me in touch with it; hence when I found out he didn't have clue what I was talking about, I was in a hell-fire which seemed like an absence of God. However I was "in touch with it fairly deeply now"! I could palpably feel as I lay there "the force" there was in him, the force that always had the power to master me. And I wanted to tell him that all he had to do in future to master me, to make me do anything, was to "shake my memory," to remind me of that day's sense of sin and sorrow. And there was no madness deep enough where it couldn't touch me.

The next time he came this was put to the test. When he said solemnly "Don't rub yourself against me Mairi," I was stricken with a sense of sinning against him, aware that daughters don't do that to their fathers! I said "I'm sorry when I disobey you," and he said "you are not sorry," wanting me to tear those offending pages out of my journal. I said I would tear them out and burn them, out of my sense of sorrow toward him. I did this, though I felt anguished as I burnt them, trying to turn the flames into a prayer.

The next day I sobbed my heart out in the church because I felt so awful about it. I was crying out *"How can you not say I'm not sorry when I'll even tear and burn my own journal to show you that I am! If ever you want any proof that I'm sorry let this pain be it!"* I felt I had hurt myself more than I could bear; I had destroyed something that was an offering to God. When I expressed this pain to my friend, Patricia replied "it is indeed an offering to God, now that you've burnt it!" I said to God "I have shown you my sorrow; by this pain forgive me for all time!"

It was beautiful when the next Tuesday night, he said thankyou for the pain I took in burning my journal. "If I burnt my journal for you, I must love you very much," I said. He said I should add "like a daughter loves a father." I replied "Well you have a daughter who loves you very much!" Yet again I sinned against him in my heart, against that father-daughter relationship. I vowed it would never happen again!

I again travelled to Kirkcraig, to confess to a priest, and I declared on leaving the church "I will not sin again, I swear it!" I thought the deepest vow I could make was to say "If I offend in this way again, I will abandon my home, leave Scotland, and never see him again!" I even had my hair cut off as a token of that vow! I was waiting for his car at 9 o'clock the next morning, intending to give him a lock of my hair, saying "this is Mairi promising I am going to act like a daughter." But I was stricken when he didn't appear!

But having found out he was going away, I caught him at 11 o'clock; I needed a prescription as I wasn't well; "you have two minutes" he said. "You have a very penitent daughter" I said; I had offended against the relationship and against my love of him; "I feel God has forgiven it, because he knows that my love of you forgives it; but I want to be fully

265

and freely forgiven by you, before you go away." He said back, smiling and kind, "I forgive you totally." I then told him about my vow, and how I didn't like to hurt him. As I left, knowing I wouldn't see him for a few weeks, I said to myself "my happiness will turn to ashes, if I ever hurt him in this way again."

Looking back, Dr.James fought like a hero, to be there for me, offering me this soul-deep friendship and this father-daughter love, fully in my need! He often mentioned that any doctor in that situation would have felt compelled to leave my care to someone else, but it was a fact that all his fellow-doctors had refused to take on my care. So he was convinced that there was only hope for me, for my future, if I had his continued help.

And I really had to bear the blame for all this! - - I was continually busy asking for forgiveness from him, for my sin in tempting him; "mea maxima culpa"; I knew mine was the ultimate blame and fault! And I know it now! And the judgement is this; such tempting self-yielding as mine should have ensnared a saint!

Chapter 66
Womb-Pain.

In the early months of '93, during and despite this beautiful soul-creating friendship, something was looming on the horizon; a destructive force was unleashed upon me in the form of a gushing mental anguish over the loss of my son.

I was able to put my finger on the pain and explore the wound. And I turned in this mental darkness, unable to comprehend it, to Dr.James, asking for psychotherapy as a help. I turned to him, as there was no-one else, and because my love of him overcame all bad things, and opened me to God's air, presence, light. I turned to him because my love of him served to dispel the darkness.

I was trying to extend a pure, cool, compassionate love toward my lost son; "I've given him life, I've started him off, I'll always be there for him if he needs me." But then intense negative feelings tumbled into me about what Walter had done to me; *"there are violations against us so deep, that they can never be forgiven in our lifetime; he abused and violated my whole being, he had a child on me, then finally he took that child away from me."* I felt it was the worst thing anybody could ever do to somebody else. I felt it as a *"dark and bitter thing"* which was impossible to forgive.

I asked Dr.James about this "dark and bitter thing." I said "Gabriel's existence is a pain to me, because he is a part of me that Walter continues to damage." He said he had come across this before, when a certain part of a woman is damaged. I said back "when they hurt and damage your soul?" "You can't hurt the soul," he replied, "the soul is unhurtable." When I pondered on this I knew it wasn't right; what is it to open ourselves to love, if not to open our souls to being hurt? Life doesn't mean very much if the soul is unhurtable! In fact the soul needs to be hurt and wounded; the "Holy Grail" text suggests we have awareness of God through a wound.

Eternal Love not only allows us to be hurt, it deliberately hurts us. And its purpose is to give us knowledge. As it says in the "Prophet,"-"your pain is the breaking of the shell that encloses your understanding."

As far as I could see, I had given the part of myself that I love the best into the power of an ogre! I had handed my son over into the same evil power that was destroying *my* soul, when he was violating the deepest levels of my being and my soul's integrity. It was intolerable unless I tried not to care. I had given Gabriel such a tender careful upbringing; now I couldn't prevent him from being under a brutish influence which was spoiling his sensitivity.

Then one day, whilst enraptured by my idea of the "perfect Yes" which should reign at the heart of love-making, I saw it all so clearly and freshly; - *"I myself have offended in conceiving a child without love, out-with love. The sin is not what Walter did to me, but what he made me do against myself."* That yielding of my integrity was out of fear and out of need, and had I now paid the price? It dawned on me with a shudder how that begetting of his body on my soul was an unnatural yoking together, disparate like the raping by a bull. Part of the price was the pain in my conscience. This "punishment" was like God's glory illuminating it, burning me!

Salt was then rubbed in my wounds by Stuart O'Sullivan, the social worker who had responsibility for the Access visits which were proceeding. He insisted that I attend a meeting with Walter, and I replied "it would fill me with such hatred as to darken my days for a month." He told me I had to "separate off my past pain," and I replied "you don't understand; Gabriel is a product of that past pain." He said something about "progress," and I replied, "Progress into what! You mean progress into pain?" Afterwards I walked along the Willow Braes seething with hatred, realising that the main point of my pain was that Walter had taken my child away from me. And as I really knew what that pain was, as I recognised it and explored the wound, I sobbed my heart out.

"I know what the pain is at last, I've put my finger on it! I loved the child who came from the wound, because I loved the wound; so the pain is that I no longer have the chance to love him, for the loving of him was healing me. It was the balm on the wound; my love of Gabriel was that balm! Being without him is a tearing of the tender tissue between mother and child; that is what the pain is; motherhood bereft of a child, when that child is the balm to the wound of its own origin."

After darkly sobbing, I sought out the man I loved, because he brought me brightness and dispelled my darkness; I waited for him an hour by his car. My psychotherapy session with him had left me very discontent, because he acted as cold and clinical as only a doctor can be. When he finally came out in a busy fashion, I earnestly said "I can't relate to you as a doctor at all; being a Master and being a doctor are two quite separate things; being a Master is a very subtle thing." Beaming and smiling he replied, "Well that lets me out then; I'm anything but subtle!" He intimated that he had indeed "put on his best psychotherapeutic hat." I said to him earnestly, "I want to be in touch with the pulse-point where you master me; it's necessary for my whole existence, for my soul's life, for my soul's breathing." I said that when he came again he should come as a Master and not as a doctor. "I'll come as a Master and bring my whip!" he joked. I went away with my soul bright again, gushing with love, thinking to myself, "the kind of Masters I'm talking about don't have whips!"

I was trying to cope with the pain inside of me which was like the howl of anguish of a mother who has lost her child. I had loved and accepted that child when he was in my womb; now I didn't get the opportunity of loving him. I hated Walter, in that he had caused the wound, and then robbed me of the balm for that wound. Was anyone so tormented by love as me? *When I wrote to my soul-friend Pater Leo, secure in his monastery in Austria, I confessed "I can't find the love of God in all this! Can you understand how God could allow anyone to be wounded so deeply? What great sin have I committed deep in my unconscious past, to merit having this degree of pain visited upon me?"*

Finally there was a Social Work meeting, on the 3rd March; and my emotions ran very high. My eruption of emotion was really due to the social workers attitude to my illness. It was when they asked for "permission" to inform Walter should I become manic that I emotionally erupted. I shouted at them that this was "petty"and meaningless; "people can do anything to me when I'm manic! Who needs to give you such permission when I'm judged to have no rights!" The word "safeguards" was used, and I shouted, "I'm the person affected the most, and I haven't got any safeguards!" Meanwhile what I felt towards Walter was that he was so mean and despicable, "so slimy and snake-like," that he wasn't worth my hatred; but I would hold his sin against me for as long as I lived! It was the social workers' naive and condescending attitude toward my "madness" that made me angry during and after that meeting. They treated it as something to guard against and protect Gabriel from; this was intolerable when I had him for 5 years as a baby! My net reaction to such prejudice was; "I want justice and fairness, and this isn't it!"

The social workers' attitude toward my illness angers me. They treat my madness as something to guard against and protect Gabriel from. That is intolerable to me, considering that I had him for 5 years as a baby; it is also intolerable in that it is like trying to circumscribe God! - - My madnesses are like the visitations of God upon me, and my life is precarious. I hate the way they are trying to make life all safe and sure and circumscribed; so that God can't erupt in upon them. I would prefer my madness any day, rather than the safe, comfortable worlds the rest of you live in! You see, my madness puts me in that universe where God can erupt in upon me!

The next morning I felt a seething hatred of social work mentality, for it was the mentality which did all this to me in the first place; the mentality which removed a 6-year-old child from his mother, and forbade me fair access, as if that child needed to be protected from me when I had looked after him on my own for the first 5 years of his life! It was an abomination! "I want fair Access," not just bits of time that suited Walter's arrangements! I decided I would fight, I would take it back to court! My mind was made up; I was going to seek for Justice! As a result of this, I first phoned up George McPherson, a solicitor skilled in mental health and child-care problems, whom my solicitor-friend Agnes had recommended to me. I made an appointment with him, but don't think I ever actually met him till that day I accidentally got hold of him when he walked into the Craigdene lock-up ward! I was full of a kind of indignation; "I want access-rights, - whole days, weekends and weeks! What we have here is an insult to my motherhood!"

I was a young and vulnerable mother with a young baby to look after on my own, coping with a stress-related mental illness, and, though I'd never married the man and was abused by him and had fled from his house whilst pregnant, the System foisted the Access rights of this man upon me, with the whole male-dominated, male-orientated system crying out "Father's Access Rights!" Yet then, when the tables were turned and the man got the Custody from the law courts, when I couldn't contest it because locked up in hospital, and I pleaded for the ability to see my son, to have a small amounts of "quality time" with him, it was denied me for 7 years, and nobody, absolutely nobody, talked of "Mother's Access Rights"!

Then one day, feeling very bitter and wronged, "so utterly wronged both by the man and the system," whilst sitting in the church with the bible doing my "penance," I had the best insight into it that I had ever had. It had struck me earlier, "my loss of Gabriel is God's judgement upon me," and that phrase from the Book of the Beloved had struck me "I wound and I heal." And it dawned on me there in the church; "Perhaps *God* has removed the balm of the wound, ie. removed Gabriel from me." Then I thought "It is a very fitting pain; like a womb-pain." I saw it might be part of His mysterious love's purpose. "He knows I can forgive myself through the pain, taking the pain as a penance."

270

*I saw something, some deep truth, my best ever insight into my pain; -
If I offended God, as I did, in conceiving Gabriel, then perhaps God
gives me this pain at the same point, - this mothers-pain, this womb-
pain, - not to punish me, but to wound me in a way that will heal me.*

And so I struggled to comprehend what I identified as my "womb-pain."
And when I couldn't tolerate the pain any longer, I was driven to go to
Iona at Easter, to seek answers there. At the same time as being in the
bliss of true love, I was in so much pain!

Chapter 67
Iona Stones.

On Iona at Easter I comprehended the two things together; my loss of my child and my love of my doctor, the cup which was the mingling of my pain and my love.

I left for Iona "on a high." For on that day itself I attended a meeting in which I was granted the right to see Gabriel "unsupervised," and the night before I'd exchanged some deep loving words with Dr.James. So that day I left with joy and hope in my heart. When I got to Oban, where it was necessary to stay overnight, I thought it romantic sitting under the moon and stars in Oban harbour; "here you could believe all things are possible."

My arrival on the island the next day was catastrophically miserable; it was pouring down, and I got my feet soaking wet getting off the ferry, and there was no kind welcome, as I had arrived too early. I approached Forbes the ferryman, and he suggested we had sex in a really cheap fashion, so I walked away from him. And so I walked in lashing cold rain with wet feet to the MacLeod centre, whilst watching my warm dry socks going off in the luggage-van in the other direction!

When I first spent time in the Abbey church I thought how I was a "young unsuffered soul" when I was there in the past, when it seemed a "place of grace" to me. I felt how I'd lost my innocence because sullied by suffering; beforehand I was "such a beautiful child". "How can it be mended?" There were a lot of Danes there; I said to one of them called Peter how "the only way to mend it" is to have another child; "it's my only chance to mend myself and put myself back together." I didn't need him to tell me, that a child must be born out of love; you can't just "get a child." I talked to another Dane in the garden, and she said to me "you are bitter." I reflected on this and saw, "I am not bitter; I am taking on a pain that is bitter, but I am not bitter." I was aware there in the abbey church that I had in me "such strong hate and such strong love;" about the loss of my son I was full of hate, but about my doctor I was full of love. I asked God to show me the way; "there must be some healing deep enough."

On Monday I wrote a letter to Dr.James, saying I was going to "listen to the wind" and listen to God there, because on Iona there was only " a thin veil of tissue paper" between heaven and earth, so perhaps God could get through to me there. I wrote that "the only thing in Kirkmichaels that isn't hell-fire is you." I wrote that I didn't have bitterness in me, and that is because "bitterness has been kept out by a bright shining heart, ie. one with love in it, because that is like armour." I wrote that I dreamt of him as much as ever, and that dreaming was joy. *"You have kept in my heart a love that has saved me from becoming bitter."*

Then I had a revelation in the Abbey church of the meaning of those words from the Book of the Beloved, "If you love me, drink." I had the same sense as in that story of being drowned in bitterness, swimming in it and unable to imbibe it. But the bitter drink was an accepting of his love; not a love demanded, but receiving. And so taking on bitter pain was a receiving of love. Then came the healing service, and I felt the holding of hands upon me like a concentration of healing power upon me. And in that lovely moment I saw how I need to accept the pain of my own life. I saw "there is joyous love in my life, and that is greater than the bitter pain."

Walking around the island after that, I saw that I was indeed working out my own healing; my head was full of a song which seemed wonderfully true; "peace, peace will come, and let it begin with me; my own life is all I can hope to control, let it be lived for the good, good of my soul." I saw that taking on the pain had only become bitter because it was too much for me; "but I *can* accept it, by the love within me." In the church again I realised that I needed to accept, to embrace this bitter pain. "If I can accept it, I may become a greater person, - sweeter, kinder, gentler." Acceptance meant "God needing my will, my consent, my assent, my Yes."

Then came that powerful Good Friday; and I realised what "tearing" is,- in the way my journal was torn, my motherhood was torn, and the body of Jesus was "torn" on the cross. Now what is torn cannot be "mended", but it can be accepted and transcended. If only I could accept my own bitter pain in the same gentle way as I could see Jesus accepting his pain on the cross! Then it dawned on me, "the tearing is not final; you can't mend it, in that you can't put it back together again, but you *can heal it.*" You can't mend these things, by resuscitating a dead body, or by bringing the journal back into being, or by having another child, but you can heal it. Christ rose from the grave, and that certainly healed his death. And so for me; *"what is torn can't be mended, but it can somehow be accepted and transcended."*

That day at 3 o'clock we celebrated by the symbolic act of writing down on bits of paper our pain, and then burning them at the foot of the cross; I wrote "the bitter pain of the loss of my son," and prayed "heal what is torn in me." I saw in that moment, that I needed to accept my own pain, my toreness, in the same way as Christ accepted his cross, with gentleness and love, and that would lead to healing.

During that Easter Sunday Vigil, celebrated at midnight in the Abbey church, with the TV cameras around us, for it was being broadcast live all over Europe, lit by hundreds of joyous candles, I experienced one of the deepest insights of my entire life. *"I glimpse a different quality of life; the quality of life that Christ offers us; that resurrection-life which is joyous, free, peaceful, hopeful, loving and loved." And I saw we can transform our lives into that Life by accepting, embracing the cross, the bitter pain, the loss.*

As we spilled out, from the bright Abbey church and away from the cameras, into the delicious darkness which was star-lit, upon the green grass around St.Martins cross, all embracing each other, wishing each other a Happy Easter, I saw this amazing thing,- "This *Life* begins now, and goes on forever!"

On the next day, Easter Sunday, I walked out to the Machair, the great sward by the Western Bay, and found my only real moment of silence. As I watched the sunset, looking over the tumultuous sea toward the thin line of the Outer Hebrides, it seemed to me as though the land were waiting, the whole of creation were waiting, for *Life*, for transformation. I had the two stones in my hand, which I had picked, out of a tray of hand-painted stones, one for Dr.James and one for Gabriel, - *one for the doctor who brought me joy, one for the son who brought me pain. I had walked a long way carrying these stones, knowing I must soon go back with them, and it slowly dawned on me that I could employ my love of my doctor which was saving and healing me, toward the loving of my son. It was a strange and mystical experience; I knew I could conduct the love which the stone represented in the one hand, because it was full and utter and complete, into the poor love and pain in the other hand.* "I can have enough love to accept my cross" because of my love for *him* that I carried around with me. Only enough love of him would enable me to embrace the transforming fire. But it was indeed "enough," it was sufficient.

So I left the island gleeful in the extreme, carrying my two stones, with a sure knowing that my life would be transformed into Life, which is joyous, peaceful, hopeful, loving and loved, because it would be Easter Life, the bliss that lies on the other side of dying, that begins now and goes on forever!

Chapter 68
The Paradise Garden.

I returned from Iona with love paramount in me; I felt I could accept bitter pain with love, and then my life would be transformed into Easter Life. But I had a miserable journey back, because I had a bad fall in Fionniphort whilst running for the bus, and was left with badly scraped and bleeding hands. It seemed so ironic; the last words I had said on the island, on the knoll overlooking the Abbey was "Carry me on wings back to those I love," and then the first thing I do is fall!

But there was new hope in me now, of good times with Gabriel to come, because there was going to be no more of the dreadful "supervised" Access. For that very day that I had set off to Iona there had been another Children's Panel meeting, at which I spoke eloquently and won unsupervised Access. I argued that, when I was becoming manic "I always put Gabriel in a safe place," and that they mustn't speak of my illness "as if it carried culpability." I argued for the need of quality time of intimacy with my son, without social work supervision, and the panel agreed with me; it was one of the best moments of my life as I listened to each of the three of them coming out with the same decision.

And so the first thing I gleefully told Dr.James was "I have him on my own now." I felt there would be a "closeness to his mummy" at last, instead of all those endless long stilted games with the social workers present and listening to every word that was exchanged. The first time I had him after coming back, he wanted to put his indoor tent up. I was so happy when in this tent he curled up close to me, with his fist in his mouth like a baby. I tried to make him feel relaxed with me. And shortly afterwards I was with Dr.James and Gabriel together at the surgery; *Dr.James' benign smile gladdened me, and I sat between the two of them feeling so very happy and relaxed, feeling bathed in love, like someone in Paradise.*

I had wonderful deep times with Dr.James after coming back from Iona. I told him of that Easter *Life* when I came back, when I spent two hours of a long communion at his house, in his study, - "that *Life* which is joyous, peaceful, hopeful, loving and loved, because it is Easter Life, the bliss that lies on the other side of dying, that begins now and goes on forever!" It was sweet and delicious to me, explaining what I had learnt on Iona, saying in subtle ways how I cared for him; and he absorbed my soul's knowledge, smiling so kindly and benignly. I wanted to say to him at long last how I loved him "completely," -"with a love that encompasses you complete being, as completely as God loves you." "It is that love that saves me and heals me and transforms me and begins Easter Life in me." I was blissful that night; *I loved him from the centre of my soul to the centre of his soul, like magnetism!*

My soul was brimful of fresh air and sunlight for a time after that. I felt happy and healed, with a head full of songs, a soul full of fresh breeze, and eyes full of light! I was busy working in the "Oxfam" shop thinking of him, because he gave me a sense of sweetness. There was a totality in what I felt for him, as if his soul were in communion with mine, and it gifted me with sensitivity. Sometimes I felt totally encapsulated by one single deep impulse towards him.

We were wrapped round in a mystical understanding. I told him one night how I had this sense of the love of God in me; and it was through him that I had realised it was there, and that I carried it with me and that it was "enough". I said in a rapture how this love enabled me,- enabled me to transcend pain, go through bitterness, and to transform my little life into *Life*. I said how there was an endlessness to this *Life*, because it was a sharing in the life of the Trinity. And he was in a rapture too as I explained how the love of the Trinity must circulate between the three persons of the Godhead.

The Paradise didn't last for long, because the next time we were in the tent, Gabriel insisted on "tickling bottoms." So once more "sexual abuse" reared its ugly head! I was astonished and asked who had taught him to do that; he said "I do that with my daddy." I said back to him firmly, "Gabriel tickling bottoms is not a sign of love and affection; you don't have to tickle bottoms to be close to someone and loved by them." But he put my hand on his bottom, and said "tickle me." This sickened me to the pit of my stomach, because this was what Walter used to do with me when I lived with him. It was in that moment more nauseating and claustrophobic in that tent than I could possible endure!

All my songs and joyousness, with which I came back from Iona, were extinguished! I woke the next morning miserable in the extreme, able to echo with Hamlet "How weary, stale, flat and unprofitable seem to me all the uses of this world!" I could only feel how this young tender child of mine was being blighted, and it was a pain beyond what I could bear. I realised I had to think how to handle it, and I decided to share it with my friend Louise, so I wouldn't carry the burden alone. So I told her, bewailing the fact that I wouldn't be believed, and it would tell against me. We agreed that I should try not to confuse Gabriel, and should let him think he could say anything he liked to me, or else he would close up against me. "The fact remains that he invited me to sexually maltreat him as a way of showing love and affection!"

At the next visit I became dead certain that he was being sexually abused by the way he molested me in the toilet, saying enthusiastically that he did it with his Dad; I was sickened to the pit of my whole being and realised something had to be done, because not to report it would be to involve myself in it. When I talked with Louise again we agreed it might be better not to report it, so that I could retain some influence over Gabriel. Obviously I felt that if I reported it, social workers would cause my access visits to stop. But I earnestly imparted the whole thing to Dr.James. It was agreed that the three of us would have a talk about it; but before that happened I was thrown into Craigdene again, with them having no better excuse this time than an ear infection!

Meantime I did my best to be there for Gabriel, and I developed with him the wonderful wise way of teaching him like my Grandad did with me. I seldom achieved it so perfectly as during those months of early Spring, as I took him for walks; I was taking him for walks so as to avoid the tent!

Then there happened that night of such deep and mystical experience that I wrote of it "I know where Heaven is, I've got there"! It was as if I had found a still perfect place that was like a "secret garden" in which I dwelt for a while. This mystical mood of mind was initiated by my ardent talking with Dr.James for an hour, when I declared "when I am really aware of your presence, you compel me into silence; talking with you gifts me with knowledge and light and brings me peace." And when he left I resided in the sacredness of that peace, of that moment.

It was like being in a sweet secret garden, "a sweetness that will pass into infinity forever," like a communion in God's love. I sat for ages afterwards perfectly still, then wrote down the words; "Love so complete, blessed, whole, that all the boundaries fuse. I am complete, pulsing, breathing, loving, at the pulse-point of the universe. All is transfigured into fire by fire, and the fire and the sweetness is love."

I was blissful on waking in the early morning-light. At first I was recalled to the present, as if my soul had been wandering; then I felt that there was a point where infinite love flowed through me; then I thought; "the most important days of our lives don't have dates"; then I felt an appreciation of that lovely sensitivity between us, when he showed me the cross around his neck. Thus I came to a sweet consciousness, and I wrote a letter to him in the early morning before the world became busy, saying how I would keep forever, unexpressed in words, the sacredness of the moment; like Ophelia tells Hamlet, "tis in my memory locked, and you yourself shall keep the key of it." *And the last thing I wrote, before being overcome and overwhelmed by the wicked world, was, "that still secret garden which was a sacred moment, I shall keep in my memory forever."*

Chapter 69
The Ear Infection.

And so it came about that, the day after I had known one of the deepest "communions" of my life, so deep and still that it was like being within a "secret garden," writing of it sanely and coherently, and obviously not remotely manic,- the evil System yanked me back into Craigdene again, and kept me locked up there for a further two months.

They rushed me off to a Psychiatric hospital because I had an ear infection!
What I can recall happening was this; -

When Dr.James came round I had asked if he would see to my ailments; *"I have a soreness between my ears."* *"Funny," he replied jocularly, "most people have a brain between their ears!"* He diagnosed me as having an infection of the inner ear, ie. inflammation of the Eustacian tube. One of the effects of this is that it makes you very dizzy, so that you keep lurching about and falling over. He gave me antibiotics for the condition, and then went away to Edinburgh for the weekend. I was getting stressed and didn't like the idea of being left without him, but I said echoing Kahlil Gibran, "I will trust the physician, and drink his remedy in silence and tranquillity." I trusted his "physician's hand," and decided I'd stay and wait for his return, trusting him utterly.

People, supposed friends, came round to see me at the weekend, and seeing how unsteady on my feet I was, phoned the surgery, and Dr.Joyce came round. She pointed out that seeing I couldn't "look after myself," as I couldn't cook or make myself hot drinks, I should go back to the hospital "where I belonged," seeing I was still sectioned and officially only out "on trial leave." I reacted to this, "No don't do that, I'm not ill, I want to stay at home!" More interfering friends came round, and the man upstairs, who had been an enemy for years, suggested he make some baked beans on toast for me. Things went on behind my back. The man upstairs insisted he would phone the doctor again; this time it was a completely strange doctor from Langport. He took one look at me, at the way I kept falling over, and diagnosed "she must be mentally ill, as she has a history of it; she is on trial leave from a mental hospital." And then the next thing I knew, the ambulance was at the door, and my friends happily waved goodbye to me as I was wheeled off in a wheelchair! *They thought I was going off to a "hospital," to be looked after; I tried to tell them I was being returned to a "prison," where I would be maltreated and more months of my life wasted!*

Nobody checked up on me; I didn't even see a doctor when I got there. It was just a nurse whom I hadn't seen before, and never saw again, who admitted me. I tried to tell him it was an ear infection that was making me act peculiarly. But he just filled in the forms; to him I was just a sectioned patient who was returning from "trial leave." He said about the wheel-chair, "you won't be needing that anymore." I said how I kept falling over; "nonsense" he said, taking it away.

Look at the perniciousness of this System! Because I was labelled as a "sectioned" patient, I was yanked back into a mental hospital when there was nothing wrong with me but a physical ailment! I was yanked back like a yoyo on a string! Let this be an outcry of protest for all so-called "manic depressives"! It is as if we carry a placard,- "Don't believe me because I am a manic depressive; if I appear physically ill it's probably because I am mentally ill; so if in doubt lock me up!"

It is as bad as what happened to me recently in May 2002, which is another chilling tale. I had at this stage kept well for 7 years, and went round to see a new GP with photophobia, which meant I couldn't open my eyes. When I finally got to Strathwells hospital in Invertay, where they had the equipment to examine my eyes, it was found that I had "corneal abrasion," but I was devasted when the GP told me "we have arranged for you to see Dr.Geddes the psychiatrist on the way, so he can check out your mental health."
I was in an anguish with my eyes, and they put me in the position of having to prove to a psychiatrist, whom I had only seen once before, that I was perfectly mentally well! They were going to put me in a mental hospital because I couldn't see! Because I had a history of "mental illness" I nearly ended up in Craigdene instead of Strathwells eye casualty department! That day I escaped by a sliver; but in '93, because I was already "sectioned" under the Mental Health Act, no such luck!

And so I found myself locked up for a further two months in Craigdene, for the whole of May and June, overwhelmed by the world's way of locking up the labelled "mentally ill" for no real reason! Oh the loss, the wastage of those years!

And so, in the hospital once again, and only yearning to get out again, I set myself to endure it patiently and keep out of trouble. *For a while I had a sense of being "robed in white light like an angel," untouchable by evil and by sickness; this was because my love of Dr.James was "like my shining armour."* But the memory of this faded as I became absorbed and distressed by the rigours and the sickness of the place.

And it was then that I met Freddy.

I thought Freddy looked like VanGogh. He used to sit there reading all the time, with his small-rimmed glasses, just keeping out of trouble and biding his time. I was taken by him because he was smitten by me. We conducted a deep and intense relationship, and the nurses counted this as "fraternisation" and were always trying to break us up. I fastened some of my affection on him, because he was there for me, and Dr.James wasn't. One day he said "Will you marry me?" And I said "Yes".

A month later, partly I think as an act of breaking up our relationship, the doctors discharged Freddy home to Glasgow, and on the same day sent me to the lock-up ward, Ward 6. Part of the reason they sent me there was because I showed my usual spirit, and wouldn't comply and act like a zombie within the ward; but I think the other part of the reason was an intention to split up myself and Freddy. It didn't work. They refused to allow Freddy in to visit me there, right enough, but when they sent me back to Morlond, due to my good behaviour, Freddy valiantly came to visit me every day from Glasgow, and they couldn't legally stop him.

And so every day, anguished by my imprisonment, I waited for Freddy to come, so I could sit on his knee, and talk, and drink "Tab"cola together. That was the only reason that I did not actively plan to escape from the dreadful place; Freddy taught me to wait and bide my time; he kept saying that it wouldn't be long before Dr.McNeill would have to let me out on trial leave again. It was like existing in a limbo-land waiting to get back to real life. *I just bided my time.*

Finally at the beginning of July, after two months of "wasted life," I was sent back out on trial leave again. This time it perhaps wasn't as "wasted" as usual, in that I came out with Freddy as my fiance. But it was no good with Freddy; I quickly realised that I didn't love him.

The nurses had been telling me that I should call it off with Freddy, before he came to live in KirkMichaels, and I agreed that I didn't have the right feelings for him. For I couldn't stand his "romantic soppiness" of sitting on knees and kissing; I hated the way he was patting and pawing at me. When I was finally given the news that I was allowed out on trial leave, he was really ungracious, saying "we can end it right now if you want to." *We thought we could try and make it work, but I realised immediately when to my delight Dr.James came round that night, how much the latter meant to me, and how Freddy meant nothing in comparison. My love of Dr.James was all subsumed into my love of God, and it made my eyes to shine; I didn't have any feelings for Freddy.*

Chapter 70
Finding Meaning.

It was the very day I left the hospital, the 6th July, that my feeling shifted away from Freddy towards Dr.James. My heart had leapt that day I was to leave hospital, for he phoned me. But I felt it unkind when he asked if I were sleeping with Freddy, which I wasn't, and then said it was important that I learned to see him round at his surgery, rather than in my house. *As I was sitting on the wall waiting for the bus, going home at long last, watching the trees waving in the sunlight, I thought to myself how I must persuade him to visit me because without him "life would be nothing worth." And I was so amazed and so grateful when that very night he did come round; and made me feel close to him again.*

That Friday at the surgery I swore how utterly I loved him, saying "my love of you is all subsumed into my love of God" and "it makes my eyes to shine." He replied ponderously, "All this sounds vaguely heretical; in the middle ages we would have burnt you as a witch." I begged him "I need you to relate to me, I just want to relate to you." I agreed that our friendship must remain platonic; "it doesn't need to be physical, because it's not"; and therefore I begged him to keep coming round to see me. "Oh I'm no coming to see you," he replied. "Oh please, give me a chance!" "You are"- he started to say, then stopped. Then he said he was going on holiday for 3 weeks; when he came back, he would see how things were. It gave me hope; I thought how often he changed a "No" into an "Alright then." I hoped he would resume visiting me; "my life without him will have no meaning."

When I thought of him in the coming days, I was filled with insatiable yearnings for him, which were indelible movements of the soul rather than belonging to the physical, ephemeral realm of the body; I recalled how I wrote from Austria "my love of you is like my yearning for God, eternal in its nature." I wrote, *"My love of you is centred out there somewhere, in the sun-drenched, wind-swept Austrian mountain-tops, where things go on in the vast marches of time, where you can never attain what you yearn for. That is why my experience with you leaves me unsatisfied, with the sense that what I want from you is far more ethereal, far-reaching, far more everlasting."*

Meanwhile my relationship with Freddie was coming to an end, because I realised I had no feelings for him in comparison. The first thing which dismayed me was Freddy's meanness; he asked me to contribute a 20p towards a cup of tea in a cafe, and after saying all along that he would buy champagne to celebrate my freedom, he produced a 30p can of "Tab" cola; I was appalled at how shabby this was. It hit me that he was not as generous as I was led to believe, and not as intelligent as I was led to believe either. There was one night when, in bitter cold wind along the West Sands, in a shelter, he started pawing at me and kissing, and I thought he must be an imbecile not to realise that I didn't like it. When we got home he tried to take me to bed with him, and it was a hateful experience, and I felt I had to put a stop to it, as I hated being with him. Dr.James told me that if I disliked him in this way, I had to tell him, rather than "leading him on."

And so, within a week of leaving the hospital, I told him I wanted to end the relationship, whilst playing with a pen on red-checkered tablecloth whilst a thunderstorm was raging. He had got me to lie down on the bed to kiss me, and I felt coerced and hated it; "my loathing of this physicality was to the nth degree." Then he asked why I seemed pensive, so I took the opportunity to say something. I stated that I disliked the physicality of this relationship, and it was making me unhappy. His reaction was to bewail the fact that he had been told in the hospital that this would happen; I said that at that time I only related to him with a fraction of myself. He said we could still get married; I said the feelings that would make it work were lacking in me. He started to cry, and to bewail, "I thought I'd found somebody to love me!" This didn't seem to me very manly or adult.

It was after that, when he harassed me, stalking me along the street and using veiled threats, that I began to see him as "a creep." He came round to my door saying "you can't just bring me to KirkMichaels and after a week discard me; all I want is a female companion." He hung on in KirkMichaels, hanging on street-corners to catch me on my way to work, and coming round to my door, in a creepy and coercive way; "I'll do whatever you want" he kept saying, and the more I saw of him, the less I liked him. He began saying that, if I didn't return his affections he would "bump into me" more often and start writing letters; I hated these threatening and sinister, coercive tactics and compared it with my ingenuous relationship with Dr.James.

Then came the night of that most horrible experience with Dr.James! He had taken journals away from my cupboard whilst I was in hospital, for safe-keeping, and he told me off saying they might fall into the wrong hands and I appealed to him "Teach me differently and I will learn differently." *But when he gave them back, I found a large section of them missing, and I felt so awful a misery about it!* Then the night he was due to leave he put a whole section of my missing journals with a thud through my letter-box at 1.30 a.m. But only half of it was there; so I got dressed and hurried after him to his house. And he was so angry with me. I stood there, so tender and innocent and undeserving of anger; following him home was an act of ingenuousness; I just couldn't bear the worried misery of having part of my journals missing for 3 whole weeks! He said with anger "you will be even more miserable in a moment when the police come and remove you from my doorstep." He said the journals he'd given were all he had, "and there's no more, and you will find the rest in your cupboard!" Now I knew I wouldn't; I had seen the completed manuscripts in his study just a few weeks before. I couldn't understand how he could be so horrible to me; *it desecrated my heart, rendered my life meaningless, the uncaring way he had said that!*

I quickly realised, in the 3 weeks that he was away, that my sense of hating him was only "hurt love," and it was up to me to find a "loving response." I felt I should say "don't be angry" and "be fair." *I could see, in comparison with the way Freddy was behaving, that my relationship with him had a "wonderful childish ingenuousness" about it.* I thought how I would throw myself at his feet, asking to be forgiven, taken up, loved and taught. I realised that because he offered me self-understanding "you hold the world in promise in your pocket." For he was like a rich soil which enabled my self-understanding to grow, and with it I comprehended the human world, the cosmos and God. I realised at that point, that though I voyaged across seas of pain because of his anger, the truth was, I loved him all the same!

Then Freddie started writing nasty letters, saying I was "unloved" by everybody else, and "no wonder my parents would have nothing to do with me," and that if I left him "in later years I would regret it." And he kept repeating this nasty veiled threat about Dr.McNeill; "you realise we do have the same consultant." I felt on the receiving end of intelligent, directed hatred. *Finally there was this letter, put through my door when I was asleep, which ended "you Ms.Colme are history."* It bothered me deeply, that he had been to my door with this kind of hatred when I was vulnerably asleep in my bed.

I became scared when the time came for Dr.James return; my friend Henry had told me I must "grovel, grovel," but I decided instead to write a very long, beautiful and honest letter. I ended it , *"Be fair! I expect of you some of the qualities that I know are in God's love, and He is always fair, forgiving and kind, and after anger, quick to take me up again. So forgive me for so angering you, teach me as you promised, and don't let go of me."*

With what trepidation I approached him that day! I prayed that he would be fair, forgiving and kind. Once in his room I said "Don't be angry ever again, as I can't bear it." And I handed him my typed letter; he read it, and then put it down and smiled. "Am I forgiven?" I said. *"Unfortunately Ms.Colme,"- I was scared of what he might say - "Unfortunately Ms.Colme, I always forgive you!" His benign kindness flooded over me; all was swept away on some great tide of kindness; I had a taste of the paradise that our souls yearn for.* "When will I see you!" he mused. I came away with an abiding sense of the caress of his kindness, an abiding sense of deep gladness.

That encounter was for me like a touch of paradise; it gave me knowledge of what God's forgiveness is like, what God's kindness is like, and the deep gladness of it. I thought then that he "focused my whole being," rather like the rainbow hues of my existence becoming fused into white light again; everything made sense and had meaning. Looking back, it is clear I loved him so much that, at the time, I had to have him deeply, completely in my life, because without him there could be no meaning!

Chapter 71
Tenderness and Tearing.

And so at the beginning of August of '93 I felt delightfully wrapped up in loving Dr.James again; I thought how the variegated feelings of alternating delight and sadness he caused me were like "the dappling of God's cloud and sunlight passing over my soul." My sensitivity to him, responsiveness to him were so acute; "my attraction to you is stronger than the electro-magnetic field of the earth." Sometimes he so astonished, silenced and overcame me, that all my thought-processes collapsed in on themselves and left "a silent light-filled sense of love."

Once when I averred "I comprehend God's love through you," and he replied that it put "a great responsibility, an enormous burden" on him, I spilt forth with my protestations of "it's not like ordinary human love, the yearnings I have are far more ethereal and everlasting, you stand for me within the pure white radiance of God's love." And he seemed to understand it all, and compelled me into silence again, and left me radiant with a deep and tender knowledge. *And when I awoke in the morning I felt in touch with God, in a silent pool of tenderness. In the coming days he always made me feel like that, "radiantly happy, whole, tender, wrapped in a womb of light."*

Then the day came when he demanded to see what I was writing in my journal. He left angrily when I wouldn't let him; I was afraid of him when his whole being was like a thunderstorm, and never could endure him being angry; so I wrote a capitulating letter, saying "I'll do whatever you say." But I was horrified when he came back and read the whole thing; I had a terrible sense of being "read", when it was only meant to be read by God. He said "carry on writing like that, but don't involve me," and left in displeasure. I had a sense of something terrible; of being read and known, and not being accepted, not loved, not taken up; I couldn't find words to describe what I felt!

The upshot of it was that I felt such a deep self-abasing desperation, that I wrote a letter averring again "I'll do anything you say, I yield to you, I am willing to be led by you and taught by you." My pain was so great; I had this sense that God loved me because he knew me, and here was this man who had read me, knew me, and wouldn't accept me and take me up. "Do whatever you like with me, but accept me; having read and known me, don't refuse to take me up. I'll do anything to please you and be accepted by you; please imitate God's love when I throw myself upon your mercy; you know how desperately I mean it, how desperately I need you."

287

It happened to be then that he found the stuff I'd written a year ago, and he seemed to throw it back at me like a manner of rejection. When I asked if he would come back to see me, he said "No; you might write it down," and it seemed a definite and absolute "No." I felt so miserable, crying on the beach; *if he wouldn't take me up, I may as well "bury myself in oblivion and despair forever." He had taken the reason for existence away from me; there was no light in this dark world apart from him!*

When I saw him briefly again, he implied I couldn't look after my writings, and my reaction became an angry one; my writings were safe in my own hands, and it was he who had lost them! I thought he was paranoid about writings; "I keep safe what I have written; I would protect what I write with my life!" Then I cried hot tears, as I felt my existence had become worthless and pointless; I had invested all the meaning of my existence in him, I was like Othello, who had invested the meaning of his life in the one ideal, and was left with nothing. Thus I felt it like one last throw, like a reprieve from a death-sentence, when he suggested to me that I make the sacrifice of destroying the offending parts of my journal. He said "What's it to be then, Yea or Nay?" I knew my life was pointless without him, so it was a sacrifice I had to make.

It was a torment to me to try and tear apart my journal! I knew that everything that I wrote was only part-true, because designed to bring me to that silence where ultimate truth is to be found. And so I seemed unable to limit or judge it; I always threw the totality of my experience at God. So if I purged my journals there would be nothing left. It was like a whole fabric; if I hacked it up it would fall apart; there would be only a few tatters left. This torment over my journal went to the roots of my being. There was a song which echoed in me, "I will do anything for love, but I won't do that." And there was a poem, "Go hack up your feet on red unending ice." I felt the sacrifice would be so sore that I would never recover from it. But then I felt a sudden release of the heart, thinking "I'll make this sacrifice because I love you; to prove that I love you even above my own journals." *And so I finally hacked and tore my journal to bits at 2 am. in the dark.*

But the sweetness of him saying thankyou to me seemed to make worth the soreness I suffered. I can remember how I put all the torn-up fragments of paper into a large card and envelope, inside of it a smaller one that read "my love of you is shown in the hurt and pain I take for you." When he said "Thankyou" it was beyond anything I had ever known of rapture! "Such rapture is sure knowledge; knowledge that is born of sacrifice, knowledge that my love of you is endless, knowledge that I am indeed kept in the rapture of God's endless love."

Looking back, he shouldn't have made me choose him, over and above the truth of my own soul! He tormented me with my own creativity; it was like marrying a potter and then proceeding to smash the pots!

Chapter 72
The Quagmire of Pain.

Since coming out of Craigdene, Access visits had been restored to me again, but they had dwindled to the 2 hours a week, supervised. The social work team led by Stuart O'Sullivan re-established the "supervised" element again, precisely because I had "voiced my concerns" about what my son had intimated to me in the tent in April, which made me believe he was being abused. *The "supervision" by which a social worker, either Stuart or Isabel, had to listen to every syllable spoken between me and my son, wore heavily on my spirit.*

I began to be dismayed, saddened and made angry, by the things I perceived Walter was teaching him, and also the way he was neglecting him. He was putting his own sick psychological imaginings upon him, about faeries and ghosts, rather than guiding him about God and Jesus as I had done. He wasn't educating him as I had done; my sensitive child was going to be stunted in his emotional growth if he never played with other children and never read books. He was teaching him to bully as he bullied, and was teaching him his own physical shabbiness. *It pained my heart to see what a "damaged child" my son was becoming.*

After two months of this supervised access I complained bitterly to Isabel that it was very unfair that I had my access diminished because I had reported sexual abuse; it told against me because it discomforted Walter, and they were apparently on his side. And they were on his side! Shortly after this, Stuart O'Sullivan came and told me that, progressing to unsupervised access again, every time he was uplifted I would be asked if I had "any concerns." *Of course if I did have any concerns, I would lose the unsupervised access again. I felt this was tyrannical!* It amounted to myself having to tell Gabriel not to talk honestly to me. Stuart O'Sullivan then proceeded to tell me that I had "no rights of Access," beyond it was given by Walter's consent and kindness; I protested that I had a "mother's rights," and that I had brought up Gabriel through babyhood. This conversation made me angrily visit my solicitor-friend Agnes, and she told me that indeed every parent has rights, that letting access depend on Walter's good graces was ridiculous, and I really must take it to court again.

I began to feel acutely this mother's torment of watching her son being "blighted." I hated what I saw of Walter teaching Gabriel so many bad things, but I felt I didn't have enough time to influence him. I remember when he wouldn't offer me a sweet once; "I taught you good things like sharing, Walter has just taught you his own meanness." He was teaching him to be like himself. Walter wasn't a good father who was adequately caring for him, but the social workers didn't seem to care. It was the greatest grief of my life to watch my child being damaged.

There is nothing worse to a mother than to have to watch the child she nurtured being gradually damaged and destroyed. This is the worst suffering known to a mother; and therefore the worst suffering known to the human soul.

I began to feel acutely how I was a mother "bereft of her child." I felt something had been done to me which was wicked, inexcusable, unforgivable, in that the one real blessing of my life, my son, had been taken away from me. When I complained to my own mental health social worker, Steven Peterson, he agreed that, as the custody case had been founded on my "mental illness" I had been "discriminated against"; I shouldn't have lost my child because of that.

Then one day I discovered that Walter had altered all Gabriel's name-tags on his school-clothes to his own surname "McKay." With pain I went to see the Registrar about it, and she informed me that Walter had a right to do this, but if Gabriel ever got married he would be referred back to the original birth certificate, naming him "Gabriel Colme." I was seething mad; "that's all that's going to be left of him for me; the fact that I gave birth to him!" *It seemed that Walter wanted to so efface my motherhood, as to take even my name away from him!*

One day Gabriel touched me by a wonderful and mystical statement he came out with about God; "It's alright Mummy, when you get to heaven, just tell him you want another Gabriel, and he'll make you one." It touched me so completely and tenderly, with its lovely mysticism; "If you can say a thing like that, you must be my son!"

I had a terrible session with Dr.McNeill; I hated listening to his soul-belittling, esteem-destroying, untrue and hypocritical, intolerable nonsense; I found myself gazing out of the window, trying not to react. He said "you get yourself into difficult situations," and "you blame other people for your mistakes," and intimated that he intended renewing my section. Worst of all he implied that I had "got rid" of Gabriel because I didn't want him; to this I finally and angrily replied. I hated his disgusting denigrating attitude. He implied I couldn't make decisions because I didn't know what freedom was. I was so angry when I came out; "to say I can't use freedom is like insinuating I have no soul!" But I converted my feelings into the creativity of writing a poem. And then the following day I got the news that I was sectioned through the post; I felt how I hated the man; "it binds me to a mental hospital for another whole year!"

Stuart O'Sullivan then came to tell me that I could have Gabriel on Saturdays, provided Walter came "right to the door" to do the handover himself; and he also wanted weekly confirmation that I was well and wouldn't be a "danger" to his son. I was outraged; I wasn't going to let seeing more of my son depend upon being harassed by Walter. I was staring at the carpet in miserable pain, thinking "I hate the System you are apart of!" I said I'd decided "No", because I wasn't going to have the destructiveness of him harassing me. Then I went and sat on a bench on the East sands and cried.

And that day I really plumbed "the mother's feelings that go as deep as hell"! It was the feeling that it was so painful to watch a child being blighted that I wish I'd never brought him into existence! I saw "I subsist in an element, a quagmire of raging pain." And it was a pain that didn't lessen; it was turning into hatred. I was only raised above it momentarily; "but it always waits for me."

Then Isabel came and said that Walter was "expressing concerns" that I had been telling Gabriel to say he wanted to come and live with me. Gabriel had indeed been frequently piping up, "Mummy I want to come and live with you." Now Isabel said that because I hadn't "made the right response" to Gabriel, access had to stop till it was ironed out. I was so angry about it; "so now they are going to prescribe how I've to respond are they!" Then Stuart O'Sullivan came, and he quite crippled me with the seething of my own dark emotion. He said I had to set Walter's mind at ease by "reinforcing reality" to Gabriel. My mind screamed out "No I won't; I'm not going to crush my son's young hopes and dreams!" I was being told that if I didn't say to Gabriel what Walter wanted me to say, I couldn't have access; but I wasn't going to be an instrument of Walter's oppression of him! I was determined that I wasn't going to do what they demanded of me, that I wasn't going to co-operate in oppressing my son.

It was about then that I began to think I must take it back to court. Stuart O'Sullivan had said that Walter had "gone through the proper channels" to take Gabriel off me. *But he had used a legal system to promote prejudice and lies with the aim of taking a child off his mother! I couldn't stand the way my "mental illness" was thought blameworthy and carried a stigma! Would I have been counted an "unfit mother" if I struggled with the difficulties of blindness or MS?* I decided I'd fight;

292

"give me a sympathetic psychiatrist, and I'll fight all this bullshit!" I decided that my rage was better in action. Accordingly I went to see George McPherson my new solicitor in Inverlang; at least he made me feel that there was some kind of rationality and fairness to be found in the law, and it put hope in my heart.

The pain of my situation was so immense that I began to feel I was walking in hell-fire flames. One day I accidentally encountered Walter in a bar, and I walked off with my hatred of him crippling me. What I really couldn't endure was the sense that Walter had taken my child off me, *after all those years when I had taught him and trained him and brought him up, just when he was old enough to become "a companion."* He had deprived me of my child! The more I went on, the worse the pain and hatred seemed to get, "until one day I'll kill the man."

My pain is the howl of anguish of a mother who has lost her child. I hate Walter, in that he caused the wound, and then robbed me of the balm for that wound, which is my child.

It was at this stage, whilst a raging pain was taking hold of me over my loss of my son, that I began writing poetry. It was really in response to my raging pain, - "the mother's pain that goes as deep as hell." In this sense it was strange that "out of the pain came forth creativity." I seemed to see the purpose of God in it.

It rapidly took a hold of me and enraptured me, as I began to feel how I could pour my mysticism into poetry. And anything and everything became for me a subject of poetry; "all you need is the one rapture of an insight." And all my poetry I garnered up to present to Dr.James; he gave me subjects, and I read my poetry out to him, and I was thrilled by the sense that I could please him like this. I felt in the times spent with him that he took my hand in friendship and gave me back myself. *He gave me wings! And to me there was nothing better in all the world than those times when he strove to understand my mysticism. For many months it was a manner of bliss that we shared. I felt beautiful and loved and complete, wrapped around "in a silent womb-like tenderness, that was a palpable presence."*

And so I communed with Dr.James, and found joy beyond telling when I carried his understanding with me. Like the idealizing love between Antony and Cleopatra, the kind of love which ennobles us though it also dooms us, I loved the ideal image; and of our talks I could say "one of them rates all that is won and lost." My need of him was like a single desire; "to burrow into you like a little furry animal trying to get as close and warm as it can! For the big wide world out there is dark and cold and heartless and filled with pain; I only feel safe in being close to you; you keep my warm love alive!" And above and beyond the "need" that keeps us alive, I desired "ecstasy," to be compelled to peace! "The more I know of you the more I love you;" it was an activity of knowing and loving at the same time; "we get to heaven on our knowing and loving"!

My raging pain over my son didn't lessen; I subsisted in a quagmire of it, and I was only raised momentarily above it by Dr.James. Endless hatred and pain were "waiting for me" and only love of this man helped me transcend it or rescued me from it. I needed him so deeply; he was like a window letting in God's sunlight. I needed him because momentarily he took the pain away; he gave me wings; I could be sprung by love out of the prison of my pain

Chapter 73
Hatred and Hell.

Then one day in the Baptist church I had a frantic sense of how the motherhood was torn out of the heart of me, and that my life was worth nothing; I couldn't continue "in a life made meaningless by hatred." I must leave Gabriel behind and try and make a new life, because seeing him was only rubbing salt into my wounds. Apart from my love Dr.James, "apart from You, my life is worth nothing." And then I saw, with a shock, that my love was "escapism." I realised then that I wasn't succeeding in keeping my head above an endless quagmire of hatred, and I'd have to go! *I ended up crying over a candle-flame out of pure hatred. I felt my hatred would increase "until one day I'll kill Walter." I realised that all my poetry and my love was an escapism from a life that is pure hatred. "And hatred leads to hell."*

"There are violations against us so deep that they can never be forgiven in our lifetime; Walter abused and violated my whole being, he had a child on me, then finally he took that child away from me. What he did to me is unforgivable; he made me betray my own love in having a child who wasn't born of love. His sin against me is far more original, older, than robbing me of my child; he violated the deepest part of me. I can never forgive him; I hope that what I hold against him damns him to hell!"

I went through a cataclysm of black despair for a few days. I grieved over my lost son. He seemed to have unlearned everything I ever taught him; for I had taught him to tuck in his vests, wash his hands, brush his teeth, love books; "have you any idea how long I spent teaching him to wash his hands!" I grieved at the thought that he wasn't even physically cared for by Walter; he was thin, smelly, had dirty finger-nails, greasy hair, and he smelt because he hardly ever had baths; "have you any idea what it feels like when you don't want to hug your child because he smells!" The Social workers had said "we have no concerns over the level of care his father is providing for him." *"Can you tell me what the word "care" means if it comprises none of these things!" I grieved so much, when I remembered him, the nice little sweet clean "biddable" boy my mother had said that he was! And it was a most horrible, gut-wrenching feeling to be as a mother not able to influence, teach, train, nurture my child! Walter was destroying my motherhood by undoing what I had taught.* I was doing the cleaning whilst I was thinking all this, but finally I collapsed in gushing tears!

I cried out in deep need, begging for Dr.James to come and visit and save from all this intense feeling, which was producing the urge to kill! He couldn't come because ill, but I met certain people that day who seemed to touch my heart with healing balm, as though they were angels. And the love within me for the man I loved didn't fail me and got me through; when I saw him I said I had "defended the universe, been to hell and back, and been rescued by angels." *I felt as though some great cosmic struggle had taken place in me and through me; and I felt that I lived newly in "a world of grace."* And I lived newly after this; I saw myself as having the inner life and the warm energy of someone who had something to give. And I saw life was about self-giving, and I began to pour myself out towards others, in meetings and discussions, imparting energy and vision. Instead of living as someone imprisoned in pain, I saw myself newly as free in the world of grace.

I was then jubilant when, due to a letter from my solicitor, Walter agreed that Saturday access should go ahead, for a longer time and unsupervised. However the jubilation rather turned to ashes when I didn't enjoy it, due to Gabriel's bad bullying behaviour and the sexual stuff that came from him again. The first Saturday I had him I was dismayed by the sexual content of his caressing of my legs; I fell I didn't want to know, because I didn't want to report it. And he seemed to have become just like Walter, always coercing, bullying, blackmailing. His whole way of relating seemed emotionally sick, saying "if you don't do it, I'll start getting upset." I felt I didn't want him with me, for he was a very unhappy little boy; *he had no sense of contentment, achievement, value, worth, creativity; he just went around in a paroxysm of bad-temper all day!*

I began to grieve all over again at the sense of this "damaged child" of mine. I couldn't stand the emotional sickness I saw in him after all the good upbringing I'd given him, nor the sense of my powerlessness; he seemed "spoilt" and damaged beyond repair. And the worst thing was he seemed to look to me to liberate him, but I couldn't. I couldn't save "my son's soul." This concept put me into a fit of despair. I thought how as a mother you hope to bear your child "to soul-life"; and it seemed I had borne Gabriel to soul-death. And I found myself beginning to feel that giving birth to him had done a disservice to his soul and to my soul and to love itself. *This was a terrible thing to think! And realising it was, I began try and think in terms of Gabriel having "a soul that could be saved."*

Then on 23rd November Gabriel said something which made it obvious to me that some kind of abuse was going on. For he said to me, "I want to go underneath you and lift up your knickers; me and Daddy do it all the time; we like doing it; my Daddy tell me that's what big people do." I felt sickened to the pit of my stomach, and I felt that the whole world had gone horrible. I felt I would be culpable if I didn't report it, but how could I when it would tell against me!

I despaired over Gabriel again after that. I watched in dismay as I saw he had learnt the same emotionally sick and bullying tricks that Walter had used over me when he got me pregnant. I felt that to watch my child being blighted in this way after the caring upbringing as a baby that I had given him, was "just about the greatest cross in the universe!" And I felt keenly how Gabriel would go on to treat women in the way Walter had abused me, destroying lives all around him; and I couldn't bear this. I had this hellish feeling that I had "propagated evil"; the evil done to me I was responsible for propagating to others.

It didn't help when I came to have a sense of his "badness", in the way he delighted in paining people. He kept playing nasty tricks, like switching my fridge off. And then he kept repeating "my Daddy says I can do anything I like!" Now what sort of a moral upbringing do you call that! Nothing I could do or say seemed to counteract the massive input of bad teaching that was coming from Walter. I grieved so much watching him, in that, after I had taught him to play quietly and creatively for hours, he now struggled and shouted at toys "this damned bloody thing!" I felt Walter was making him "twice as fit for hell" as himself! I went and sobbed my heart out by the sea.

I felt that I'd wasted my life! I had wasted ten years of my life under the destructive domination of Walter, and now I was wasting my life grieving over a lost son. I felt the only real thing I'd ever done was destructive; for in giving birth to Gabriel I had spread destruction. My friend Helen tried to help by suggesting "forgiveness." *I replied that it wasn't a matter of forgiving a thing of the past, but of what Walter was continually doing to me through Gabriel in the present. "How can you forgive an offender when he is still offending you, when the act of violence is still being carried out against you!"* She asked if I "loved" Gabriel; I replied "how could I when he was the spitting image of Walter!" but I did try "to lovingly accept him, over and beyond liking."

As Christmas approached I began to see that this nine-hour Saturday marathon with Gabriel had to stop; it would be better to see him only occasionally, like once a month. When I suggested this to Isabel that at least the nine hours should be limited to two, she came back with Walter's answer that it had to be nine hours, so as to "suit his

297

arrangements." I was angered, in that he made my access times "suit his arrangements." It seemed to me so ironic that the whole idea of increased access times was enunciated by the solicitor as a way of "getting my son back." It struck me now that he was so damaged that I didn't want him back anyway! It struck me with pain at Christmas time that everybody was cosy and warm, with families, husbands, children; "and I have bloody nothing!"

I saw Dr.McNeill again before Christmas. At this stage the sweetness of my life was entirely collapsed, and I wanted to go away somewhere, acutely aware that my house had lost its warmth. Because I was obliged to stay there by the section he had signed, my house now felt like a prison-cell. So when Dr.McNeill said to me that he was fed up of my "hostile attitude," I said back; "given that you have made my home into a prison-cell, and given that you helped to rob me of my child, why should I not have a hostile attitude!" He replied that clearly we had different ideas of what a prison-cell was. I said "a prison-cell is where you are forced to stay, where you are imprisoned." And he replied "Nonsense, a prison-cell is where there are bars at the window." And I went away cursing that he was a "stupid bastard!"

Then on Christmas Eve something terrible happened. I went to the Registrar to get a copy of Gabriel's birth-certificate, because I had lost it; the only one she would give me was one with the information entirely altered, naming Walter as the father, and altering my son's surname from "Colme" to "McKay." I went bananas with pain; she had told me earlier in the year not to worry, because Water could never alter the original certificate without the mother's consent. But somehow or other he had pursued the matter to the source, in Edinburgh, and got the birth-entry changed! *I walked out of there in the cold snow, beside myself with pain and hatred and wrath. It was like the "last straw," the last straw breaking my grieving mother's heart!*

And having got a copy of this new certificate, which was now the only one I could get, I wrote on it, "this piece of paper makes you, my son, a bastard." But I added, wanting it to be a piece of paper that he would keep forever, to contradict what it seemed to say; *"But you are not; for you are born of Love, out of your mother's love. He wants to own you, but I owned you first; he wants to have you, but I did all the giving to you. This says "I let go of you"; love lets go. And because I loved you at the beginning I love you always."*

I never saw my son for a long time after that. And so having voyaged through seas of raging pain and hatred, out of my mother's anguish at seeing my once-tender child so damaged, this was all I was left with; nothing but this piece of paper, and memories.

Chapter 74
The Divine Energy.

I reached a crisis point at the end of October. Life seemed so bitter to me, my soul full of hatred as it was toward the man who had robbed me of my son, that it seemed not worth living; I cried over a candle-flame; I saw that I took refuge in that love of Dr.James as an escapism from life. I needed help, as I had the urge to kill; and when Dr.James didn't turn up, it felt like the universe's cruel joke. "When I really need you, you are beyond my reaching," I bewailed, though finding out that he was ill. I wrote to him, "the universe needs you, there's the sick to heal, the devil to fight, me to save." But what happened was that I encountered several people that day, who made me feel "helped and rescued by angels." When I next saw him, I told him of the vast voyage I had been on, being saved by angels, and that I had never doubted my love of him; it was that pure love I clung to which "called the angels down"! And he said "I often come here like a sponge that is wrung dry, and you fill me up!" *And I saw then, "my love isn't escapism; it is the highest and the best in me."*

I was transformed by that experience. I had been in a prison-cell full of hatred, and now I was in a different world of "angels." "The world in which angels encounter you is like an open blue sky; there are no prison-cells in such a world." Suddenly I blossomed and came out of myself, attending endless discussions, pouring my mystical and poetic understanding into the world around me. I was suddenly open unto life. *My love of him was suddenly like an energy on which I rode!*

It was then that we talked about "kelpies"! He explained one night that a kelpie was a water-sprite in the shape of a horse, who absorbs all the love that can be given, then rides off out to sea; he said he was like a kelpie in that he couldn't return love. I replied "bear me off to sea then; you can never take all my love because it is inexhaustible!" My romantic notions about the kelpie increased when I researched it in the university library; "I'd love to be borne off by a kelpie!" I wondered "Why do you identify yourself with a kelpie who is incapable of loving, when you are so warm!" The thing I loved most about him was that he had such a warm, living, responsive soul! I would love to be carried off by a kelpie, because it was like a quick way to heaven, a giving of oneself to love measurelessly; it was a reckless act, giving oneself to a love "when it demands one's life, one's all." For what happened in the myths to the victims of the kelpie was, that they were found drowned!

I found I was waiting on him a lot; I felt I could take on the pain of "waiting for him forever," but I felt it was wasting of my time, efforts and gifts, when I had other things to do these days. Sometimes waiting was like pain; I had a grasp of "the love that will wait on the beloved forever". "Forever" had the same sort of quality of time "as the angels waiting around God's throne."

Once I really needed him, because I felt I was riding on too much energy, and was "about to explode like a supernova." I told him of this briefly in the car-park, adding that I was sorry for always needing him so much. But he readily responded in that true need, as he faithfully and always did. I poured out my ecstasies to him, and the pain of the love I was comprehending. And he absorbed all of my soul-energies, and, as always, compelled me to peace. And the next day, overwhelmed as I was by the mystical sense of the "ecstatic intertwining within the divine energy which is God, of giving, needing and taking," I wrote a card to him. *I wanted to express my sharing in the loving activity of God in the present; so I wrote "Today I am loving you, so endlessly and so deeply."*

That day I lived in the bliss of the supernatural depths that aren't touched by the surface of life. And I wrote the card carefully, shot through with the piercing light of comprehension about a present, loving, active God. But he rejected it, as I had put on the envelope "to the best Master in the world." "What are people to think!" he said, so the next day I tried to explain to him what I meant by the card, and how it was an expression of mystical bliss, and how I felt part of the divine activity. I said "the knowledge that dwelt in me was bliss; I felt like an angel trying to hide its wings," and he laughed. I explained about this divine energy which is both giving and receiving, *and felt there was nothing better in the world than his understanding of my mysticism!*

Then a bit of a catastrophe happened between us, and he was angry with me, storming out one day in wrath; something like a "wad of reality" had come between us. And so very contritely I went to the surgery the next morning; and after a two hour wait for him, just as he summoned me by name, I found that the thought of something "touched and stirred me, like an angel's finger." And my attention was thrown; *I had wanted to say "don't let this wad of reality come between me and you, because I love you and would wait for you as angels wait."* But I found I couldn't speak, as he shouted at me, "don't play that repentant nun routine with me!" I was bowled over by the sense of him as the "totally other," being the subject of his wrath.

So I walked by the sea, wishing I could adequately say "I'm sorry" and "I love you." So I wrote a poem for him, sensing it was the best gift I could offer; it began "I would throw at your feet an ocean," and ended "the heart I yield you is an ocean of love." I thought how the bliss and the pain are together in love, and "if you take the anger lovingly then the pain creates and saves you." I reflected that I would say on seeing him, "well you could hardly have found a more repentant nun if you had waited a hundred years! I'm sorry for arguing with you, sorry for angering you." But he didn't come; and I comforted myself with the thought "I'll wait on you forever, even when it's pain."

Then he did come, but it was painful, because his attitude was so prohibitive. He said "stop talking about me, stop trying to tempt me, stop writing about love." It was so painful to me when I felt my intense flow of self-giving toward him was "a ready roadway into God's heart." It was as if he put shutters on it and tried to glue it up with concrete! I protested that I had always talked of Love, I was talking of the divine love I was riding on; I was a mystic, trying to comprehend God's love; how could I not talk and write about Love! I felt how much hurt I got through him; "timewise you hurt me far more than you make me happy." *But I knew I had the love in my heart to take both the bliss and the pain; for ultimately the bliss surpasses all the pain!*

Then one day I found myself walking in the snow with my heart as cold as the snow, for he had said something that had pierced me like a piece of ice. When I had earnestly explained to him about the bliss of God, he had said "all life is vanity." And when I had sat on the floor earnestly averring that as a mystic I wasn't capable of understanding anything but love, he walked away imparting to me the cold pain of "I know that"! "Why were you so cold?" was my reaction. I couldn't understand why I seemed to have gone cold towards me; was it all over and had he had enough of me? But I felt the alacrity of love within myself to stoically bear hurt; "even though you don't love me, I still love you." *In that cold and horrible snowy world, I said "I've a heart that warmly beats in the heart of Love for you."*

And it was then that I discovered "Deep Peace"! The way it happened was a mystery, in that, in that snowy cold world, completely uncharacteristically, I phoned him from a call-box; it was like a mute appeal into a cold wide universe, waiting for a responsive God. And he came round, and showed me an understanding warmth. It seemed to me in the deepest darkness and coldness the Easter fire was lit; the warmth of God's love lit in human hearts. I realised he wasn't at all and could never be "cold"; I loved him so much for the way he was always so warm and understanding and benevolent! *And the next day I hastened to get a card for him, a Celtic benediction, to give to him before he should go off to Skye! I suddenly comprehended the concept of "Deep Peace"; "deep peace of the running wave to you, deep peace of the shining stars to you, deep peace of the Son of Peace to you."* I wrote on the back; "This may be a rune to ward off the kelpie, or it may be a way of thanking you for the deep peace with which you gift me, or it may be a benediction on your travels; but take care and come back safe." But unfortunately he had already set off!

Whilst he was away I comprehended a wonderful and new idea about "Pleasure." I realised that Pleasure, our pleasure in each other and God's pleasure in us, saves us from pain; not that we don't know pain, but that pleasure triumphs over it. I realised how I was employing this Pleasure in loving him, to help me bear the pain of loving my son. "Pleasure in that aspect overcomes, triumphs over the most terrible, senseless destructive pain; not the fractional pleasure of the senses, but the Pleasure which shares in Christ's pleasure, which is total and sacramental and redeeming."

I sank into a despond again whilst he was absent; I recognised how these periods of darkness corresponded with his absence, as if a supernatural darkness enveloped me, and I wanted to shout "bring back the light because it's gone dark!" My love of him was the light in me which dispelled the darkness. I ached with waiting for him, reflected that one day I would "die waiting for him." I reflected that this wasn't a way to live, existing in a life-situation which was painful and destructive, depending on one man for any salvation from it. I seemed to take pain immeasurably, and hardly ever find joy! I was possessed by deep dark feelings that went as deep as hell. Thus my despair was absolute, until he returned and I expressed it to him and got beyond it!

And he spoke to me that night little truths which seemed like pools of light in the darkness. And I saw in explaining to him that pain is always fractional, in that it doesn't embrace the whole being; therefore the Pleasure and Bliss which are all-embracing triumph over it. I had quoted to him Dame Julian, "to bring us to bliss he lays on each one he loves some particular thing"; *and I saw that the pain that we take serves to bring us to that Bliss, that total pleasure which we find in Christ in the end. The Bliss takes us through to eternity, but the pain is transcended and left behind.* I felt that on that beautiful night that he gave me vision of this saving truth; the song came true for me "You put me on a pedestal, so high that I could see all of eternity."

The "Deep Peace" I knew the next morning, I wished I could experience every morning, but unfortunately it only lasted one precious day! I quickly felt the pain and restlessness of the world again. I thought how Christ "tempts us" by giving such moments of Deep Peace amid the earthy restlessness; by giving us a taste of heaven He makes us to desire it. I explained to him about the "Deep Peace" next time he visited; "Deep Peace is in the moments when I transcend, when I am so aware of you that I cease to be aware of myself." I told him *"I want more of the Deep Peace, because I live on it, it has become my spiritual bread-and-butter, the only thing that fulfils me, and the only thing that I desire."*

I told him "You always raise me high upon a pedestal; in my coldness you give me warmth, in my darkness you give me light, in my despair you give me saving truths." I said "I hold you as in the middle of my heart," and he beamed at me. I told him I loved the way he compelled me to silence; "what bliss it is for someone like me to have a completely quiet soul." I told him that Deep Peace was like "finding a home for the heart." And when I was in it I was unhurtable, for I could say "my soul is a lamp whose light is steady, burning in an abode where no winds come." But when I felt hurt again it was the end of the oneness and integrity of this Deep Peace.

As my 40th birthday on 11th December was approaching, I sensed again the encroaching of meaningless supernatural darkness. I felt that nobody cared enough about me to take note of my birthday; presents and cards should be a matter of warming the heart and showing you care; "care whether someone is dead or alive for God's sake!" And the cry was wrung from me "Who cares about me? I've been in existence for 40 years, and no-one cares about me, - except for Dr.James that is!" In contrast to the warm family atmosphere exuded by Christmas, I felt keenly that I had no son, no husband, no family; my parents who forbade me to visit them pained me immeasurably when they sent slippers as a present instead of the gold ear-rings I had begged for. I went to the chaplaincy to pray there for a while, sensing only the emotional poverty of my life.

He came that day, my birthday, but he didn't comfort me; he could have made me feel rich when I was poor, but he didn't; it was a black and miserable day for me. I thought I would drown in tears the next morning, because I had the sense that my love of him had no hope. But I thought there was always a way through for a soul loving enough to take the pain, and I wrote, "I'll always love you, no matter what." But he came back, and for the first time ever, he said to me "I'm sorry." *I responded "you could have made me rich when I was poor." And for the last time, that night, my dreaming was filled with winged and happy thoughts.*

It was ominous that I wrote the next day that I felt how my mind always disintegrated towards the blackness of Death without him; "without you something in me collapses." It was as if he gave me the "desire to live" to keep me out of death. A lot of Death followed in '94, as this "beautiful friendship" broke up and dissolved.

But it shall remain treasured in my soul forever as my life's "one beautiful love-affair;" it wrapped me up so intensely in the pain and bliss and tenderness and rapture of God!

305

Chapter 76
The Heart's Winter.

On the eve of the 18th December my eyes seemed opened about the truth of this mystical friendship which had absorbed me for the whole of the year of '93. For he chose a moment when I was praying "may this moment last forever," to speak of the possibility of what was so beautiful to me "becoming sordid," and I was hurt immeasurably, and protested that this friendship was "the source of all that was strong and pure" in me.

When he was gone, I went through a marathon of feeling. Tears came as I reflected, "that was the year that was; it started in January and ended in December;" and I slowly realised what it meant. A miserable awareness hit me when going to bed; that he wasn't offering me a pure whole soul. A quote came to me; "Love is a heart that offers itself to love totally, that is pure; the essence of sinning against purity is to offer, or seem to offer, a spurious love, a love that is not and cannot be whole." *I realised, grief-struck, "he never did offer me a whole heart." And with that came the knowledge, the seeing into his heart, that he never did really care! And I sat there on the edge of my bed, my face in my hands, as if in the direst moment of my existence, realising that this was the end of all my happiness!*

Most of the night I thought and felt miserably, continually resurfacing to consciousness, revolving it in my mind. "You make me feel like someone who makes you guilty; I am not guilty, but *you* are, because the gift you offer isn't whole." I felt it was far worse than what Victor did to me, when he took me up to love for a few weeks then threw me aside "like a dirty old rag." It was worse because I had invested my whole soul-life in this year-long friendship; by taking me up and then throwing me aside, he had wrung my heart and extinguished all its hope. Then I found myself thinking where to go and how to go, for it was no longer true that I had "a home for my heart" in him. I slipped into a horrific nightmare, in which he said "it's not me, there's two of me; I am the one who murders you." I woke, aware, "this is a living nightmare from which I cannot wake up."

That day I listened miserably to the wind howling in the chimney, and felt the world to be a wasteland. I ended up sobbing my heart out in the church, until the priest came in and cruelly turned the lights off; it seemed allegorical, saying to me "no light and warmth for you anywhere!" The cruelty of the winter's weather made me want to cease to be alive. I felt too heartless to maintain my being in existence; everything I had lived for had gone!

So forlorn I saw so clearly into it; "I gave my all to him, and he gave nothing of himself to me." I felt that he had his fill of me, and then threw me away, threw me down into the gutter. He had said he was a "kelpie" who was incapable of love; at least a kelpie consumes until death, but he was throwing me back out; "it is trolls that spit people out."
I reflected on how I had rejected Matty and Freddy that year, who could have offered me some future life, because I was too busy loving him! "That makes me moral and you immoral!" He had tempted me to invest so much of myself in him, only to destroy it. "I offered you a whole heart, a pure heart; and to you it was sordid because you didn't offer anything!"

Christmas was approaching and I couldn't stand the thought of it; it had no meaning for me; I felt I was "shut out in the cold forevermore." Christmas was about the warmth of human hearts; but no-one seemed to invite me in. I felt I had reached the winter of my life; I began to desire to go to a place where the winter outside would match the winter in my heart. I just wanted to go somewhere, to get over my quick life with my death; I grimly thought how there was "nothing out there for me."

And then he came to visit me, and seemed grace-less, never even saying "Don't go!" There was no reprieve and no miracle happened. I pleaded "I will go anywhere on earth where I can leave a door open to you," but he didn't respond. He said "I never had anything to offer" and "you demanded too much." It hurt when, believing always that he felt a sense of loving responsibility for me, appealing to him "do you want me to go?" he curtly said "it's up to you." It hurt when, after what seemed like millions of hours of shared understanding, he left saying "we don't speak the same language."

I was outraged when he had gone; "he gets me involved in total self-giving, and then rejects me after tempting me into it! How dare he say I demanded too much!" I had said to him, cutting to myself; "I will not have warm memories of you; I will see you as the man who has made a winter in my heart." *I had said he had made my life meaningless and left me with nothing; I might as well go, and choose the meaningless. What hurt me most was that he didn't even care enough to say "Don't go"!*

Then around midnight, on the 21st, I had a kind of revelation, a conversion-experience; I saw that instead of "going out there to die," when I didn't have the right to take my own life, I could choose "a better way of dying", - *I could "become a hermit."* It was the way that would conserve the most meaning, because it was a choice of "sacrifice," of a life "given over to God."

A night of another marathon of thought and feeling ensued, in which I had an insight into what he had done to me; he had made such a winter in my heart, that I could never love again in human fashion. I compared him with Philip; when I declared my love of him, he replied "I cannot love you back"; he was true to himself and therefore true to me. "But you, you took my total self-giving then said "you can stop now" when I can't stop! You seemed to say Yes, so that I invested the whole of me in you, gave you "all that I am." You should not have let me invest all of myself in you, and given nothing of yourself! I'm not saying you misused me; but you rejected my love."

Yes, I would make myself a hermit, "sacrificing in order to offer a whole heart to God." I would make myself alone, "out in the cold" with those who are out in the cold, going to those in need, giving my heart to the lost and lonely, loving the unloved, "giving up the world." I would "wait on God's time," doing nothing to hasten death, making my dying a long sacrifice. My heart like my door was no longer open to him; he had made a desolation in my heart that would never offer itself to human love again, but "if ever you seek my understanding, I'll be there for you." From now on I had a consecrated heart, "and it was a heart no longer offered to you." And so in the morning-light I was left feeling "wise."

In the next few days I realised fully and talked and wrote of how "being a hermit" meant "the rejection of the world and all its values, in order to offer oneself to God." A hermit was not someone who stayed solitary, but someone who retired constantly to his cell to offer himself entirely to God there, and then shared what he had learnt with others. A hermit was someone who didn't want anything for himself, and to achieve that, he had to cease to live for himself, and was accounted a dead person. My knowledge of the writings of the "Desert Fathers" flooded in upon me, and became illuminated with understanding. I began writing down "Rules" about how to behave as a hermit, the attitude of the heart that it was necessary to preserve.

And so I turned, converted what was a bleak, crushing, winter of the heart, from which had been wrung all hope, and which tended toward despair and death, into a rich and meaningful renaissance of spiritual life, into a conversion-experience, of turning toward God. I used to have a "pure heart" offered and consecrated to Dr.James; now I had a true "consecrated" heart, turned to God alone.

The day before Xmas Eve a memorable thing happened. After I had averred that my heart was "no longer offered to him," I melted with a rush of the heart, when he came and presented to me the much-desired golden ear-rings, saying "they are from your Grandad!" and "If I treat you like a daughter will you treat me like a father?" I hugged him with heart's gratitude, and I felt looped in a golden moment.

And on Xmas Eve, because of the accident of having been found by the police in the snow at night, I found myself back in Craigdene. I obviously wasn't manic on this occasion because I had written that very day perceptively, succinctly, carefully about the meaning of being "a hermit"!

Chapter 77
The Black Year.

1994 was the worst and darkest year of my entire life! It began in a mental hospital, with the pain and meaninglessness of being put there when I was essentially well, and ended with a near-death experience and the horror of being put out of there "maintained" on a psychiatric medication which made my existence and my mind "like concrete."

The year was characterised by the "dissolution into the meaningless" of my first encounter there on Christmas day of a man shuffling along the corridor. In that previous week I had known a powerful "conversion" experience, which had "consecrated" my heart to God; I'd comprehended a whole concept, as if fresh from the mouths of the Desert Fathers, of how the call of the "hermit," was to dwell "out there somewhere," rejecting the values of society, dwelling prayerfully in a "cell," but always being there for those who "seek his understanding." A whole host of "Hermit's Rules" had flooded into my mind about the attitudes which could be maintained in order to live such a holy life. Sometimes "my manicness rides on the back of my enlightenments," but not in this case; I was perfectly "sane," healthy in my mind when the police lifted me from my walk in the snow that night. Having lost the key to get myself back in the house, and having the police set on me, they tracked me and arrested me, thinking that as I was "sectioned," they would just "return me to the place I belonged."

And so I met this man in the lock-up Ward 6, who was shuffling back and forth along the corridor, like the pacing of some caged animal. And trying to express the new meaning and purpose of my soul's life I greeted him with the words, "I am a hermit." He replied out of a world of petty, common and atheistic thought, a world of meaninglessness, "I'm a hermit too!" All he meant was that he liked living alone. And it hurt my heart immeasurably.

The ideal of "the Hermit's Rule" lived in me those winter months, and every chance I got I wrote about it, trying to make it into a whole. Dr.James graciously came to visit me, which made me feel that there was still some "care" there; and I showed him what I was creating. He laughed when he read "- -otherwise you are a dead duck." He laughed again when he read of the vow of silence, "- - you can always speak in Latin." Shortly after he had been to visit, I escaped to Edinburgh, carrying with me a rough copy of this "Rule." *The original rules which I'd written at home, were far more benign and wholesome, but because of the lurid touch added to my mind by the drugs, and because of the*

*element of coercion and fear in which I lived, they became a really
awful mixture of wisdom and madness.*

I was brought back from Edinburgh and again Dr.James came to visit
me on a lovely Spring day. This time I alarmed him by saying that I
couldn't abide eating apples any more after writing the rule of "you shall
not throw away your apple cores." For I suddenly rolled an apple
across the hard floor. He confided in me then about how much he
hated mental hospitals. On this occasion, seeing I had carefully for
weeks created the completed "Hermit's Rule" lovingly, with real ink and
an italic nib, I presented to him the finished copy, secreted in the
pocket of my hermit's jacket, asking him to "keep it safe." It has always
been a matter of great chagrin to me that he could never present it
back to me afterwards, and he said something to make me believe he
had burnt it! I held his hand and followed his car as it rolled away, and
he said "every time after I have been, you run away." "It's not running
away," I replied, "it's escaping." And I did it again, this time only getting
to the local village of Nethercraig.

All that winter, really crucified in that lock-up ward, stifled beyond my
endurance, I wrote very intense "black" poetry, about the "cage-like
walls" and about the rooks that hovered and circled over the roofs like
some ugly apocalypse. Finally, liberated on Good Friday by a removal
to Morlond Ward, I took my opportunity and escaped from there,
gloriously on Easter Sunday. And for a whole month,- for I had to be
absent for a whole month in order to break the power the section had
over me,- I gloried in my freedom in Lytham-St.Annes! Though I
suffered rather physically, not having enough money for the food and
warmth to keep me comfortable, I gloried in my emotional and spiritual
liberation, writing poetry every day about the boats and the beach and
the lovely way the light played on the sky and sands. I was so happy
for a while.

On my return, feeling fresh and free, I got involved with the tragic,
tortuous breaking-up of my friendship with Dr.James again, and ended
up heart-broken and tortured. I went on a trip to Iona to try and come
to terms with it, but couldn't. I also suffered mental ravages in the
continued efforts to get access to my son, as Walter used his
"domination games" to torment me at every turn. I was also making
efforts to leave my home and live in KirkOswald, as I sensed the "threat
of living in Dr.McNeill's territory" hanging over my head. Because of
these things, because of the pressure on me, I couldn't hold my act
together, and ended up sectioned in Craigdene again.

And so, for the whole year, I was only free May, June, July! I had tried to establish my freedom, by breaking the power of the mental health law, and only won 3 months of it! "You didn't last very long" was what Dr.James cruelly remarked.

At least it was Morlond ward I was incarcerated in for the last 5 months of the year, but they were long months which were a monotonous burden on my spirit. I never escaped this time, partly because I got the measure of the place, and made it my home. I had weekly visits to the dentist, because I was tormented by teeth problems. I tried to keep out of trouble. And I wrote. Finally I had "an argument" with a nasty nurse, a bathroom, whose steam was a danger to my manuscripts, and several syringes loaded with Largactil. I was overdosed; I had a nasty reaction and nearly died. They used that as an opportunity to establish me on a new, different drug, a depot injection called "Clopixol." I came out of there like a zombie at the end of the year. I remember when I visited Dr.James he drew a finger across my make-up to see how thick it was, and I knew that he knew I was existing with something like concrete poured into my brain; I was "deadened."

So that was the black year of '94; *the year when the doctors earnestly and threateningly declared; "you have a serious mental disease, and it is getting worse." They intimated; "we are thinking of taking away your house, and keeping you locked up in the hospital permanently!"*

I only narrowly avoided such a fate! If it weren't for my tenacity in escaping from the System, and for the much-appreciated help of dear Dr.James, such a fate would have been mine! Instead of these past 8 years of "real life," of soul-life, I would have been a "dead zombie" in the hospital!

Chapter 78
The Hermit's Rule.

I have become a Hermit,
and am given a Rule.

1) *Strive to keep quiet when your Master is thinking or speaking or listening.*
For-- In waiting for him strive only to answer his questions.

66) *Only when your deep need drives you to seek his understanding should you seek the   resting-place of your Master.*
For-- You need a good excuse.

3) *Therefore whatever you see your soul to desire according to God, do that thing.*
For-- So shall you keep you heart safe.

4) *Infinite bending of rules is always permitted, for they are rules-of-thumb;*
Don't do as I do, for -- I am a bad Hermit.

2) *Strive to attain the silence that is beyond words;*
For-- that is what you strive to attain.

5) *Maintain silence according to your Hermit's Vow, unless you can't help it.*
For-- Silence wastes words, and Words cost the silence.

20) *Be a good Hermit.*
For-- All your Rule is your penance, in being convicted of sin, and dying.

21) *Say to all your Friends, "I have failed you, but I will strive by grace of God*
*   not to fail you again."*
For-- The curses that are not forgiven before Death go on forever.

22) *Never sacrifice your integrity at the cost of your needs.*
For-- you must never use the right thing for the wrong purpose.

25) *It is not wise to arrive at someone's table hungry.*
For-- Custody of the senses lapses whilst one eats.

26) *It is not wise to enter anyone's dwelling as they may hold you to ransom.*
For-- You will pay with your integrity unless your trust is complete.

27) *It is not wise to confront anyone at any time for any reason, either in charity*
  or in anger,
For-- At best they will betray themselves and at worst they will kill.

24) *Strive to be first to God's love, and never let others come in behind you.*
For-- Otherwise you'll be a dead duck.

28) *Never ask hospitality of a member of a family whose needs are strained to*
  serve you.
For-- Hermits don't enter other people's houses.

29) *Never intrude on a Friend's heart or home.*
For-- Hermits dwell in the solitary spaces.

30) *No foundation for your cell; safe places only are permissible for the taking*
  of a roof.
For-- The only real "roof" is the stars!

33) *According to this Rule, Once you are committed, you go through with it.*
-- Think pure thoughts, and Evil shall not harm you.

32) *According to this Rule, You can pinch and you can beg all you like, provided*
it is in a good cause.
-- Not for the benefit of the self.

34) *According to this Rule, Custody of the body means when writing don't lose*
your head.
-- When writing on stone don't fall whilst walking down mountains!
-- You can't be saved unless you are a sinner.

35) *According to this Rule, Your humility lies in the custody of God's good gifts*

of the earth.
-- You shall not throw away your apple-cores!

80) *Hermits are allowed to speak in Latin at all times, for it is a holy language.*
-- Absolves from the vow of silence!

82) *Hermits are allowed to be resourceful;*
for -- they must rely on wits as well as God.

83) *Hermits are allowed to dislike people:*
for-- people can be evil, and God doesn't like Evil.

84) *Hermits are allowed to keep their heads and feet warm;*
for-- they must strive to keep well.

85) *Hermits are allowed to go to bed together and to cuddle like teddy-bears,*
provided they don't sleep; for the providing of warmth.

86) *Hermits are allowed to wear make-up; to keep the skin against the environment.*

87) *Hermits are allowed to glance in a mirror just momentarily; to make sure of*
their appearance.

88) *Hermits are allowed to chew gum; for the health of the teeth.*

89) *Hermits are allowed to comb their hair, only if someone combs it for them;*
for they aren't allowed to be vain.

90) *Hermits must conserve Everything.*

109) *According to this rule, I am only allowed to use what I am given.*
For-- You should honour the origin of the gift.

100) *Always strive to obey your Master.*
For-- He is God to you, and to be feared as a Father.

101) *It is wise to take care of yourself, of your whole being.*
For-- Only one body is given and your time is short.

107) *A hermit is only allowed to use or eat or accept or take what is genuinely*
   given from the heart.
For-- The vow of poverty must be absolute.

108) *Strive to take with you all you value and possess when you leave your cell,*
   and always be prepared.
For-- You never know whom you might meet: for "Often goes the Christ in the stranger's guise."

110) *Be prepared to eat whatever you touch.*
For-- It may be holy or it might be an instrument of death: for "I the Lord your God
am Holy."

104) *A hermit should never hasten over meals.*
For-- Manuscripts and water don't mix.

125) *A hermit strives to take what he is given, and to eat what he takes.*
For-- It is a judgement of God upon you, and may kill you.

126) *A hermit never loses anything.*
For-- If you can't remember where it is, where you put it, you don't deserve
to have it.

127)*A hermit never takes his feet off the ground, nor rides on wheels.*
For-- A hermit is an Earth-walker.

142) *The Privacy Rule: Hermits do not steal; they are honest among one another; there is to be no usury, borrowing or begging.*

143) *The Self-control Rule: Hermits are sincere individuals, seeking and loving Christ, caring for one another and for others, and blessed.*

144) *The Cleanliness Rule: Hermits keep mind and body clean; no impished behaviour, ablutions only in the morning, careful use of water.*

145) *Second Self-control Rule: Hermits outside their home must be controlled individuals at all times. For this explosion from a centre must be controlled.*

146) *Custody Rule: Hermits strive not to leave things half-finished, but to complete one thing before moving on to another; to "do it, drop it, and move on."*

147) *Rule of the Rune: Hermits strive to peace of mind, happiness, Nirvana, and "Deep Peace."*

148) *Rule of Achievement: Hermits allow access to the right kinds of people, in order to be taught.*

149) *"Be Cool" Rule: Hermits keep close, and have someone always there, and don't get excited at all in the company of other people.*

150) *"Be careful" Rule: Hermits are good custodians of their cells, and allow only trustworthy friends in the door.*

103) *Beware the Devil who goes around seeking whom he may devour, steadfast in faith.*
For-- Nothing worth attaining in life is easy.

154) *Make aims that are viable;*
For-- Otherwise you sin.

156) *When you make Mistakes, you pay for them, and Walk on.*
For-- God always forgives.

158) *Be true to your Vocation, true to yourself, true to others,*
And strive to be a good Hermit.

Chapter 79
Escape to Big City Streets.

I believe I was put straight into the lock-up ward, when I was re-admitted at Christmas '93, in order to prevent my escape attempts, because I was becoming well-known for my "escapes." When I once heard them referred to as "running away," I replied with indignation that it was "escaping," because indeed they required as much planning and as much guts as a POW escape from the Nazi fortress of Colditz! For you were watched all the time! Not only was every door locked before and behind you, even the toilets, but it seemed there were more nurses watching each patient than there were patients in the ward! I heard it said that it was supposed to be "one-to-one care," but I remember the sense of an endless bevy of female nurses all watching me and being my warders!

I remember how, when I'd only been there for a week, I felt violated to the core when all this bevy of female nurses, at least five at the one time, all leapt on top of me on my bed, and held me down and injected me with one of those horrible long-term drugs. Its technical name I can remember was Zuchlopenthixol Acetate, or "Acuphase," and it was designed to give a long-term shock to the mind, to make it adapt to a new phase. I knew I was well at the time, and wasn't manic, and the sense of being so "robbed of my right mind" by this drug was a horror to me. When they let loose the pressure of all kneeling on top of me, I leapt up and tried to "beat them up." But it was no good, they all hid behind the closed door, holding it shut by the pressure of their bodies. Now this was the very room where I had been incarcerated and maltreated during my pregnancy. According to the new Mental Health law it was illegal to "lock you up" in such a room any more; this was made a nonsense of in that they all stood at the door, watching me from its window. I tried to block this window with a towel, but they kept removing it.

From that very moment, motivated by my sense of outrage, I started hatching my plan. I remember trying to stretch a longer and longer lead, by getting them to let me out on the patch of grass, watched by them from the windows. I tried to win a moment when I wasn't watched, a moment, a chance, a slim opportunity. I can't clearly and completely remember how I ended up in the local village of Nethercraig in the dark, carrying my essential clothes in wash-bags, but I believe I went for a mad dash through the fire-escape of the female bedroom, having planned this for a time when there was a hand-over of nurses. At hand-over time they were vulnerable, as they were less vigilant. I think I managed to get in the bedroom, usually locked up, by saying I was going to collect something, and I had planned my clothes and bags to be already packed. It was very scary, feeling I would be "punished" if my attempt failed; I must have walked swiftly down the main road for a mile in the dark, hoping I would make it due to the nurses'disorientation. It was even more scary, having got to the village, realising that the only way out of it, was to carry on into a wide unknown and unlit darkness.

Now what was I to do? There was only one unlit country road in front of me, and very soon it would be crawling with police cars, combing this country area for me. It was miles to anywhere; even if there were any buses I couldn't catch the bus back, which passed through Craigdene; besides which I only had one £ coin on me; where could I go with that? I was so intent on just the "escape attempt," that I hadn't planned any further ahead!

A car came towards me with blazing headlights; I realised it might be a police car, but I would make one desperate throw. I stood right in front of it, waving my arms; and when it stopped I asked the young man, trying not to sound suspiciously like an escapee from a mental hospital; "Please could you give me a lift back to the main road, as I've missed the bus back!" The ruse must have seemed plausible; I got a lift to a bus-shelter along the main road to Inveroth. I walked along that road for a bit, still wondering how to get as swiftly as I could out of the area. I was along another dark country minor road, when I took another risk of stopping a car again, standing in front of its blazing headlights. They dropped me off at a major roundabout. I saw the sign to Inveroth and there hatched out my plan of trying to reach there and get to the house of Matty, whose address I knew. A bus came along; I practically stood right in front of it, trying to flag it down. When it stopped the female drive was furiously angry with me, saying it was a dangerous thing to do; realising I only had one miserable £ coin, I presented it to her, saying I'd pay the rest on getting off. Once in Inveroth I played this trick again, saying to a taxi driver that my "boyfriend" would pay the fare, once he got me to that address.

And so I ended up knocking on Matty's door in the middle of the night. Once in that flat I felt trapped there. Asking Matty to take me in, I let him partly make love to me, without intercourse, and then found the next morning that I was flooded with blood; I couldn't understand so heavy a period, and was scared by it. To be fair to Matty, he tried to look after me, giving me food, and warmth and a bed to sleep in; he even, being penniless, obtained food like eggs and bacon from his mothers; I remember how I had a terrible "fear of open spaces" when he took me to the supermarket. But he was very bad-tempered with me; I remember him shouting at me whilst doing the hoovering; and because he was worried about all this blood, I was afraid that he was going to insist on getting a doctor.

After staying for a few days, I felt really "enthralled to him," and wanted to get free; so when he was out once, I made my attempt to get away from the house. The thing was, I didn't feel "safe" there. I managed to find my way to the bus-station, but became fearful there of meeting any Craigdene nurses, and I had no money, so I walked on to a petrol-station, where I found a "nice bloke" filling up his big-wheeled AA truck. So I bravely asked if he could give me a lift; "I'm going to Edinburgh," he replied, "hop in." Basically my "need" was so great that I was willing to throw myself at anybody who would enable me to stay out of that ghastly hospital!

So I rode with this "nice bloke" to Edinburgh, in his big-wheeled truck, and I remember feeling terribly glad and grateful to him when he finally paid the toll over the bridge. I felt "I'm out of Kirkshire; I'll be safe now." Partly out of gratitude I gave him hugs and kisses, before getting out of the truck, saying that I would meet him at that same hotel where I alighted the following night. I went into this hotel, with that strange touch of "unreality" in my mind, convinced that I could walk in, in confidence like my Dad used to do, register at the desk, and it be accepted that I pay later. Now I had secreted in a secret compartment in my handbag, not only that rough copy of "the Hermit's Rule," which was so precious to me, but also an old check-book. I felt that somehow I might be able to survive on this check-book; so I flounced past the receptionist, got shown a room, and was convinced that I could somehow pull this off. But when I went back out, to get something to eat, the receptionist challenged me to "sign in." Apparently I aroused suspicion, because when I came back to the hotel I found my belongings thrown out onto the street, and a burly man saying to me "we don't want your sort here." It then struck me forcibly, with a blue hat on my head and my stuff in carrier-bags, I must have appeared like a "bag-lady." When I went into a pub, and asked a man, "would you like to buy me a drink," I got the same reaction from the bar-tender of, "we don't want your sort here."

Chagrined in the extreme, I spent the rest of the night, for it was now very late in the evening, trudging back and forth along a certain street which was replete with B &B's and guest-houses, trying to obtain a roof over my head. I felt sure, convinced, that if only I could get a foothold

320

in Edinburgh, I could then stay there for a month, and write out my "Hermit's Rule." I felt sure that if I could just convince somebody else to trust me, and not reject me as a seeming "bag-lady," I could solve the money problem later. I thought that if I waved the cheque book in the air, and say "I'll pay the £20 in the morning," everything would be alright! But it wasn't; everybody rejected me at the door. I even went to one guest house, which had a pub, showing to the landlady, not only the cheque book but also my copy of the "Hermit's Rule," thinking that this would convince her. But she told me to "get out," probably thinking that rough little book was some kind of secret esoteric manuscript belonging to the Freemasons; she certainly took fright.

Then at 2 o'clock in the morning, tramping the streets forlornly, a sudden accident occurred. My foot slipped on the edge of the kerb, and my ankle fell over. It was very painful; I couldn't walk on it any more. So there I was limping along the pavement, in a quiet deserted street at 2 am., when a man came behind and said "Are you alright?" "No," I replied, "I can't walk; I think I've broken my ankle." "I'll help you," said this kind young man, and he supported me as I limped along the street. He asked me where I was going, and when I said "nowhere," as I hadn't been able to find a bed for the night, he offered to let me stay in his flat. This was a wonderfully kind young man, a genuine "good Samaritan." He helped me up the stairs of this flat, explaining that he shared it with others, and making me comfortable in the kitchen. He was wonderfully kind and gentlemanly, even offering me a clean towel. I saved this towel afterwards, taking it with me, in memory of this lovely kind man. That night I painfully hobbled to the bathroom, and managed to wash my hair there, hoping no-one would mind my using of some shampoo.

In the morning all his flat-mates trooped in the kitchen, and, on seeing my ankle which had swollen enormously, they insisted on taking me to the hospital to get it looked at. I wasn't terribly afraid of the hospital, as I was more afraid of having a broken ankle. I was left at the hospital with a student who spoke little English explaining the circumstances in which I was found; I was hoping this group of students would give me the means of returning to their flat, but no such luck! I think my great downfall in this new atmosphere of the Edinburgh Infirmary was that, in pain during a long wait, I recited all my prayers, such as the Credo our Father and Hail Mary, in Latin, which was my custom. I think this alarmed the staff into thinking I was doing strange incantations or "speaking in tongues." For, after they had done an X-ray, finding that the ankle was "smashed up," but without a broken bone, and strapping it up, they then wouldn't let me go. It could have been that I couldn't give a proper address, or couldn't give them a birth-date to match an NHS number on their computers. Whatever the reason, they called for a psychiatrist to examine me, and then forwarded me to the Edinburgh Royal which is a psychiatric hospital.

I remember very well how I wasn't sure that this was a psychiatric hospital when I went in there; they just shoved my wheelchair into an empty smoking room and left me there. I remember being very aware when seeing a female doctor that I must not under any circumstances seem "ill," or "mentally distressed," that I mustn't put a foot wrong. And I didn't; I replied to all her questions carefully and calmly, but without giving her my real name, birthdate or any means that they could identify me; because I obviously didn't want to be sent back to Craigdene! *And she said to me, "start from a hundred and I want to you to tell me the successive numbers, taking off 7 at a time!" So I proceeded, doing it correctly, having a very quick and agile mathematical mind; and because I got this difficult task right, she concluded "you are ill."* It was rather like that doctor in that hospital in Aberdeen once, saying "you must be ill, because no-one can remember the exact words they spoke a week ago"!

I managed the best I could there; the boss-nurse soon took away my wheel-chair, saying I was getting in the way. I was determined not to give away my true identity; social workers were sent to interrogate me, because they couldn't find any medical records for me; I gave my name as "Marie James," wanting to belong to Dr.James. Apparently the reason I finally got found out was because I mentioned to one of these social workers the name of Philip Davidson, who was a known social worker in the Edinburgh area. And so one day, about 4 days later perhaps, I looked down the corridor to find "big Rob," the charge nurse of Morlond ward, together with a nurse called Denise, coming toward me. I had just been sitting on my bed, balancing my handbag on the one finger and my glasses on the other finger, and the girl opposite had commented "she's new, she's a bit strange." *The point is, I had begun to feel "safe," which meant to me, safe from being taken back to Craigdene.*

And they stuffed me in a wheelchair and wheeled me along the corridor at a great pace, and I cried out "mind my best dress in the wheels." But they paid no heed, and hastened me into a car in the car-park, and I remember my strapped-up leg wouldn't fit into there, but they just stuffed me in unceremoniously, as if something important depended on the haste. And I felt violated, before we even began the long journey back. I felt tragic as we went over the bridge back into Kirkshire, and as we wound along its country roads in the dark I screamed with a kind of terror. When asked why I was screaming I said I had in my mind the fright of going along those roads, of standing in front of car's headlights in the dark.

And so it was all in vain; the "grand escape" was all in vain; I was taken all the way back! I remember how I was man-handled when we got back; I remember how they rushed and carried me through to Morlond ward like carrying a carpet between them. And I remember being injected in a bed with Largactil, Rob saying he would try to keep me in Morlond ward, but I wailed and cried, so they said they would have to return me to the lock-up ward, as I was "disturbing the other patients." And I remember being put into a position facing the wall, in the very room I had escaped from, and I turned into a foetal position for comfort, but they gave me more injections in my backside. *And so I was back, faced with enduring again the long "daily dying."*

Chapter 80
Escape to Village Claustrophobia.

I licked my wounds for a while, after the failure of my Edinburgh escape. For those long dark cold winter months I "daily died" with the stultifying effect of being incarcerated in such a "prison." I remember writing of the boarded-up taped-up and smashed-up windows, "what chance or what hope is there for us when we are not even allowed to see the sky!" They wouldn't take the risk of letting me out onto the green patch of grass any more; I spent my time trying to negotiate round the mental mine-field that existed, between the nurses forcing me to take medication on the one hand, and the small group of hostile sometimes-violent young men who were incarcerated with me on the other hand. But I tried to spend my time creatively at least by carefully writing out in real ink and italic pen the "Hermit's Rule" that I had created.

I remember I was doing this once when George McPherson, my new solicitor came past my door; apparently he had been to visit one of the young men about their sectioning. Surprised to see me there he came in, and I asked him earnestly what chance I had of ever getting my son back. *And he replied "there's not much chance for you of any sort whilst you are in the lock-up ward of a mental hospital! Don't you realise this is the lock-up ward you are in!" He told me I had to get out of there and out of the "Psychiatric System" before he had an opportunity to fight for my rights by taking the thing back to court. (But he was true to his word and did fight for me after I had got "out of the System" in '95, winning Access rights for me in the late'90's.) But back then in that winter I felt I had no hope!*

Then one day a social worker took me on a trip to my home, and hope surged in me when I clandestinely got hold of money! What this new social worker and Steven Peterson had done, early when I was admitted in January had outraged me. They had gone to my house, used my keys to gain entrance, without my knowledge, and brought bags of clothes away, together with some old handbags containing things precious to me, like treasured cards, jewellery and crucifixes. When I had accidentally seen these handbags in the valuables cupboard, I had screamed out "they're mine, they're mine!" And when told Steven Peterson had uplifted them from the safety of my own home, and put them in such a hospital cupboard, I was outraged; "How dare he do such a thing!" But I was told that the social worker had complete and utter "responsibility" over my house and possessions when I was sectioned in hospital! This was why the hospital always took the house-keys off you and locked them up!

One thing I always dreaded was having my house-keys locked up in the hospital, as it meant if I escaped I couldn't get back into my own house. So when Dr.James came to visit me, that time that I handed over to him my completed "Hermit's Rule" manuscript, I managed to get these keys handed over to him. Then one day, having finally managed to persuade them that I needed pants and tights and underwear, a trip was organised to take me to my house. What followed was really stupid. After going to the post office I proceeded to walk to Dr.James' surgery, believing he had the keys. And they stood in my way along the street, and manhandled me, saying I wasn't allowed to walk along the street, because I was sectioned. But I had lived in that area as a "sectioned patient" since '88; so how could being "sectioned" make a difference! They refused to let me go to the Health Centre, choosing then to reveal to me the fact that Dr.James had handed the keys back in again; but unfortunately they had gone off without them! This was farcical! So there were no keys and we couldn't get in the door, so I sat down on my doorstep forlornly. And they physically grabbed hold of me and tried to force me to get back in the car. I used "passive resistance," saying "Why can't I sit on my own doorstep!" But they threatened "if you don't come now, we will get the police to remove you!"

I was badly shaken up by this event, by the way I was maltreated, by the way I was thought to have no "possession" of my own house, or ability to sit on its doorstep or walk along the street, because I was "sectioned"! It made no sense when I'd lived there "sectioned" for the past 6 years!

The occasion made me change my feelings and attitude toward the nurse who was present, called Ritchie, who up until then I had really liked. We got a chance though of going for my underwear on another day, and it was then that I happened to find an envelope containing a £100 in my cupboard, next to my DSS documents. I remembered the sense of silent awe on finding it, and the way I quickly secreted it away in my handbag, whilst the nurse was calling on me. It was that money which enabled me to escape all the way to Lytham-St.Annes at Easter. So I was ready to make another escape attempt; not only had I given over into the "safe hands" of Dr.James the manuscript I treasured, but now I had money!

I planned it meticulously. This time I intended getting on the bus, so that I could escape from the surrounding countryside quickly, and not be left trying to get lifts along country lanes in the dark! The nurses, although they let me sit on a seat by the green patch of grass, to write my poetry, yet checked my existence there every two minutes. So I only had this "window of two minutes" to be gone and get clean away. I found out the bus times and watched for their regularity day after day. I worked out how I could pack a blue wash-bag of valuable things I wanted to take with me, especially my poetry, and carry it always with me, so they would get used to the sight of it by the seat. I also timed everything the nurses did, to try and work out the best opportune moment.

Finally I hit that opportune moment; I had layers of warm clothes on, I had my bag with me, the bus was due imminently, and the nurses weren't in that moment watching. I got up and made for the bus-stop in the dark. Unfortunately that 64 bus was that day a little late, and it was still heading in the Nethercraig direction; it was due to turn round there and come back past the hospital, before offering me the freedom of an escape from the area. With adrenalin passing through me, I decided I'd get on it there and take the risk of coming back past the hospital in five minutes; I thought that the safer bet. As I hurriedly got on it, shielding my face, that nurse Ritchie whom I had for ages liked, got off. *There was a quick glance, a quick flash of recognition between us; he had seen me!*

Now I was running scared; I didn't dare stay on the bus for its journey back, because they would surely be waiting for me, when Ritchie reported it, so I got off at the far end of the village of Nethercraig. I went feeling scared into someone's back garden; there I tried to calm myself down, looking at the stars, and trying to relax my adrenalin-pumped consciousness. I wondered whether I could perhaps stay there till the morning, sleeping outside. There was a boat in this back garden; I put my wash-bag in there, intending to climb into it. "Oh no, it's full of water!" A paroxysm of fear grasped me, for my manuscripts were in the bag! I couldn't get over it; "what a stupid thing to do!" I was too shook up to think of staying in that garden after that.

I had to find somewhere I felt "safe." I could only relax, feel OK in my mind, or ever be able to go to sleep, when I felt "safe." This was always true of my escapes, and why I was sometimes driven so far away, to find refuge in strange hitherto-unknown places. This had been the reason why I couldn't stay at Matty's when I was in Inveroth; I didn't feel "safe" there. *Really I always had to flee far enough away so that I felt Craigdene couldn't grab me and get me back. I always felt Craigdene was like as spider on the map of the countryside!*

So I knew I had to get away from the area, before the streets should be filled with ambulances and police cars looking for me. I latched onto a couple of mothers walking along the street with their children and dogs, thinking that this would divert the police attention away from me, as they would look for a solitary figure. I asked these women if they knew of a taxi service in Nethercraig. I was told there was a taxi service from a house nearby, across the street from where this woman lived. I enquired at the door, and was told I must come back in a half-hour. This woman invited me to wait in her house. Waiting in this house was horrible; it was disgustingly dirty and smelly, with lots of tumbling children and cats and dogs. Then a dog did a shit in the cat-litter tray, and the stench filled the room; I couldn't endure any more of it. I looked across the road at the taxi-driver's house, and saw a commotion of police around the place, with blue flashing lights.

Why I did what I did next, I really don't know! I somehow felt that if I walked straight through them it wouldn't harm me; that I was unhurtable, untouchable, that God would protect me. I had in mind that notion of Pater Leo's when he sent me back from Austria; "you shall walk through fire and it shall not harm you!" *I really thought I could walk through this mass of four police vans and umpteen geared-up police officers with their walkie-talkies, all of whom were looking for me, and pass myself off as another person! It was rather like the unreality of that belief in Edinburgh that I would be able to get lodgings, a roof over my head that night, by waving a dud check-book! There was certainly, perhaps due to that initial "Acuphase" injection, a certain fog of unreality surrounding my mind!*

So I tried to walk straight through all these police-officers and flashing blue lights, and one of them challenged me, "Mairi? Is that Mairi?" "No," I replied, marching straight on, "my name is Theresa." Again I was challenged, and again replied the same. I thought I could pull it off! It didn't work of course; I was stopped, stuffed in a police-van, and returned to my "prison."

327

Chapter 81
The True Death.

The poetry I wrote in my Craigdene prison that winter was harrowing. I wrote of a place that is "eyeless, roofed-over with an eyeless mindless deadness," containing souls that were "eyeless," stunned in psychiatric sickness, with my "poet's mind, poet's responsiveness" incarcerated in it. I had the image of the continuously circling crows that perched on the rooftops "like an apocalyptic swarm ready to peck out the eyes." I called upon the "Saviour," who "created the eyes to let life and love in," to "rescue me from the true Death."

And this "true Death" to me was to exist in such a place were minds were made deadened and unresponsive. It seemed to me like a torture-chamber where minds were mercilessly processed; you were forcibly "treated," every movement of your thought or feeling was checked, stamped on, overcome, until you were reduced to a thing feelingless and dead. It seemed to me you were robbed of any individuality, any spark of resistance or soul-life, until you were made into the "sameness" of your persecutors. I had so much sympathy, such "primal sympathies" with the violent, rebellious young men in there, who shared this incarceration with me, because they represented the "dispossessed of the earth." The System devised by the privileged and free was concentrated into controlling them and crowing over their spirits. I seemed to see it all so clearly. *And then having forcibly overcome and beaten them, they claimed, nodding heads wisely, "we have made you better, you are settled now." I had a sense of outrage reaching to the skies!*

"There is no life here"; life was stamped out. There were all around me minds in torment, minds abused, minds suffering; and no life or hope anywhere; "hope dies its daily wreckage in me." Such imprisonment was "a long daily dying;" "imprisonment wraps its long and lonely, deadly fingers around me." We weren't even able to see the sky, that small blue square which to a prisoner can give hope; for the windows were all boarded or smashed or taped-up; "each window-pane nailed up to the cross-beam of an insane mockery."

Even the sight of the occasional crocus or daffodil, on an occasional nurse-accompanied walk, could barely cheer me; "whilst I daily die, the mad wind burdens me with the daffodils." They made me think, momentarily, tenderly and sadly of my past love-affair. But there were no wings existing in my soul that could flutter, or raise me above the "death" of the place.

328

And this "true Death" seemed to have no connection with the death of the crucified Christ; it was "a living death that has no connection with Your death in its nobility and saving power and love." This living death that I couldn't tolerate seemed to me worse than Christ's dying; instead of "something meaningful, soul-life and real," it was a "dissolution into meaninglessness which makes a soul meaningless and Void."

My soul screamed in anguish when I wasn't allowed to go near a church, or in any way to celebrate Easter; I felt how I'd missed one of "seventy seasons given to us to celebrate our Saviour's risen life." On the Good Friday I was moved to Morlond Ward, and it seemed to me I had "merely moved from one prison to another." For Dr.Dawson who supervised Ward 6 had spoken to me and said how I wasn't going to be quickly let out and returned home as usually happened; they were planning to slowly move me from Morlond Ward to the long-term rehab ward, and then out to the cottages which were attached to the hospital. They were intending to take my house away from me, so I could be "kept in the hospital permanently." Why? Because according to him,- and the words yet ring in my ears, - *"You have a serious mental disease which is getting worse."*

And so, that Good Friday, I made a resolution that I had to somehow at all cost get away and keep away for a month, in order to break the power that the mental health law, and the System and Craigdene had over me! It was going to be "a daring death-defying act," but I was going to strike a blow for freedom! It wasn't only for my own sake, to escape from a system that was closing around me and intended never to let me return to life and be free; it was also for every body else's sake. I believed that in doing this I would light a beam of hope for everybody else, for every other suffering soul stuck in the System!

And so I planned an escape again, this time having it well planned, with a proper waterproof bag, good shoes, a black woollen throw to keep the rain and chill off my head, and money in my purse! I planned it to take place on Easter Sunday at lunchtime, when people's attention would be diverted. That Mental health law was designed with a loophole in it, the assumption that if you could prove yourself well enough to keep free for one month, then you must be "mentally well" enough not to be in hospital. This was what I was aiming to prove.

Thus I found myself writing on a seat at dusk the night before my attempt, trembling at the sense of the risk to my life, health, safety, and the degree of punishment should I fail, telling myself "Be brave, my soul, be courageous." For I was going to "take destiny in my hands, assert my self as free master, captain of a ship that steers a course, and has an inalienable right to be free."

Chapter 82
The Great Easter Escape.

Easter Sunday lunchtime arrived; the time I had set to "assert my right to be free." The nurses were serving tasty chicken-legs in the dining-room; I remember thinking I would have liked to have stayed and had some. But a greater purpose beckoned me. I was wearing many layers of clothing, with that black stole round my shoulders, and carrying a new proper transparent kit-bag I had obtained, containing my poetry and a change of clothes; I intended to travel light. I had got the nurses used to seeing me always carrying this bag around.

Morlond ward was easier to escape from than ward 6; though the front door was relentlessly watched, there was a back door behind the dining room which led onto the patio, and there was a stiff wooden garden gate opening from this patio onto the grass beyond. I chose my moment, and quickly slipped out of this patio door. Once on the green grass, I headed for the farm, as I was relatively safe on the farm road. Having experienced several failures getting stuck in the village of Nethercraig, I had decided to head the other direction, to the town of Kirkcraig; as the trick wasn't just escaping from the hospital, it was escaping from the surrounding area. I intended to walk to Kirkcraig. It would have to be as quick as I could, as most of it would be along the main road, and nurses would probably be using that road on the way to work and back, as the handover time was approaching. But the thing was, once in Kirkcraig, I could get away from the area by bus or train.

I was so scared, especially when the farm-road joined the main road and I faced the risk of nurses in the traffic; I knew I would be punished if found escaping; I would be put back in the lock-up ward with injections. I kept thinking how, if I were caught, I would pretend to be just going for a walk to write my poetry. It began to rain. I pulled the stole around my head, and held the bag under my arm, trying to keep my writings dry. I walked as fast as I could in what became pouring rain, until I reached the railway station. I had a £100 in cash with me; I didn't care how much money I initially spent on escaping. When the ticket man asked me where I wanted a ticket to, I replied "Where is your next train going to?" But I afterwards thought what a suspicious thing this was to say, and sat miserably on a seat waiting for the train to Invertay, scared that at any moment I was going to feel "the long arm of the law" take hold of my collar!

I'll never forget that wait for that train, because in my scared frame of mind it seemed interminable. *I sat on the seat in the rain, feeling this was such a "brave attempt," but so afraid of capture, gazing placidly into a rainwater pool. The water went drip, drip. And my mind was steeled to be "caught" at any moment. I was such a picture of patience, of waiting endurance, with "the slow slipping of time into the sad mind."*

I got to Invertay, and there felt scared again, as I believed the ticketman would phone the police to say I was on the train; I expected the police to be waiting for me at the station's entrance. But they weren't, and I breathed a sigh of relief and headed for the bus-station. Again I made the mistake of saying to the ticket-man "Where's the next bus going to?" It must have sounded suspicious, for he replied "Are you in trouble, are you running away or something?" So I found myself getting on the bus to Glasgow. I got to Glasgow and there felt scared again, as I felt it would be reported that I was on that bus. It was dark in Glasgow by now, and there were a lot of police about the street. I decided that what I would do was catch a bus to England; I would be safer there once "over the border." I was a bit hazy about whether the Scottish Mental Health Act would apply in England; I just wanted to get as far away from Kirkshire as possible. So I caught the overnight bus to Manchester. I had a hazy idea that I would go to hide for a month somewhere in my native county of Yorkshire, to somewhere I knew like Ilkley. I couldn't go home to my parent's address, obviously, as the police would go looking for me there; apparently they always did. But I felt it would be a comfort to be somewhere near my parents' Yorkshire home.

But waking in the middle of the night from a horrid and fitful sleep on this bus, I once again felt scared, dreading that the police would somehow trace my movements. I decided there and then that instead of waiting till the bus hit the vast city of Manchester, and instead of branching off to the right into Yorkshire, I would go off to the left into Lancashire; largely because I had some kind of knowledge of Lytham-St.Annes, some happy memories of holidays there with my Mum and my Grandad when I was a child. The bus was in Preston, stopping there briefly at 4 a.m., and I suddenly decided to get off. And providence seemed to offer me a helping hand, because there stood a taxi, a people-carrier, with the driver shouting "Anyone for Lytham-St.Annes?"

And so I arrived in Lytham-St.Annes at about 6 on a cold grey morning, hungry and tired, on a Monday morning at the beginning of April! The man who was the taxi-driver, called Gus, was basically a kind man though I came to dislike him later. When I let him know that I had nowhere to go, he offered to let me stay in his new flat, where he was living on his own, having split from his wife. He provided food and warmth for me when I first arrived, but I didn't like the way he tried to get sexual in the bed. So I straight away started to seek alternative accommodation and some kind of job, as I wouldn't have enough money to keep myself for a whole month.

I remember one day I wasted money going all the way to Manchester on the train to obtain Lithium, believing this was necessary to keep me well; I had to go far away because I believed they would trace these things through the NHS computers. The chemists would only give me an "emergency dose" of five days at a time, so I had to go round to lots of different chemists, lying to them all, to get a month's supply. I got to be quite good at lying! I went to the Jobcentre in Blackpool, walking all the way and making my feet very sore, and told a pack of lies about my situation, and my background, and they believed me. I remember I was quite astonished when I got that job in the holiday-home hotel, because the employer believed me when I wove a story which was a pack of lies!

This live-in job was onerous, because they treated me like slave-labour, were very mean with the food they provided, gave me half the minimum wage, and were extremely unkind to me. I was the kitchen skivvy. But I was proud of myself, because I supported myself; I was fighting for the life and freedom that was mine! I wanted to come back saying "look what I did." *If I could survive on my own and hold down a job for a month without anyone suspecting that I am a psychiatric case, then I didn't deserve, didn't need to be locked up in a psychiatric hospital for that 6 months which was threatened; I just wanted to prove that point!*

I suffered but was determined to endure. I remember, being bent towards this endless kitchen scrubbing, and urged round cleaning the rooms so fast sometimes, I looked out of the windows wistfully at the sunlight and the sparkling sea, wishing I could be out there. Gus didn't help, though he had kindly lent me a small TV, by offering me a £100 as well as free board to go back to him; "what a creep" I thought, because it amounted to making me a prostitute. But soon I couldn't stand this job any longer; my ankle had become very painful, because I was always on my feet, so I used this excuse to say "I quit"; in a sense I was sacked at the same time. My employer Colleen said that if I left the room in five days, then signed something and left the keys, she would give me £50 in wages. I would have ten days left that I needed to stay, and only £50 plus the £20 I had left to spend; how could it be done? Again Providence seemed to offer me a helping hand, in that I asked around in the local Catholic church on the Sunday, and a landlady agreed to let me have a small attic-room, with no food at all provided, for £50 for that ten days!

My employer Colleen treated me badly and shabbily that day I left; I remember struggling out of the door with my TV with no help and not one kind word; I offered my hand, trying to be nice; "I hope we don't part with hard feelings; I've learnt something from the experience, and I've done some good writing." But she turned away saying in a broad accent "I've learnt something an'all." I felt like one of last century's maidservants leaving in disgrace!

I was hungry at the other place! I didn't have enough money left for food, and ended up combing the shops and supermarket for anything with reduced prices, even if it were a tin of cold sausages when I am a vegetarian. I was in the mentality of "if it's cheap I'll eat it," like a human dustbin! I had no means of course of heating anything up; when you don't eat hot tasty nutritious food for a long while, something inside of you wilts. And in this hungry state I faced real temptation in the form of Gus. For he offered me again the invitation of free accommodation with him, plus £100! Now no-one has known real temptation until they have been tempted by riches in a state of hunger! I was disgusted that he should make that offer to me; it was wicked to offer to someone hungry the chance of selling their body to gain money! I said "I don't want to mix money matters with a matter of integrity"; he replied that really it was "not only sex, but love and friendship," and that afterwards I could go back up to Scotland "with no harm done." I said No. I didn't choose that option because I felt it betrayed the love in my heart; my love of Dr.James.

For Dr.James in that place was always present to me, guiding me and directing me, and keeping him to the fore of my mind and heart gave me wisdom. "I've kept myself pure for you," was the truth of it. And so I struggled, and suffered to earn my freedom in that place. I'd always been in bondage there; first to a man, then to slave-labour, then to hunger; but I had a sense of my soul as free, both by its power of love and by its poetry. My love of Dr.James got me through it; whilst crumpled on my knees, he reigned in my mind and heart. I could say "for the sake of the prize set before me, I've run a straight race"; the prize was the hope of happiness restored; thinking of him gave me the stamina.

And so having first checked up with Dr.James on the phone that I would return liberated for my section on that date, I returned on the buses on Monday 2nd May. I threw a backward glance, writing, "Land of Light, Coast of Grace, Lytham I shall remember you."

For in that place I had come "alive" and been transformed. Writing journals, poetry and lively conversations, studying and typing in the library, an awareness of beauty,
had returned my mind to its usual well-stimulated state. *How could I deserve to be locked up when I'd lived a creative and meaningful life for a month! I so readily returned to a real and creative life when put out there in the world! So what justification was there for making me spend lost months of my life locked up!*

The outside world of sand, sea, sky, with its magnificent interplay of light which had inspired the painter Turner, the sunsets and stars and moon, and the Spring with its churches, daffodils, blossom and bursting buds, had entered in my soul and altered me. *When I arrived, the trees were bare, the wind cold, and I was huddled away, collapsed in myself, uncreative, full of the long ache of fear. But after a month there, I was replete, rich in love, and brave, my soul singing its creativity to the skies. Beauty had opened up my heart, gifting me with happiness, poetry, freedom, worth. So I left Lytham with sadness.*

Chapter 83
The Ultimate Freedom.

The first poem I wrote in Lytham-St.Annes expressed the belief that *"Ultimate Freedom, silver-sea-freedom, rainbow-freedom, star-freedom, exists, and is worth the striving for."* I found it! Through my suffering and endurance I found it, in that land of Light and Spring!

I found there was "a wild majestic world out there," of sand, sea, sky and starlight, outside the circling of men's lamplight, of the orange lights which circled the promenade, and it became a world which intoxicated me. I watched the sunsets, the moon-rises, the stars wheeling and the wide expanse of sky and sand in all the changes of the light, and I sensed the "glad movements of creation" like some complex dance. It took me out of myself; the beauty gifted me with Freedom, and the freedom with happiness.

I was possessed at first by an intense hatred of Dr.McNeill, reflecting on how he saw me as "mentally lame." He had put a report in to the Children's Panel; "she has had a relapse into schizo-affective psychosis." It was like saying "she has a lame mind," like treating me as a "sick thing," when really I was a living whole creative person with a small defect; and that was the very "defect" that informed my creativity. He saw me a permanently sick with brief interludes of sanity. So how did he think I got a degree?! In actual fact, if I got into a manic state, it equally quickly abated. I was someone capable of flaring up, but equally capable of returning quickly to a normal and creative life. What I minded was not my illness, but the prison of other people's minds that it put me in. My illness was not my cross; other people's attitude toward it was.

But there also existed in me a capability of appreciating beauty, and a devoted love of Dr.James. And gradually in that place the Beauty and the Love gained the upper hand. And I was transformed and became really "alive." I used to wander amid the birds and boughs, daffodils and blossom of Spring, remembering him, yearning for him. And that love indeed kept me alive; it was "the inspiration of all that is purest and best in me."

It was that love which made me make the choice I made; of suffering slave-labour and then suffering real horrible physical hunger and need, rather than accepting a roof over my head and a free £100, offered by the taxi-driver Gus. I felt this offer of his a "nasty deed" because it was such a dire temptation; without hot tasty food inside of you for a long time, the spirit wilts; I could have eaten with that money! Yet I turned the temptation aside; "I kept myself pure for you."

It was so hard in that place to "earn my freedom," but it was by my love of Dr.James that I got through it; for he was always present to me, guiding and directing me. His presence reigned in my mind and heart, giving me the stamina. It was "for the sake of the prize set before me," that I endured; that prize was "the hope of happiness restored," the happiness of being with him. "I've won life and freedom because I loved you; love of you has given me life."

The whole reason I endured it was to earn my freedom! I hoped that "all things would be given back to me," my house, my son and my love-affair. I was glad to think I would no longer be on the section, so I would no longer have a home as a prison-cell, able to go where I wanted. It struck me that in order to really achieve something there, to protect that "ultimate freedom" that I was about to win, it would be best to move home and build a new life; otherwise, if ever sectioned again, I'd be more "punished" than ever, and I might lose the advantage I'd gained. I was glad to think now that "ultimate freedom" was approaching; when the month was up I would be a genuine "free agent," able to go wherever I liked!

The weak part regarding this "prize" of happiness, I realised, lay in whether Dr.James would still be "there for me." My desire was so pure; all I wanted was that he accept the self-offering of my soul; "I ask so purely from you; I don't ask for anything but yourself, your listening ears and your listening heart." Yet I couldn't know how he would respond, and so was shot through as my return approached with a sense of "absolute uncertainty." I was scared of returning; not so much scared of the police, but scared of him! I knew how he might reject me on the grounds that I was a temptation; and I couldn't counter that except by stressing that my love was pure.

I was scared of phoning him. But he endeared me by his laughter when he said he'd told Dr.Hughes, who had stupidly asked me "where are you?"- "she may be mad but she is not daft!" When he said "Don't go manic on your return," I had a sense that he cared about me and my well-being. I felt that he was positive about seeing me, saying "save it, you can tell me about your adventures later." It was like a communion when, after a period of silence at the end, I stammered "I love you so much." He rejoined "you don't mean that at all," and I protested "my love of you keeps me alive." I wondered afterwards why he found it so hard to conceive of the fact that I really loved him.

I had to phone back to check with him that that it was indeed safe to return on Monday 2nd May, that the 28 days were indeed up. On this occasion I lost money on the faulty phone, and I cursed it, as I could ill afford to lose money. Then suddenly I was through to him, and what I wanted to say tumbled out with passion. "I've come through such temptations and hardships loving you all the time; it's some strange quality, rare, refined, pure and subsisting, and nothing stops it." I had in mind the concept of "perpetual adoration," a prayer that was going on all the time! *My love of you informs my being, it goes on forever, subsisting across rifts of time and space; it's so pure that it keeps me alive!*

I managed to say that to him before the phone cut off, but afterwards felt badly, stricken with the sense of uncertainty. For he had expressed the "I'm not coming near you" sort of attitude. I felt rather stricken with doubt of him, rather as when I was returning from Austria; I had been kept going by my belief that the happiness I had with him could be restored; but supposing he wouldn't be actually "present" for me, supposing he wouldn't love me back?

That night, the night before I set off to return, it was as if my heart were continually speaking to him, telling him tales, loving him. And I saw that my sojourning there had been a proof of "Amor Vincit Omnia," which is Latin for "love conquers all things." What kind of love was it?- "the love I have for you, so pure and so strong." It was "Absolute Love." *This love had carried me through my suffering, and through it I had earned the Ultimate Freedom I had wanted. "And when I awake,"*- when the following morning the section was broken and I could return free,- "when I awake, I shall have won it absolutely!"

When I was in Lytham-St.Annes, struggling and suffering to earn my "ultimate freedom," inspired by a pure love of Dr.James which I kept to the fore of my mind and heart, I espied a large framed photo outside a shop. It was a photo of a most cute baby with a baggy nappy trying to stand up between its mothers legs, and I thought "that would appeal to you." So even though I lacked money to buy food with, and had to go hungry, I decided after passing it many times to buy it for a present. And so I ended up carrying this cumbersome and breakable photo all the way home from the bus-station, when I arrived back in KirkMichaels on Monday 2nd May, the day when I knew my section was lapsed.

When I got in the door and before I had even been to the toilet, a policeman came and arrested me. Apparently I had several times been in the front pages of newspapers, as a "missing woman," and before I had walked that small distance from the bus-station hundreds of people had contacted the police! And so after all my talk of "winning my absolute freedom that day," I found myself behind the grill of a police-van! At the police-station they didn't treat me very nicely, trying to interrogate me on a chair, saying "you are an absconded patient." I protested "surely you know my section has lapsed," but they said they would have to enquire about this Section 18. I said "you don't even know your own laws!" After two hours, and after calling in a local doctor who checked me over and said I was mentally well, they finally let me go.

In Lytham I had no great desire to go "home," having decided I would have to move house to get away from Craigdene's jurisdiction; I saw KirkMichaels as a point on the face of the earth where I could find a bath and something to eat and a rest. The bath was now in jeopardy, as it was now too late to buy power-cards, and I had to wait for someone to come round in a van to switch my electricity back on. And just after I managed to have this bath, Dr.James came round; I remember it was luke-warm scummy water. So then we talked of all my adventures, whilst he kept looking at this cute picture of the baby which was my gift to him; and it ravished me with its sweetness, though he left me feeling sad.

The next day I rapidly found I hated the place! For people kept saying to me "aren't you that missing person." I kept saying "well you needn't bother reporting me; they know I'm back." I couldn't stand the sense of inhibition from the people and minds around me; I felt I was being treated like a criminal or a fugitive from justice, or a freak at a zoo or a side-show. Instead of being glad that I'd won my freedom, they seemed to be all plotting in terms of depriving me of that freedom. Gone was the sense that "I am a free agent" that I had in Lytham! Only my best friend Louise seemed to be glad for me, and to understand me when I explained how freedom is necessary "for the soul to be alive."

I thought it pitiful, what I had told Dr.James the night before, in that I had in no way expressed the spiritual reality of what it was really like in Lytham; I had only told silly little tales. What I really wanted to tell him was how loving him had inspired me to fight for life, and to have courage and integrity and purity and endurance-power; these things I should have said. And I wanted to tell him of that "purity of my love." I also wanted to ask him the burning question "if I move to Edinburgh, can I still see you?" So I wrote "please come back" in a note.

So the next night, on the Wednesday, he did come back, but I was stunned when he said that, if I lived in KirkMichaels, he was never going to see me again either; "you have got to wean yourself off me." I argued as passionately as I could, "you are the reason for my being alive; I won life and freedom by loving you." But he asserted "it doesn't do you any good, and it certainly doesn't do me any good; it can't go on." When I protested "my love of you kept me alive," he said "it is imaginary; I'm just an idea in your mind; now I see that you can survive without me." I protested all I could, but he was unsympathetic. "You reigned in my heart and soul when you weren't there," I appealed, "if I don't love you, something in me will die!" But he was unrelenting. And then at the door he said of that picture "a photo of a baby between its mothers legs; what am I to think!" I replied with pain, "But you liked it when I gave it to you!"

My reaction when he'd gone was, "if this is true, if he won't change his mind, I have nothing to live for!" He was the reason for my being alive! It was a matter of; "there where I have garnered up my heart, where either I must live or bear no life!" I had fought for life against impossible odds for a month "believing in the happiness I could have with you; and now you say, just on my return, that I can't see you any more, can't love you any more!" It wasn't a very kind thing to do. "If you can cut me off like this, how can you pretend to care, or to have ever cared about me! How can you so reject me after the long self-offering of all my mind and soul to you! How can you be so uncaring!" It dawned on me how my greatest fear had been realised; that "absolute uncertainty" I had in Lytham, that he might reject me as a temptation and not take care of me. The pain sank into me that night. I felt this was the greatest single blow to my mind's stability that I had ever suffered; "he is the cause of all the stability and staying-power that I have!"

I immediately slipped into one of my nihilistic frames of mind, a bottomless black pit of depression. "If you reject me like this, when I have invested the meaning of my soul in you, then all there is left is Nothing!" When I talked with my friend Patricia in the Wine Bar, she didn't understand this black mood of mind. She stated that my doctor probably "pulled out" because he realised I was a danger to his career, but in any case I had still won my "freedom" from Craigdene. I replied with passion that "if you relate to someone so long and deep that they invest the meaning of their soul in you, and then pull out, it is culpable," and "I gained that freedom by my power of loving someone, and if I can't go on loving that person, the freedom means nothing to me." When I desperately stated, "I'll go find an Austrian mountain-top to throw myself off," she didn't realise how utterly I meant it!

I couldn't comprehend what had happened, and I went round in a daze; my outcry was still "How could you do it!" I couldn't comprehend how I was so jubilant just two days ago, saying I'd won life and freedom by my powers of loving, "and now there's nothing worth living for." It was so ironic; I'd kept myself alive believing in that hope of happiness; and I came back to claim it, only to find "absolutely nothing." I had hopes of creating a new life for myself, and now there was nothing before me. My cry became "how could God let this happen to me!" It was the annihilation of everything I'd lived for and all the meaning and love garnered up in my heart. *"I achieved that freedom, believing in the happiness that love offered me, and I come back, and there is no happiness, no love, nothing to live for; absolutely nothing!"*

The next day I went to speak to Dr.James at his surgery, hoping for a reprieve from the Nothingness. When I asked "how can you pretend to care," he insisted he had his say; "it is for your good; you've got to wean yourself off me; I've done it on purpose when you are strong; I'm willing to support you during a weaning-off period." When I said how the meaning of my soul was invested in him and without him I had "nothing," he replied, "you will find other things to inspire you, other people to love; it's like a vacuum and will pull in other things and people." I was at my wits end, and wanted to reply, "nonsense, the soul's nothingness ends in annihilation and Death." I said earnestly "my poet's mind only functions because I love you." The plaintive sadness of it was apparent in the way I said "you are the single greatest sorrow of my life," and "I wish you could give me back everything I ever gave you, but the gift of myself you can't give me back; my poet's mind and heart's love you can't give me back; and the pages of my journal I destroyed for love of you, you can't give me back."

And he came back that night, insisting on the finality of it. He read all the poetry I wrote in Lytham-St.Annes, and he wasn't pleased with it, because he said it showed that I was "besotted" by him. He pronounced that there were two roads in front of me, one broad way leading to life, and a narrow one leading to a cul-de-sac with him in it. I protested "loving you gave me life, inspired all my poetry and creativity; how can you do this!" But he sat down close to me and said "this is absolutely imperative; you have to free yourself from me." He said I was "in bondage" and I had to go "out there" and find new life. *I protested at the door, "But without loving you there is nothing in me; without my love of you there is no life!" But he left, saying he would never come back!*

After that single greatest cataclysm of my entire life, I spent a completely sleepless night, in which I scribbled away out of my pain. My soul was screaming "I offered you the best part of my heart in those poems, and you use it as a further reason for totally rejecting me!" Everything he had said seemed untrue and wrong. He was under the illusion that pulling out of this relationship was giving me life, saying "you will find it liberating, you will find new life," but as I was trying to tell him, "you can't make a new life when the soul has no love left within it." "I'll never be happy again, never love again, and he claims to be doing it for my good!"

That night I wrote that fateful letter, which began, "There is a danger I shall remember you as the bastard who destroyed my powers of loving." It said, "You know full well that you were so deeply a part of my soul-life that to get you back out of it would destroy me; would completely destroy the core of me, my powers of loving. For years I've only kept my integrity and wholeness to offer it back to you. So it doesn't matter any more does it! I might as well embrace the life of the meaningless." And because I felt so destroyed myself, I suggested that if I ceased loving him there was nothing to prevent my destroying him; "I'm going away, before I hate you enough to want to destroy you." Determined to go away for a bit, I went to the surgery the next morning and pressed it into his own hand. *That letter, unread by him at the time, lay as a minefield for future anguish and pain!*

That void of nothingness into which my soul collapsed was caused by him, by that cruelty of rejection when I returned from Lytham, vulnerable, recently escaped from a mental hospital, dependant on him

342

for my happiness. He seemed to spend the rest of the summer trying to take no responsibility for me; but the hospital waited for me, and ultimately his was the responsibility for driving me back.

Chapter 85
The Wasteland.

After putting that letter into his hand, I had determined to go away for a while, to Abbotsford Abbey, but I found I couldn't get my act together well enough to make a meal, or even get out of bed in the morning. I realised then that that without that power of loving in my heart I was indeed Nothing; "I bend toward annihilation."

I did something very stupid, something meaningless, in this nihilistic mood of mind; I got involved with Walter. For he showed me some loving kindness in those following few days, for which I was grateful. I sobbed my heart out at the supermarket to him, saying how I had believed in Dr.James and loved him so much, and now there was "Nothing but a big hole where that love was." I said he had made me feel so unique and loved and cared for, but he was "a sham," and life was meaningless to me. And Walter listened and seemed wise when he commented "there's never any greater hate than that of broken love."

When I was incapable of setting off to Abbotsford the next day, Walter took me together with Gabriel to Magusdean Forest. I was aware of the essential meaninglessness of what I was doing, but for a short while I saw the idea of getting back with Walter and Gabriel the only thing that could make life worth living. My son said sweet and plaintive things like, "you just come and live down here mummy, you'll be safe here and you'll have a nice life." I didn't understand how I could so lack the integrity as to get involved with Walter, but I needed him to be kind and supportive to me.

A sense of hatred for Dr.James was building up inside of me; "you can't wean me off from loving you; it will convert to hatred." I depended on my love of him; "either it lives in me forever, or my heart is annihilated along with it." I knew this fact so deeply and wanted to scream it out to him; "the existence of my soul depends on my loving you." You couldn't wean someone off this kind of love; "by freeing me from loving you, you are not giving me life, you are giving me Death." It was hatred that is the bondage, not love. I was screaming out "I'm not going to let you destroy the core of my soul where love reigns." He had given me soul-life, so he had responsibility for me. Stopping loving him would send me towards destruction and death; "and what destroys the core of me will also destroy you."

It was stopping loving him that was going to put me "in bondage," it was already putting me in the immediate bondage of getting involved with Walter; all my integrity was gone; it made me do something so meaningless as to be an effective death-sentence. It was Walter who stood "in the cul-de-sac," whilst Dr.James opened me out into life. Rapidly I felt Walter's emotionalism and bad-temper, his coerciveness and domination, closing in upon me, and I felt disgusted with myself that I let myself be kissed by a man who had destroyed and rendered vain the greater part of my life. *It was a descent into Death and the meaningless. It was indeed the most meaningless five days of my life, for I knew that getting involved with Walter would spell the death of my personality utterly.*

I decided to go along to the surgery at the end of those five days, to appeal to Dr.James. I wrote a letter to read out to him, about "the Void that will destroy us all," but he wouldn't let me read it. He pronounced "once a child has learnt to swim, you must let go of the chin," but I protested that my love of him was upholding my soul, and I reminded him of how I once said "you keep in me the warm love that keeps me alive." I finished by saying "unless you can come up with a remedy, you might as well put me in the dustbin!" He joked "what size of dustbin will you need?" "Will you give me hope?" I kept saying. He finally stipulated, knowing that I had an invitation from Maggie to stay for a week in Ayrshire, "Go away for a week, and I'll come round to see you on the Tuesday night."

Life and Hope surged in me! Just the hope that he would continue to relate to me was fluttering in me as with wings; it brought me back from soul-death and the brink of destruction. And so I set off for a week's stay at my friend Maggie's, who lived in a place called Hawkeshill in Ayrshire, with a sense of hope. I left revolving thoughts like "he cares for me really," and "my love is pure and strong, centred at the highest point my soul can reach." I said to myself, "in 40 years it's only you I have loved from the core of my soul, and it's an illusion to think there is someone "out there" to love, so don't destroy the deepest spiritual connection I have ever known in my life; you must allow me to continue loving you."

And Hawkeshill seemed a wasteland to me; because I had come there with a devastated heart! Maggie didn't help, in that I couldn't talk about it with her, and she kept comparing it to her own love-affairs; and her constant yelling at the kids, and her denigrating instructing of me wore me down. In addition it became obvious to me there, whilst talking to people and looking at council house swaps, how impossibly difficult it

345

would be to make "a new life" for myself. When I climbed up the hill called "Hawkeshill" one day amongst the gorse-bushes, so I had a good view of the hills on the horizon, I reflected that I couldn't understand those two days when on my return from Lytham he welcomed me and then rejected me! It didn't make sense! "When totally involved in loving you, you gave me a light-enhancing heart," and the light of the world seemed like light; "without it, it's coal-black!"

Then one memorable day we went on a trip to Whithorn Priory and Ninian's cave. On the way back from Ninian's cave through the woods, a lady preached to us about "destiny" and "life's meaning"; and I became angry saying, *"I tell you, life can also be empty and meaningless and Void, and perhaps that's the ultimate truth about it!" I had a most terribly overwhelming awareness in Whithorn, seeing all the graves and skeletons, of "the dissolution of life towards the meaningless, towards Death."* I reflected how I had had the belief that he would always be there for me; the way he used to say "you are always forgiven" meant I was always accepted and loved. And then I remembered how he had said to me "nothing lasts forever"; the words suddenly came to signify the mortality of our friendship.

That night a religious experience grew upon me, thinking as I had been about entering the religious life. *I reflected on the total investment of all my soul in a friendship that is in one day destroyed; "I am left with Nothing; I gave my All and am left with Nothing."* I thought "Not that I was wrong about friendship, about total soul-love getting us to heaven; but that you were shallow and fickle-hearted." And it then occurred to me, like a moving from God, "perhaps He has shown me the mortality of human feeling for a purpose." And that purpose was most certainly not to go and find someone "out there" and to love someone humanly again; it was rather a complete rejection of human love, of the world and all it contains. The following morning, during a service in a church-hall, I realised how really disillusioned I was about human friendship; I declared, "there is nothing left for me in human love; it is empty, defunct!"

I couldn't see beyond that Tuesday which was coming up; it was like an ominous brick wall to my comprehension. Maggie urged me not to go back to KirkMichaels, asking "what chance of life" was there for me in such a place, when all the minds along the streets believed me to be an "escaped patient" who should be in Craigdene. She was right, but then again, I had to go back and face the truth about this relationship, I had to get past that Tuesday. I saw clearly that last night there; "there is no new life "out there"; if I had clung to my love of you I might have tried; without it, it's a wasteland!"

And so the five days at Maggie's had been bad for me; there had been filtering through to me "the reality of the death of love." The friendship between us I already saw in the past tense, and it was already damaged too deep to be mended; "you are destroying my belief in that friendship; I think it is destroyed already." And so I returned with a heart full of hatred, dead and closed up to love; I felt "the bondage of not being able to believe in human love." *So I was left with a wasteland; "how can I go off with all the love in my heart destroyed, and all the world meaningless and void before me!"*

Dr.James effectively trashed my soul-life, by rejecting me, when my mental state was vulnerable, and fragile, and I had all my meaning invested in him; "you have trashed my heart and put me in a rubbish-bin!" Coming back on the bus my hatred was speaking; "If you think you can trash my soul-life like that, I'll call you to account for it! In that hole where love was, will be a creeping, menacing, meaningless Void, and it is that which will destroy you!" And I reached my door, reflecting on how difficult it was for Freddy to break off from me when he had invested for so short a time so little, and I just wanted to shake my fist and yell, "I gave you my All!" *He seemed to trash my soul-life at will that summer!*

And so that fateful Tuesday arrived which was like a "brickwall" that I had to get past. I had arrived back from Hawkeshill feeling full of hate and with a nothingness inside of me; "you destroy all the life of meaning I created, leaving a world in front of me that is empty, meaningless, void." I didn't believe in the love I had for him any more. And yet he chose that night to make me feel overwhelmed by a sense of being loved and accepted! *It liberated me from a dissolution towards death, making me feel that I was attached to him, and I'd love him no matter what! It seemed to me like God performing a miracle for me!*

After that I went around happy in a daze of non-understanding. I felt I didn't understand what happened or anything about him; all that mattered was that the love in my heart was restored. I had the sense that life was a mystery. But I wouldn't trust human love so much ever again; I had been disappointed by its mortality. He had left my soul in the chains of death for two weeks; that he could do that to me was something I wouldn't be able to forget. My love put a halo around him; but I was aware as never before, since seeing those skeletons in the Whithorn dig, of the precariousness and mortality of it. "I mean love can die; I know; it nearly died in me."

Though the next Tuesday was one of the sweetest and most aesthetic experiences of my life, when I said all I really wanted from him was "his listening heart," when he left I felt I didn't know where I was with him any more. I never asked him "why did you reject me?" and he was as much a mystery to me as ever; I got no clarification. The trouble was I had a feeling that at any moment he might reject me again; I now felt the relationship was precarious. The bottom line was; *"I trusted you, trusted you to always forgive me, always accept me and love me; but after that experience of love dying its death in me because of your rejection, I don't trust you any more; I've lost my trust of you. I trusted you, I rested my soul as on a rock; I can't do that any more!"*

It caused a crisis in my faith. I said next Sunday at the Baptist church, "I don't think I believe there is a God." Everything about my life was broken and ragged; it didn't show how good God is; it made it hard to believe there was a God. That experience of the Whithorn dig shook my faith; "if you can give your All to human love and be left with Nothing, if life can be as meaningless as that, merely a dissolution towards death, then there isn't a God reigning!" I was living a precarious existence, "saved from that, but only just saved from that!"

And so I had lost faith somehow; faith in him and faith in God, because they were connected.

The next Tuesday was one of the most morally-charged occasions of my life, as I was feeling; "I can't live in this degree of precariousness; tell me what you intend with me; if you are going to trash the whole of my soul-life I want to know about it; I've got to get some answers." "Let me ask you something," I said, and he came and sat close to me. "I trusted you," I said, "why did you reject me?" I said what I wanted was my trust restored, for him to tell me that he would "never let me go." The only thing close to an answer was "I thought the time had come for you to stand on your own two feet." Otherwise he left with, "I think I understand what you are saying."

But I didn't think he did understand what I was saying; and the next morning I wished I had shut up and let him go away content. But it struck me that the spiritual life had to be both precarious and morally-charged. What I couldn't abide was the sense of him caring for me and accepting me, if he might just stop again; "if you intend trashing my soul-life the next week, it's not genuine." I reflected on how I had said "I can't live in this degree of precariousness." *But "everything is precarious!" I concluded;* "perhaps being-in -existence itself is precarious; does that mean you have to live without trust, because everything is too precarious to trust, even human love? Perhaps you are not supposed to comprehend life, but must learn to live in it, as something precarious and incomprehensible." I needed an acceptance of the precariousness!

Then on the night of the 7th June, he came with that letter that I had written in my nihilistic mood of mind overnight when he had just rejected me. It was the greatest catastrophe of my life again, the same one! How ironic that I was just going to tell him how completely he could trash my soul-life, and he does it again! How ironic that I had written just before he arrived "my love of you is fastened to the core of my being; it lives with me or it dies with me!" *For he came in like a whirlwind, and waved this letter in my face, claiming that it had been found and read by his fellow-doctors, and shouting that he could have nothing more to do with me!* I was shocked and horrified; I had always feared this letter might turn up, because he had never responded to it at the time. He wouldn't listen to my protestations; finally I stood in front of the living-room door, preventing his angry exit. "Do I have to physically throw you out of my way!" he shouted, throwing me forcibly aside. I couldn't stand the awful sense of his coldness; a horrible nullity or non-feeling swamped over me.

With my soul screaming out into the universe for help, I went to the public phone, to tell him "I'm so sorry." I tried to tell him that I wrote that letter when I was overcome by intense negative emotions, and I had a sense of a menacing void destroying me. But the coldness of his reply shattered my dreams; "you can't control your emotions, you can't control your writings; if you want to see me come to the surgery; my surgery door is always open to you." All this struck a chill in me; for the door of his surgery wouldn't be "the door of his heart."

When I awoke the next morning my pain and the sense of my aloneness were extreme; my soul's scream was, "Why do you keep doing this to me! Every time you do it I die a thousand deaths!" And I thought of all the times he had done it; "all my soul-life came to grief again because of that letter." It was a dangerous letter indeed, but I had carefully given it "into his own hand" before leaving! He was thinking I was a dangerous person, but "I'm only dangerous when I stop loving you." *I wanted to explain to him, that letter was the mere expression of emotion; "something passing, it's nothing, it had no meaning."* I had been struggling with emotion, with the recognition that it was my soul-life he was destroying, the desire to let him know how I felt before going away, the need to involve him in the destruction that was going on in me; "believe me, it was an emotion!"

After a few days I had this perception of it, though not necessarily a true one; "I can't go on like this! You accept and care for me one week, and the next week throw me away! How often have you done it now! I'm fed up of this; I deserve better than this! Though it is strange I should say this after so long connecting my love of you to my union with God, I can't go on with the spiritual torment you exercise over me. This relationship has destroyed me more than it has created me. This isn't friendship, it is emotional terrorising!"

What is true, as I judge it, is that he seemed to toy with me cruelly that summer, with no real sense of care; with not one ounce of care for me, for my real welfare, or for my mental health which was taking such a beating! I said at the time, "Don't pretend to care for me, because you don't!"

Chapter 87
Domination-Games.

When I returned having "earned my freedom" from Lytham-St.Annes, I found the problem that Walter and Gabriel were posing, unsolved. At first Walter allowed me in his house to see Gabriel, and I was going through the ravages of a break-down in my relationship with Dr.James, so I clung to the two of them like to a raft in a storm. I can remember holding my son in my arms, thinking "there's nothing worth living for." And in that nihilistic depressed state, Walter was very kind to me for a few days, and I was grateful for the kindness he showed; he said "you do have something to live for, you have Gabriel."

Walter continued to be kind and supportive for those few days when my interior life had collapsed into a nothingness; he took me out in the car and made me meals, and let me get close to the son who was a comfort to me. I can remember walking along the sea's edge with Gabriel at Kirksbank, and I was hoping as my son was, that the three of us would go back to living together; it was clear "what the dream of his little heart was."

But rapidly I felt Walter's coerciveness closing in on me; I felt like a slave when he bullied me into washing up, and I felt disgusted with myself when I let him kiss me. When he didn't understand why I "seemed down," I was appalled that he thought my love of Dr.James was "such a shabby affair as to require only a day's sobbing." I realised love meant nothing to him but coercive sex and fleeting emotions. I was disgusted; "how dare he compare this cheap and meaningless relating to him with that all-encompassing love of Dr.James!" I couldn't stand his sick emotionalism and bad-temper, the same old coerciveness and domination. I realised when I went to Hawkeshill that I had really messed my life up, getting involved with Walter; I was disgusted with myself, and felt it to be the most meaningless five days of my life! I had so embraced Death as to let the man kiss me!

When I returned from Hawkeshill, the world in front of me seemed meaningless and void. When Walter pressed me about "arrangements," I erupted, "that's rich; you say that when you are established here with my son, and I don't even have anywhere to go, with a world empty in front of me!" When I gave Gabriel his present saying I would have to move house, I was astonished and hurt when he replied "but what about my toys mummy!" He seemed to care more about his toys than he did about me, and I felt I didn't matter to anybody!

On the 21st May the whole "cosy thing" with Walter and Gabriel exploded wide apart. An anger had been building up in me, because I felt intimidated by Walter and "under his thumb," and I was fed up of him waltzing into my house as if he had the right to be there; "after the price I paid to get him out of my life I'm not having him waltzing into my house!" And so when I went to collect Gabriel, our mutual niceness blew up in our faces. "I demand to know where you are taking him; I'm coming to get him from your house," said Walter. "Are you saying it's not safe for me to walk him along the street," I responded. "I'm responsible for him" he shouted. "I'm responsible too as his mother!"I replied. Walter shouted "Right I'm taking him back!" And I said crossly, "I'm not having this; I'm not dancing attendance on you in order to have access to Gabriel." And I went away saying to myself, "I want proper access arrangements, I have rights as a mother"; *for Walter's behaviour was saying, "if you don't please me and be dominated over by me, I won't let you have access."*

In the following days I realised again how Gabriel was different from the nice little boy he used to be; he used to like helping, to like pleasing, to like being constructive and creative; now all he did was tear around destructively. He jumped up and down on a clean bed with dirty shoes, for example. And what really undermined me as a mother was his sexual harassment of me. He used to feel my legs and say over and over "I want to go underneath you." I felt the only way I could put a stop to this was by a sense of complete rejection, and a mother's role was based on acceptance, and so the whole relationship was being undermined. I began to feel he was a wretched child that I wanted no responsibility for.

In the Catholic church one day the photos of first communion were being shown, and I was pained to find Gabriel's picture absent. I said to myself, "I gave him an upbringing, a biddable child who was a credit to me, and now Walter allows him to do whatever he likes, without any discipline or teaching." My pain was immense as I watched other mothers with their kids, "and there was I with the motherhood torn out of me!" I remembered how I used to be in that church with that little baby hung around my tummy in a pouch, and I thought, "I am a destroyed person!"

At the end of May I went to see George McPherson, my solicitor. It wasn't too good. The first thing he said was that my escape to Lytham-St.Annes had "harmed my case"; I protested that I had gained for myself "six months of real, creative, meaningful life." We got into deep and murky water when I tried to explain I didn't want access to depend on "pleasing" Walter. He tried to tell me that I didn't need to "jump into bed" with Walter; I tried to tell him "all that Walter can understand is a sexual relationship; I don't want any relationship with him at all." We got into even deeper and murkier water when I tried to explain I hate the way Gabriel is sexually attacking me, as it undermines my motherly acceptance of him. When he said "tell me exactly what he does," he failed to understand how it was an inappropriate way of showing love and affection to an adult; I thought crossly on the bus afterwards "it's bloody obvious if you ask me." Finally I told him "I'm willing to always hold out a hand to him, but I don't want him back," and he said he'd investigate the possibility of Saturday or Sunday access. I went away feeling that we basically liked each other, but he made it seem that I had no moral insight into my own emotional condition; as if he were "treating me like a moral imbecile."

Then, Gabriel's birthday approaching, I had an argument with Walter over birthday cakes. We agreed I wasn't going to the party that Walter was going to throw, "but," said he, "you will make some birthday cakes though, won't you!" I replied that seeing he was throwing the party he could make his own cakes. "But you're his mummy!" came the reply. I could have shot or whipped him! I had a deep perception in that moment of what he had done to me; after trashing me when I was pregnant, saying "a baby would ruin my life," he went on year after year using every dirty trick and insidious move he could think of to take that child off me, so he could claim "he's mine," and possess him! *I was angry; "you've pinched him from me, you're responsible for him, you changed the birth-certificate, you are throwing the party, so you can make the cakes!"*

It became worse a few days later when I had to wait fifteen minutes on Walter's doorstep, then he returned saying "Stuart O'Sullivan is coming." He was reintroducing the social workers into it again, having enlisted their support, for I knew Stuart O'Sullivan was no friend of mine! He at that moment arrived, saying he had an appointment; I retorted "well you don't have an appointment with me!" and walked off down the garden path. Walter after this insisted that I had Tuesdays and Thursdays access-time in order to "suit his arrangements"; I was angry, because he was just using me for child-minding! I began to hate Walter again; he had already said that I had to "make arrangements" for continuing a liason with him, in a creepy fashion. He was saying "If you won't have a sexual relationship in the way I want you to, if you won't child-mind for me in the way I want you to, I'll cut it back to handovers with the social workers;" he was a creep and a bastard! "I won't be bullied and coerced and used and manipulated in this way!"

Gabriel's 8th Birthday, on the 5th June arrived, and it was a day I went bananas with pain. It began with my raging impotently in church against the sense of unfairness at what had been done to me; and I felt "I'd rather not remember that birth." Walter played out his domination-games at the party; when I'd gone to fetch Gabriel from there, he said loudly "you will wait a minute Mairi," and I felt like a spectacle in front of the other mothers and kids. And when I brought Gabriel back he had me waiting fifteen minutes at the door before he returned, scoring another point over me. I was angry, feeling I no longer wanted to be involved with the two of them; *"I'm not interested in your domination-games."*

And I had a terrible time with Gabriel that day. I had carefully arranged a birthday pile of presents, food and a card, but he didn't care about anything, and just rolled about on the floor. He seemed to me "uncivilised, undisciplined, unappreciative, ungracious"; I saw the difference between the sensitive child I nurtured, and the "brutish boy" he was now. And my heart cried out that "8 years ago I gave birth, and I wish I hadn't!" *And I remembered how Walter used to say "I just want to see him," and how this escalated to "I want to have him completely, changing his name to mine and having custody."*

"But you see with Walter it was only ever a domination game. With me, having Gabriel was an act of love. Keeping him in me and giving birth to him was an act of love, as was all the nurturing afterwards. That is why it is so heart-breaking, that a domination-game should have beaten my love."

The next day I felt sore, I felt only the pain of what Walter had done to me; his getting Gabriel had been done by bullying and coercion and insidiousness, for that was the way Walter operated. *I felt how there was nothing worse to a mother than to watch the child she had nurtured being gradually damaged and destroyed. This was the worst suffering known to a mother, and therefore it was truly the worst suffering known to the human soul.* And I reflected how I must stop the access visits because it was filling my heart with hate, and I didn't want to see him any more, and I didn't want him back. *"Having a child is not a matter of possessing him, but being able to educate and nurture and guide and teach; if I can't do those things any more, I don't think I want to see him again."*

Filled with the sadness of this decision, and meantime absorbed by the horribly painful breaking-up of my relationship with Dr.James, and being advised by a wise and moral man to "come apart" for a while to "ponder" on my mistakenness, we then come to that wonderful Summer solstice, when for 3 days around the 21st June, I won to a real peace and gentleness. And in that "gentleness" I realised I had to "let go" of Gabriel; that the best way to "fight for him" was a letting go. And Walter and the social workers chose a time within that few days to hold a "case conference" about Gabriel; I declined to attend. This was partly because I couldn't face Dr.James being there, partly because I was getting ready to go away, but really because I understood this; *"that real strength lies in gentleness, and not in opposing power against power, argument against argument, force against force."*

I believed that my "letting go" was the best way to fight for Gabriel, if I loved him. " For if I now continue to fight and damage Gabriel by crying "mother's access rights" then I am not in accord with my giving up of him which was a real act of love."

So I didn't attend the conference, but went the next day to give Gabriel a going-away present; this occasioned one of my most horrid encounters with Walter ever! Insisting that he talk with me in the bedroom outside of Gabriel's hearing, he said "there is a another case-conference, to arrange that you should be stopped from seeing Gabriel at all." I was angry, sensing that he had used the case-conference to get everyone to gang up against me. "I'm not listening to your threats" I said, and tried to walk out. But whilst Walter was saying "you are not to come back in this house any more," Gabriel got in the way; so I assured Gabriel that he would get letters from me. And Walter shouted "there'll be no letters." I said in anger "you are trying to cut me off from my own son." *And he said back "you can have nothing more to do with him." I shouted in uncontrollable anger as I stormed out of the door; "Do you know what you are? You are a bloody bastard!"*

But I held to my belief that "the real strength lies in gentleness." I was still convinced that going through "domination games" to force the world to give me access to my own son was not the way to fight, and I believed that if I had been at the conference the outcome wouldn't have been any different. *To the social workers limited understandings, to love a child meant to have, possess and keep; but 3 years ago I had insisted that my mother-love should "let him go"; and that remained my best insight.*

I refused to struggle over him; I'd always said "I love him enough to let him go." *"I feel that I can now have the gentleness and real love to let Gabriel go, rather than tearing him apart in a perpetual squabble."*

Chapter 88
The Black Hole.

So after the cataclysmic event of "the letter," after he had insisted that I see him only at his surgery, I had an appointment on the 9th June. I spent hours waiting to see him, but he wouldn't even listen to me, and after two minutes threw me out! I tried to say it was a "passing emotion" in that letter, and that it "arose out of a destructive Void," but he said he wasn't interested. I tried to say how I needed his presence in my life, loving and accepting me, and I had taken a letter that I had written from Austria to prove the point; but he didn't care to listen. He just said "you write down what you should not write down" and urged me out; it seemed to make a mockery of his saying "my surgery door is always open to you"; it was not open to indwell and to listen, it was open to throw me out of!

I didn't think I could be stoical enough to wait for another week for a repeat of such a shallow event. My friend Harriet said "leave it alone, give it time." I tried to cling onto some faith that he was still worth my loving, but I rapidly felt an emotional complexity that was like hatred. But I knew the hatred was an "emotional complexity" within the love. I thought "if I'm not loving you I'll be hating you," when I glimpsed him in his car. He seemed now so insensible, graceless, cold; "you can't involve me in loving you so deeply, then pull out to my destruction." It suddenly came home to me, "if you were not really involved with me and caring for me, then you were misusing me." And that thought remained in my mind to torment me. I began to wonder whether this was "a completely wrong relationship."

This thought really drove me into a "black hole," for I saw the whole ethos of my life as invalid. I began to see my whole path of life, of being "a contemplative in the world," had been invalid and meaningless. *I wrote to Pater Leo, "if my relationship with the one person I've loved all these years is breaking up, leaving me with a life that is meaningless, then my whole way of life is meaningless and invalid, and always was."* The whole way of the last 25 years was invalid. Pain was "breaking the shell of my understanding!"

I thought I would appeal to him; I felt that if I were contrite enough he would take me back. I would appeal "I'll do anything, but please don't punish me any more; forgive me, I'm only little, I'm only a child, and you have more experience than I have; I am redeemable; with you I am redeemable, without you I'm lost." I had a strange sad yearning on the beach, thinking how I would say "I am your spirit-child attached to you, don't throw me away." I remember how I'd once said he was "worth going to the ends of the earth for;" I thought how I could climb Mt.Everest and bring back something from the top, or perhaps polish for him an Iona greenstone; I sought a way to plead with him deeply enough. I just thought I had to touch something in him which would make him say "I forgive you," which would restore the relationship, the love and the trust.

With this attitude I went to see him at his surgery, and he said cruelly to me some of the most awful things! What he said on the surface was reasonable and kind, saying "I'm not throwing you away, for you can come here to see me." I said with appalling sadness it was no good; "If you never come into my home, my life will be so empty; it was only a home because I met you there." But the real sadness which made me later sob was his attitude of "before it went wrong," as if to say "my loving of you was all a mistake." *He said "I used to come because I liked listening to you; I used to have a great deal of affection for you, before it became so overwhelming." My pain hit the roof! It implied that he no longer had affection for me, and could in effect now "throw me away."* I hated his glib, self-assured mood. I continued to idealistically rant on about how my love of him "came over the mountains and was deep and everlasting," *knowing this was nonsense in the face of the fact that this I-You relationship was breaking up!*

The pain, once home, made me disintegrate into tears. "If you were toying with me, when I had my whole soul engaged in loving you, you were misusing me!" What he said implied that whilst I was doing my total self-giving and commitment to him, he was in fact ceasing to care for me! What was the point of my seeing him in his surgery, if he was really saying "I don't want to be further involved with you; this is a way of fobbing you off!" Worst of all was the moment when he threw me out of his room, and I thought "So that's the way it's going to be!" Observing that moment remained to haunt me, for I saw I wasn't loving him any more. "I'm not really loving him any more, am I, when I see him as an "It"!" He was an "It" I could observe, not my whole soul responding to "the mystery of my You." This hurt me more than anything, as I dissolved into tears, for I could see my feelings for him were deeply changing, and it really was breaking up! And I sobbed my heart out in a numb fashion.

I cried all night with the painful perception "you have misused me." *Worst of all those words burnt into me; "I did have a lot of affection for you until it became so overwhelming." I thought the pain of this more than I believed I would have to go through in a lifetime, concentrated into a lump!* "So when I was growing to care for him more, he was ceasing to care for me!" I felt he was so glib, and it was all re-interpreted and relegated to the past! He was no longer open to me; this was such pain, when he used to say "I like coming to see you," and my door was always open and receptive to him! His attitude was that it "had to come to an end," but meaningful relationships don't come to an end; if it wasn't "the responsibility of an I for a you" that goes on forever, it was always meaningless. I thought I must try and "salvage something," but it had disintegrated too far. I felt my soul was dying; it was like being starved of Oxygen. *I was collapsing into a "black hole."*

And hatred lay in this "black hole!" I was outraged when I felt he had misused "his position of care and trust," and wanted to "call him to account." I felt he was being immoral, trying to relegate it to the past! But my better instincts rose to the fore, and I was determined to be "moral" about it; I wasn't going to give up so easily, convinced that the relationship could be "rescued and redeemed." I saw that I had to be "willing to be more hurt"; it was best to be open to more hurt if it meant "salvaging something here." So I went to the phone-box, intending to say "come and talk with me, honestly and deeply." But he put the phone down, and I stood there pained with an expanding apocalyptic awareness of "this is the end"; it seemed like the end of everything for me.

I then phoned from Henry's home, but it was a horrible, extreme and raw experience. I said all my deep feelings, saying we had to salvage something. His reaction was to say "you aren't trustworthy; you said you would never write something like that , and you did; tell yourself you are a very stupid girl, and you are paying for it." I said I had to talk for my healing "and if I don't talk with you, I'll talk about you," and he said it sounded like blackmail. I said ominously, "what destroys the core of me will also destroy you, in that the love which was upholding me was also upholding you!" When he told me to come round to see him in his surgery for a couple of months, I again felt that he was "fobbing me off." This phone-call showed how the relationship had really descended into the pits!

I was cross that he all he saw was the fact of that letter, and he was trying to punish me for it. "I don't have to pay with the ending of a relationship because of some stupid accident of a letter!" He treated it as a sin against him that I had to be punished for, but what about the fact that he caused it, by so rejecting me when I returned vulnerable from Lytham! So he was taking no responsibility for causing that letter! And why did he say I wasn't "trustworthy" when I had been so for years!

Was he "true to me" when I came back from Lytham! Was he going to say trustworthiness lay in not writing down a dangerous thought, but not "being true to someone" when they had staked so much on you! "You can't say that letter annihilates all my trustworthiness!"

I thought that if we talked long and deep, we might yet salvage something. And when I found a note from him at my door, hope surged in me for a moment that he might be willing to talk, but he wasn't. My heart cried out "I thought you were a moral man, with some understanding of things!" But now I felt disillusioned; it seemed he had no understanding of moral matters, and a punitive idea of things, and no sense of responsibility, and an ice-cold heart! "Love is the responsibility of an I for a You, but you never could understand that, could you! "

I felt "we need to talk now" because the hate and destructiveness inside me was increasing day by day; every day the "black hole" got worse. How could things go so utterly wrong! It was a communion that used to radiate like the sun in my heart, and it was ending in such a black and painful destructiveness! "There's nothing for me here but a black hole!" I couldn't face staying here any longer, because before when I saw white cars like his along the street they seemed like miniature suns; now they were all like "black holes," reminding me that my sun of meaning had collapsed!

It was because of the fact that I needed to talk for my healing, that I decided to approach Prof Gray, because he was "the most moral man that I know." I was intending to tell him, "the deepest, most loving and most meaningful relationship of my life is destroying itself; I'm trying to rescue it, but he won't talk; he's no longer open to me, his heart closed against me. And the more I am offering that openness, the more I am getting hurt."

Chapter 89
The Gentle Moment.

So I went to have a long to talk with Prof.Gray, "the most moral man I know," and he made my unbearable pain more "bearable" by his listening and his wise advice. He freed me from "the burden of an enormous aloneness," by going along with me in that time when our moral paths and understandings were shared.

I told him, without revealing Dr.James' identity, that in the horrible breaking up of this relationship the pain was making me hate him; *but I wasn't really hating him, it was an "emotional complexity," caused by the way he was so coldly rejecting me and taking no responsibility.* He pointed out sagely *"the opposite of love is not hate, it is indifference."* I said I was trying to transcend it, and salvage something of a meaningful relationship; he said "I can see you have great strength." It was the trueness of his moral insight which really helped me. He let me explain about the relationship, and when he asked "how much did he mean to you," I unhesitatingly replied "everything." *He didn't speak of the "mistake I'd made," but sensitively said "there was something wrong in it, which meant the pain had to be." He said it was "too intense, too isolated, too all-consuming," as if it had a hint of "idolatry" about it.*

I trusted Prof Gray, the more I heard of his reply, because it seemed sage, moral, wise, non-condemning, and true. He said I had to understand the man's "fallibility." When I protested "I don't understand him," he replied "perhaps he doesn't understand himself." I replied "I can accept into my love his fallibilities, because I know him so deeply; what I cannot accept is the way he is trying to relegate me into history." He pointed out that I mustn't destroy his career out of hate, because that wouldn't be acting out of strength but out of weakness; "make choices that are for your healing."

He offered a twofold advice. Firstly, I had to "reflect on the relationship, and understand why the pain had to be"; recognising there was something wrong in it, but salvaging the good out of it; "for your own healing, look back and see that you were investing too much." Secondly it would be wise to "withdraw and give the thing time"; we should always "throw away the things that don't work," and this bickering between us wasn't working; we could try and salvage something when the relationship was able to be tranquil and non-threatening. I took up this advice to "come away and ponder."

I felt very sore about the subject of "responsibility." He was busy blaming me for responsibility for that fateful letter, taking no responsibility for the fact that he caused it and he lost it. "You will take no responsibility for how much I invested in you, how much I've lost because of you, how deeply you engaged me in loving you." Now I was having problems with my Lithium medication, and went through was a long, painful and lonely anguish that lasted for weeks. I needed him to take responsibility for me as my GP, but I felt intensely that his cold rejection meant I couldn't approach him in my need; for he would think I was deliberately involving him in that responsibility. "You are busy denying responsibility for what you've meant to me, or what you've done to me, or where you've left me; but though you coldly reject me, I'm not denying responsibility for you, or the need of my love to uphold you." I felt he was being "like a kelpie," not very human or moral!

However I decided to approach him that afternoon, taking the "moral letter" I had written, with that compassionate understanding of his fallibility shown to me by Prof Gray. It detailed the finer points of my feelings, saying I was going away to Ireland for a month, and wanted to talk with him when I got back. It said I didn't want to destroy his career, as I really was still loving him, and I needed to go away where I could talk in a way that was needed for my healing; I hoped he would have a better sense of things like trustworthiness, and forgiveness and responsibility when I got back, and would stop trying to relegate me into the past; "I will meanwhile ponder on my own mistake." I wrote that he had to keep the letter, ending, "you know I will assert beyond my dying day that I will always love you." I decided I was going to read out this letter to him, without pause, insisting that as these might be the last words I had to say to him, he mustn't lose or destroy it.

One of the best, most soul-wrenching moments of my life followed! He listened intently as I read it out, and that letter which "cost" me so dearly in terms of the destructive emotion I had to transcend in order to write it, must have impressed him, for he bent forward and laid his hand on my wrist; "don't" I said. He solemnly promised not to lose or destroy it; I said "you must promise to ponder on it, whilst I'm doing my own pondering." And I grasped his arm, saying "God I really love you! I'm only hating you because I really love you!" He wasn't self-assured and he didn't throw me out; I went to the door, and turning back, saw him sitting there looking like a child, so lost and lonely and pained. And I went back and said "Goodbye," touching him again. That moment's image of him remained with me; I could say after that, "I love you very much and will forgive you for anything!" *For it was a gentle moment in which I saw and loved his "humanity."*

This tender experience with him took place on 21st June, and I walked along the beach that powerful Midsummer's night, sensible of the fact that it was exactly three years to the day that he had first overwhelmed me, and feeling that my situation was "too intense to take." I felt I couldn't possibly sit opposite to him during the case-conference about Gabriel which was scheduled for the following day. And I wasn't willing to struggle over Gabriel and to fight Walter's domination-games. So I wrote a letter for Dr.James to take, so as to represent me, the crux being "at last I feel I can have now the gentleness and real love to let Gabriel go, rather than tearing him apart in a perpetual squabble." *That night felt like a great watershed; I had both withdrawn from the man I loved and let go of my son, and this was a very free-ing thing. I felt wrapped round in the goodness of God, and I attained a real "gentleness."*

When I gave him the letter the next day, asking him to speak on my behalf, he invited, "come and speak with me a moment," but I shyly and sensitively replied "No." During the rest of the day whilst I was busy in town getting to ready to leave, whilst he went to the case-conference, I felt how my feelings had very much changed towards him since that "moment" in the surgery; I now felt such fondness for him! That evening I phoned my friend Rachel, whose mother ran a retreat house in Cairndale in Argyllshire; I thought I'd rather go there than Ireland initially, because I would have more comfort and solace. I told her how I needed to "come apart" for a while, and I received the good news that I was invited to stay there.

I was looking forward to seeing him on the morning of my departure; I just wanted to stand there in front of him "in gentleness and real love." This encounter was initially sweet, but didn't seem too good on reflection. I had had a really bad experience with Walter, and held to my belief that "the real strength lies in gentleness." But Dr.James started arguing about it, and didn't seem to have any understanding of the real "gentleness" which allowed me to let my son go. We said a few deep, explanatory things, as if for a long parting. I gave him a card, which said from the heart, *"may God wrap you safe in his goodness and whatever the future holds, remember that I too always uphold you in my love."* I told him it was "always valid." I had taken a huge flowering plant round with me, thinking it symbolic as it had grown during my pain, wondering whether I would be returned before its flower died; "well at least he accepted the amaryllis!"

I see the human and emotional complexity of it all; and he seemed to be struggling with it no less than I was. I shall always remember that "gentle moment" when I saw him burdened and sad, when I was looking back from the door, and I loved him in all his fallibility and humanity.

And so I went away, as Prof Gray had suggested, in order to ponder over this "one great passion of my life" and how I had been mistaken about it in some way. A flood of emotion went through me as I reflected on that morning's encounter with him, on my way to Cairndale; though a temporary sweetness, it was not important next to the pain he left behind in me.

For I felt it was "cheap"afterwards, when I reflected on the journey on all the things he had said that morning. "I wanted you to be free, so that you could make an informed choice; I didn't reject you, I just wanted you to be free; when you came back from Lytham I thought you had the strength," he had explained. This was rubbish; "we don't make an informed choice about whom we love"; we don't make a rational choice; "rather God or Love grabs us!" And I felt I couldn't easily forgive him for the pain he had put me though; we might need to go through pain, but there was "arrogance in prescribing it for somebody else!"

I reflected, arriving and waiting in a lonely fashion at Cairndale station, on all that it had meant having him as my "Master"; if I couldn't have that kind of communing friendship with him I didn't want anything; "I don't want anything less than that." I had mentioned to him how my love had been "so total, so absolute;" stupidly destroying that totality and absoluteness of my love, didn't make it any more or less of a choice. *"He has destroyed the totality of it, the absoluteness of it," and I sensed that it couldn't "mend." And alone and forsaken at Cairndale station, I found myself shouting into the emptiness; "you've destroyed my total love; and for what!"*

These were the feelings with which I arrived, and upon which I was left to "ponder" in the coming days. I wondered whether I would really be able to re-orientate myself; *for I was aware that I had lost my sense of my "aloneness before God."* I was aware of the sadness of it; of this "mistake of my total self-giving." For I could never do it again; I could never love as totally ever again. I realised painfully how he had "got into the relationship which is between me and God." I felt the one thing I couldn't forgive him for was the ruining of the integrity of my journals. I found an analogy for it; "it is like spoiling integrity by getting a finger inside a bubble." He came out of it with his integrity and I hadn't, but he never "gave" like I did. And so I got up to face the world the next morning with the thought; "that you pierced into my soul-life is something I find hard to forgive you for, though I forgive you the pain."

The following days, as I tried to talk with my friend Rachel or her mother or other guests about this matter, were painful and sad, because of their deep misunderstanding of it. They were busy morally judging it, and finding it "culpable" because existing out-with marriage. I tried to explain how its "mistakenness" didn't lie in this, and it was a kind of "spiritual friendship" on which marriages aren't based. Rachel's mother in particular came out with an angry moral condemnation; but I fared forward untouched by all these wrong judgements, because I knew that we invest our life with meaning by choosing where we love. I watched how these people were investing the meaning of their lives in information about the personal revelations of Our Lady; I believed I had chosen a better path in centring my life upon the friendship with one man. In their talking they were all "in the shell of their own aloneness"; I began to feel better about the fact that I had enjoyed a deep sharing of my soul-life.

I dwelt upon the "mistakenness" of our relationship, which the wise and compassionate Prof.Gray had pointed out. Was the mistakenness in so losing my aloneness before God? Then it dawned on me; "I let him in; I can't say I don't forgive him for piercing so deep into my soul-life, when it was my choice to let him in." I seemed to oscillate between trying to reject him, and dreaming about him. I thought I would write to him to say, *"you may not be my Master any more, but please continue to be my friend. I don't regret your getting into my soul-life in that it was my choice, and I don't refuse the pain of it, but please continue some kind of meaningful relationship with me."* I reflected that though I'd left myself nothing to live for, the poet's words were true; "tis better to have loved and lost than never to have loved at all."

I wrote lots of letters, to everyone whose lives touched mine, but in particular I revealed to both my Mum and Pater Leo, how I had experienced this total absolute love for one man, and it had absorbed me totally and left me empty; "I gave my All and am left with nothing." I told Pater Leo that it was it was a total, intense and absolute friendship, and it was only a pity that it wasn't absolute in time. I said he needn't tell me that I was mistaken in staking so much on the one person, because I knew it; "I threw my absolute love on the one man, when it should have been reserved for Christ." And the tears rolled down my cheeks as I gazed out of the window, writing, "he was everything to me; how can I continue to be alive without him!" And then I finally wrote what seemed the worst thing for me; "that my absolute love should came to nothing, because apparently having his fill of me, he threw me away." *This was the sorest thing; "it's as if he's exhausted his care for me, and throws me away." And I cried inconsolably.*

After this I found my extreme emotions were calming down, but I felt confused, and I felt sad and alone. I was trying to "take on the pain of my aloneness;" I thought I'd try and beg him, "please continue to be my friend," because otherwise my life was waste and meaningless. This appeal of "I want you to be my friend" was plaintive and continual in my mind. I began reflecting on all the things he had said to me which were pain, and seeing them differently, thinking "perhaps he didn't mean what he said," and "I'm sure he does care for me really." Perhaps this was a failure on my part to accept the pain of reality, or perhaps it was my gaining of a more compassionate understanding of him. I felt that I was gaining a more compassionate insight into his "human fallibility."

Then finally one day in the chapel after reading though all the rolls of pain in my journal, I had my "one best insight", which was this: *I had said it myself, "I love you with the total love that should be accorded only to God." Such a love was wrong, whether he was fickle-hearted or whether he was a saint. I based all my soul's meaning on the one man; and because of the weight it couldn't bear, it came unstuck. As Prof.Gray intimated, I had to purify my love, establish it on a transcendent Christ. It was mistaken not in quantity but in quality, for it was "total love." For that reason perhaps it had to be destroyed; I had to "understand why that pain had to be."*

So I finally wrote that long four-page letter to him, which I intended taking back with me. I said "for the sake of keeping my life meaningful, please remain my friend." It said I was convinced he cared for me really, "though you haven't been open to me because you are angry with me." It said "I hope you will see that I can't stop loving you, and I'll want and need you always; take me back into your heart." I realised I wasn't accepting that it was over; but was thinking in terms of getting him to care for me again. That was it, basically and finally; "I can't believe it's over, I won't let it be over."

And so the last night before leaving for Iona, as I had arranged by phone to travel on and stay there, I found myself sitting on a rock halfway up the hill, looking at the mountains on which the clouds rested. *And there came to me words as strong as if it were a voice; "Hold to that belief that it's not over; hold to that belief in love; hold onto it."* It was partly an echo from the words of Dame Julian of Norwich; *"hold onto it, comfort yourself with it, you will grow to understand it, but you will understand nothing else ever."* I looked at the pink clouds over the mountains; *"it was a complete total love that I experienced and my soul was ravished by it; hold on to a belief in it."* I saw how we are *"crowned for our belief,"* for the belief we hold in our hearts, and the only thing that mattered that would define my future path, was that I *"hold onto a belief in that love."*

Thus my revelation on that hilltop the night before I travelled to Iona. Somewhere on my journey I said to myself; "hold onto a belief that it was true and real; for it was the best relationship of my entire life, perhaps the only knowledge of human love I'll ever really have!" I arrived at Iona abbey, "that place of grace," reflecting on how "implacable" he had seemed, and prayed there that I should be able to "touch his heart." The community at Cairndale had given me as a parting present a kind of rosary of pearl-like seven-fold prayer-beads; and I took it out when I was in the abbey, and solemnly said; *"I take this as a symbol that I hold onto a belief in that love, in its purity and strength and everlasting nature."* (I used those prayer-beads daily for my prayer for the next 8 years, constant to that belief.)

The Abbey people didn't really help, in that they kept telling us about the need of "letting go." There was an Abbey service that first Sunday in which we were all told that we must "let go of other people, to allow us to move on." I had already decided that I couldn't let go of this love, and establish my "aloneness before God" again. At the end of the week we were supposed to throw a stone into the sea at Columba's bay, in order to signify some letting go of something we wanted to leave behind, in order to walk away from it and make a new beginning. Now I had been told, in a talk with the warden of the abbey, that I had to "let go and let God," that I had to "let it go inside of me," in order to establish my integrity again; she told me that I had to throw stones into the sea over and over again until I could achieve this. But when I threw my stone into the sea that day, I did it saying "I don't mean this!" *I had already decided that it was the one great friendship, the pure true love of my life, and I would hold onto it.*

Another theme of that week was that of disabilities and stigma. I felt wretched when they talked about his subject with their endless sessions, because, although I owned to the fact of having a "disability," I felt I couldn't reveal what it was, because I would be so condemned and ostracised. And it was so sore, realising that I was so stigmatised by society that they had taken my child from me. I went around feeling solitary and pained, not even able to tell the friend I'd made why I was so miserable; I was fed up of having my wounds probed!

Partly for this reason I was talking to the warden of the abbey instead of attending the sessions; she was helpful in pointing out something out about men, especially intellectual and spiritual men. She told me that they like the adulation of someone sitting at their feet, but they can't cope with love being "human," physical and real. Why? Because it forces them to recognise "their own feet of clay." I found this helpful. I was still going around aware of his "implacable coldness" and the pain of rejection, but I began to think more and more "all he has to do is forgive me, all I have to do is earn his forgiveness." I was hoping it could "mend."

Finally I had an inspiration and an insight on Iona. It happened during the healing service on the Tuesday night. Hands were placed on me with the words "Spirit of the living God present with us now, enter you, and heal you of all that harms you." And I wept, aware of the pain in my thought "How can I let him go!" And in that state of vulnerability and tears, a man called Jim came up to me to comfort me; and he told me it was apparent that I had a "particular talent in showing warmth of heart." And he suggested that I use this particular gift by employing myself in some way to show that warmth of heart to all those who were genuinely poor, to those who have nothing, all those who are rejected and unvalued and unloved. The thought inspired me, lifted me on the wings of vision and insight. For I saw this was "somewhere else in which I could put my heart," a cause rather than a person.

And then this idea inspired me. I was told during the pilgrimage around the island that I was "a very warm-hearted caring person," and I saw that I could go back to the ideal of "caritas" that I used to have, previous to the 8 years when all this happened, when I used to work with Mother Theresa's nuns among the down and outs in London. Instead of a love of a particular person, "caritas" was a universal love. *Seeing then how the loving of one particular person came to grief, I decided I would give myself to that ideal of "caritas."* And then the last night, during the communion service in the Abbey church, there was this song; "here I am lord, is it I lord; I have heard you calling in the night; I will go Lord, if you lead me; I will hold your people in my heart." And I was shot through with the swelling sense of some great vocation.

And so I returned from Iona with vision and insight. I travelled back with the sure knowledge that "there are two particular people I am committed to loving, even through hell!" - my son Gabriel and Dr.James.

Maybe it was a big mistake during that trip, not to go through the pain of "letting go" at the time. But I judge that the opposite is true; that my salvation came from holding on to belief!

Chapter 91
Polishing and Forgiving.

So I came back from my "mountain-top experience" in Iona Abbey. *And I bought presents returning through Oban, of blue crystal candle-holders for those "two particular people I've broken my heart loving," my son Gabriel and Dr.James, as a sign of the light burning in my heart. It was to say that I was committed to loving them and would "go through hell with them." I saw that the relationships were in earthly terms over; "the best I can do is to be toward them lovingly open-hearted."*

On my journey I felt I had achieved that aloneness and "letting go" that had eluded me on Iona. But I arrived in KirkMichaels sensing it was a hell and a sea of pain; "all I've got is a desire to live differently, an aim to be in this world other-worldly." I thought I would "walk on through this hell, trusting that God would walk with me." But I felt immediately how the man I loved was no longer "a presence in my life"; my existence was hell because it was the absence of what I knew heaven was. The bliss of human love had vanished from my knowing.

I wrote a letter to him, saying I would remain lovingly open-hearted; "it may not have been everlasting on your side, but it is on mine, so if you ever want me to walk through hell with you, let me know." I gave him the letter and the present of the candle-holder by his car, saying it meant "I am committed to loving you in everlasting terms." He replied "no-one has ever said that to me before."

But "I didn't think being lovingly open-hearted would be so hellishly difficult!" I went through miserable awarenesses late at night; "the bliss of human love is over for me; I have torn you out of my heart at the price of putting myself in the pain of hell for as long as I am alive." I didn't want to go to him to get my ears syringed, because I didn't regard him as my friend; indeed I began to see him as my soul's enemy. "I offered you my whole mind and soul, you took it shallowly and never pledged your own; so you trashed my soul-life and left me with a life that is sterile and empty. You said I will love again, but I won't, because you've closed my heart; I'll never share my soul-life again." And so I came close to hating him again. I had brought back an Iona stone for him as a present; but I polished it with silicon carbide paper, saying "I don't know why I bother, I don't love you anymore."

Then he came very late one night, when I was polishing the stone; I showed it to him, and I read him my letters that I'd written when away, whilst we handed the stone back and forth; these letters had asked "will you remain my friend." "You always have my friendship" was his reaction. But he meant "mere friends," and I was aware as we hung about at the door, "I don't want anything less than total friendship, and that kind of friendship includes human warmth." I was leaning towards his arm, and he was saying "stop it, this isn't friendship." And it left me cold.

Something he had said really hurt me; "you forget that when everybody else rejected you, I stood by you," and he was referring to keeping my antenatal care when I was in Craigdene. "What's the use of saying that 8 years ago he cared for my pregnancy, if now he trashes my soul, and doesn't care about me now!" And he was still saying he was doing it "for my good"; "how is it for my good if it robs me of every shred of happiness I ever had!" *My emotional hatred went beyond words; I didn't want to keep polishing, "in case it will infuse hatred into the stone!"*

I found myself in the dentist chair in Invertay, feeling again that I hated him, feeling how my ideal of "caritas" was tumbling down because caritas was nothing without a warmth of the heart; "and I only had love in my heart because I loved him." As I realised this warm tears gushed over my cheeks as I walked though the streets of Invertay. I thought how my insights on Iona could make no impress on the reality of this emotional pain. Hatred was taking root in me; "When I loved him it brought life to me, now that I hate him it brings death."

To Edinburgh I went, in this hating frame of mind, in order to gain insight from both Philip Davidson and Paul Thompson. I happened to see Dr.James before setting off, to see about my ear-ache, though I really didn't want him to doctor me. When he said to me "everything is connected to everything else," *I replied earnestly, "they are all connected with the love in the heart, and when that goes, everything goes to pot!" At this he smiled at me with affection, saying "Mairi you're mad!"* I tried to tell him of the emotional pain I was going through; "won't you come and see me, as only you have the solution." He said affectionately "that's blackmail," but he promised to come; and I felt it was a touch of grace on the whole venture of my Edinburgh trip.

I hated the business of Edinburgh; it was like going through "a wad of reality." I was struck by the big difference between the limited human understanding of Philip and the warm divine comprehension of Paul. Philip was cold and judging and condemning, sitting in a chair watching the movement of my hands; and he seemed to take no responsibility for me, saying "this is your journey, not mine." But Paul took responsibility for me "as a priest," and it cost him something. Philip spoke coldly of "the threshold once crossed," and "if you drop a vase on the floor it can never be put back together again." Then he said it was the same as "other experiences of loss and bereavement" in my life; and I had to learn to live with it, "like learning to live with your leg off." *I didn't find this helpful, as it didn't give me any solution for turning hatred into love, which was what I was looking for!*

The warm divine energy of Paul swamped over me and inspired me. He said I was trying to love "as God loves," everlastingly. But for human love to come near divine love it need "a framework of expressed human commitment," and without that commitment it hasn't got a chance! I said I thought I did have his commitment, unexpressed, in that Dr.James took me up to accept and love; Paul pointed out that it hadn't been there on his side. He ended up banging his head on the cabinet, saying "put yourself in God's place." He added with wry humour, "I know you are quite capable of thinking that you are God, but please refrain from doing so at the moment!" *I shall always remember him banging his head against the filing cabinet, in his anguish of trying to give me real answers!*

"The answer is forgiveness" he suddenly pronounced. He explained "Sort out your end first, your bit; don't go in for blackmail; as soon as you try to force him to do something, that's blackmail. Find a way of loving him whatever." I said I didn't want to lose such a meaningful soul-connection "and would preserve it at any price." He pointed out that Christ said "he who would save his soul shall lose it"; he laughingly said "Don't go in for the preservation-business; forget Rentokill!" It was amusing when I tried to leave and couldn't get out of all the locked doors I found; I had to return to him saying "there's another wad of reality in the form of a locked door downstairs!"

I left Paul feeling touched by grace; I realised that my emotion had also been a "wad of reality." "These wads of reality get in the way of the real reality, which is always the reality of divine love." On the way home I was capable of an act of pure compassion; I began talking with a homeless person, and invited him to live at my address. It was the responsibility of an I for a You in a pure Jesus-like manner. I realised that love is a matter of going through life taking responsibility for other people, and love isn't blackmail. And so inwardly in a day I turned from hating to really loving! My thoughts were now loving; "we were committed to each other; I am totally given over to you; if you were in hell and having you would deprive me of heaven, I'd still choose you." *I would say to him, "don't let this wad of reality get between me and you; the only real reality, in the light of divine love, is that I love you."*

Then came the encounter which was deep and strange, but left me glad with the sense that we were taking responsibility for each other. That night he talked more deeply with me than he had ever done before: "I treasured it, that soul-connection with you; I gifted a lot of time to you; we shared a lot, we shared thoughts; I treasured that and would keep it; but anything beyond that must not ever be." I tried to explain how I had committed my whole soul-life to him. He touched my wrist, and I couldn't carry on with my explanation after being made so self-aware. He told me to listen very seriously; *"I couldn't commit my soul-life to you, because it wasn't mine to give, and I wasn't free. It's like this difference; you have a horse to give, and I have a house; you can offer me your horse, but I can't give you my house; I couldn't match what you had to give." He added affectionately, "no-one can match you spiritually any way; I can't equal your intensity."*

He stood up and I said I was sorry if my love ever hurt him. "You never hurt me," he said, and it seemed to me like saying "there's nothing to forgive you for." And I treasured that, and it remained sweet. But then again he said "you've loved other people before me." And that caused pain to remain with me, because it wasn't really true, and I felt incapable of loving anyone after him. But I was happy when he left. *I continued polishing the stone after that, valuing the one day of happiness I had got. My happiness lay in the thought "he seems to have forgiven me."*

I went round to his surgery then, to give him the finished stone. And I said to him earnestly, "it's only with you I've shared my soul-life, and I'm not capable of offering it again; I gave you something I can't take back and I can't give again." And I pointed out to him, "you talk as if I had many horses to give; but I only had the one horse!" He replied that I had freely offered my knowledge. *But the loveliness of offering the large polished stone from Iona remained with me; for I said, thinking of the way he is always losing pieces of paper, "you can keep things under it that you don't want to lose," and he leaned forward and placed it on my head!* I couldn't help laughing, as it seemed like him saying "I don't want to lose you." It made me feel that his coldness had changed to affection; he seemed to have taken me back into his heart.

That was the day that, filled with happiness, I made my first trip to KirkOswald, to see if I could find a house-swap there, riding on the top of a bus, singing, and revelling in the day's beauty. I had a successful day there, thinking it would be ideal to live there as a writer, as the solitariness was magnificent. *I could embrace life, now that this relationship seemed mended, redeemed, healed; it seemed my loving-devotion had been rewarded. How it had happened was a complete mystery to me, but we seemed to have forgiven each other! In the same few days that I was enabled to forgive him, he also forgave me; and it seemed strange and wonderful!*

Chapter 92
Loss and Sadness.

I returned from my trip to Iona, with a blue candle-holder for Gabriel to signify that I would always remain committed to him and "lovingly open-hearted." But I found on my return that Walter was true to his word that he would allow me no more access to my son; "you will have nothing more to do with him" he had said. I was busy for a while struggling with the breakdown of my relationship with Dr.James, but the loss of my son weighed upon me with a sadness.

Then I got a report from the case-conference I had missed, which said the social workers supported Walter's position and that I should get no more access. I was angry; *"they had argued about father's access rights, well what about the relationship with his mother! The law says the child has a right of access to both parents; now when Walter says "you'll have nothing more to do with him" everybody supports him! It was I who stood by him in the womb, I who stood by him when he was a baby; I want to stand by him. It is important that we should continue a mother-son relationship, and officialdom should be helping to make that happen, not obstructing it. Why don't they ask Gabriel if he wants to see his mother!"*

I had a miserable awareness of the whole story of my life in KirkMichaels; "I never had a choice or a chance since I moved here." It felt indeed as though my walls were soaked in pain, in my own pain; this was part of the reason why I was determined to move to KirkOswald, if I could get a council-house swap. *I saw how, as an unmarried mother everything was stacked against me. My life had been blighted by Walter and by his burdening me with a child!*

I knew what I wanted now as regards Gabriel, after enduring all that pain and domination-games earlier in the summer; I wanted one day a month of access, and no more than that. I could only cope with my loss of Gabriel this way, without regularly witnessing the damage that Walter was doing to him; I could better come to terms with losing him if I didn't see him much. But I wanted to see him occasionally, to let him know that I was still his mummy and still loved him.

On the 2nd July I happened to see him at Jack's house, and it was a lovely experience. "Walter is here" said Jack as he answered the door; "and Gabriel?" I asked, catching my breath. The next thing I knew Gabriel had pushed his way past him and was standing there in the hallway. It was like one of those slow-motion films; there was just the two of us in a timeless realm, running towards each other, hugging and kissing. And it was stolen, a stolen moment; we both of us dreaded at any moment Walter coming. But it seemed endless. "When will I see you?" he asked, and I replied "Walter won't let me see you." "What do you have to always remember?" I said, and he replied the words I had long ago taught him; "always remember my mummy always loves me." *It was for me a moment exquisitely sweet and excruciatingly painful at the same time. I went home feeling my heart tugged to bits, and the pain of my helplessness.*

That same day I saw Dr.James before he was due to go away for a fortnight, and I realised how, as regards both of them, I must wait; it may be a long time before I saw the two of them again. It seemed to me that I would never find fulfilment, because the two people I loved, I hardly ever saw. Everybody else around me, my friends and the holiday-makers on the beach seemed to have some family-life, some emotional life in which they had invested their self-giving, but after all my complete self-giving to these two, I seemed to be left with nothing; they had totally absorbed me and left my life empty. "Every body has somebody," through their self-giving building ties of love that last; only I seemed to be all alone. *I grieved over my sense of loss; I felt my happiness in these two was something I wasn't going to find again. I wasn't able to walk on, because my anguished sense of loss disabled me.*

The social workers became a bit more of a help when Jackie Bennett stepped in. When I first went to see her in Kirkcraig, I found she had an enormous sympathy for me. She said "we are aware of the games Walter plays, we are aware of how damaging it has been for you." Her sympathy came over in the way she finally said, "I am aware of how appalling it must be to have a child by a man who is abhorrent to you; I can't even imagine what it's like, but I feel for you." On 1st August I had a good experience when I went to see her again; I told her and Stuart O'Sullivan of the "unfairness" of the whole situation, and they said they could see it was important for Gabriel to have access to his mother, and they promised they would try and facilitate it for my desired one day a month. They said they could see the relationship between myself and Walter was "unbelievably destructive." I commented that *when I had said when pregnant that, no matter what the suffering I wouldn't kill a baby, I had not realised what never-ending suffering it would entail.*

A short while later Stuart O'Sullivan returned to me, saying Walter absolutely refused to let me see Gabriel; it occurred to me with sadness that the three months I hadn't seen him amounted to a thirtieth of his whole life. I said it was ludicrous *how Walter got what he wanted by operating through threats, bullying and harassment; now that I was being good, reasonable and law-abiding, I didn't get anything.*

One night I had an insight into what a "bastard" Walter was! *"All he knows is possessiveness. I tried to share Gabriel, Walter wants him all to himself; because he knows nothing of love, only of possessiveness, and the coercion, bullying and domination that attains his ends. I allowed him to see Gabriel when a two-year-old baby because I thought it was fair; I had some notion of giving and sharing, even the giving and sharing of my own child. Walter took advantage of that to take him off me, and when he gets him says, "you will have nothing more to do with him," wanting to have him all to himself!"*

I had a phone-call with my solicitor George McPherson. He seemed to have faith in the system and the reasonableness of the law; I felt we were worlds apart. I said there was "something evil and wicked in the system" that allowed Walter to do this to me. He told me to stop harping on the past; "you will get all these things at the end of the day if you are reasonable." I replied in grief and rage, "how can I get custody back, when fighting against a man like that!" *I felt "the futility of it"; the futility of fighting against evil in this world; for evil has a ruthlessness, and the good that is loving always gives in.* I felt it was evidenced by Christ on the cross. However an elderly and wise man, who came to see about a house-swap, restored some of my faith in a "transcendent love." Evil may have its way in this world, he said, but the love that gives in, the love which sacrifices, wins ultimately.

I was struggling with my anguished sense of loss that summer, trying to come to terms with it, but losing ground. I tried to open myself up to new life, with the hope of obtaining a council house swap and moving to KirkOswald, but it was having no success. I had thrown myself into a summer-school event in Kirksferry; I had talked there in such fresh and surprising ways that they told me I should mount my own series of lectures, but it ultimately made me realise how "unacceptable" I was to authority and to society. So the net result was that it didn't open life up for me, but rather closed it down; I became heartless about starting a new life for myself. Also the cold "platonic friendship" Dr.James was offering filled me with a progressive despair, and I seemed to walk through a long loneliness of pain beyond what I could endure. I was struggling, but losing ground.

Then I collapsed into a suicidal state overnight, when on the 15th August Dr.James came to visit me, and was very cold to me. I walked on the edge of life and the edge of sanity for a while. At first suicidal, I then determined to "give up the world and bury myself in death" by returning to my primal roots and entering a convent in Austria. When I was about to set off, having changed my will to gift Dr.James with all my writings and make him Gabriel's guardian and trustee, I found I couldn't leave the will with him; he told me to be "humane" because he was ill with flu, and asked for some "time" to consider it.

Whilst I was "waiting on his understanding," I decided I'd stay in the East Holme. Having found a B& B in Kirksferry, I wrote there a letter for the coming case-conference, insisting on the fairness of allowing me Sunday access. I decided there that I would wait "in transit" for a few months, partly to get an understanding with Dr.James, and partly to "save" whatever I could for Gabriel. I thought I could arrange for things to be saved for him out of my house, and make sure of some quality time with him between then and Christmas. From there I journeyed to the case conference, which was chaired by Stuart O'Sullivan, refusing to stay to be bludgeoned by Walter's domination-games, insisting on just handing in the letter I had written.

Very soon after that, because of the way the police were harassing me and making me fearful, I ran off, down on a train to England, intent on getting to that convent in Austria.
But I saw Gabriel one more time, to give him presents when I was on the point of leaving. Walter was still determined to put into practice the ruthless decision that I should have nothing to do with his son, and he behaved abominably. When I found them out in the back garden, he tried to stuff Gabriel into the kitchen, despite the child's frantic attempts to reach me. I reminded Gabriel of "always remember my mummy always loves me," and read him out a card which said, "even when I can't see you, I love you just the same." I left with a cut-up heart, whilst Walter was yelling after me, "this is your last chance."

Chapter 93
The Long Loneliness.

In the middle of July I found it strange and wonderful that somehow Dr.James and I had been able to forgive each other. I was glad that I had persevered in my loving-devotion and had never said that he "wasn't worth loving"; for we seemed to be "mending and redeeming" the relationship. I was delicately happy and filled with love and hope for a while, aware of his "being around"; I was enamoured of the song "love is all around." *However rapidly what gripped me was an awareness of a "heaven lost," and its sadness; "all I'm aware of, is what I've lost."*

He came one night to say he would be away for three weeks, and he didn't seem in the mood for me; I tried not to mind, having said to him "at least I know you are around." I was brave enough to then use the phone-box, to ask him to set me some task of writing for when he returned; and he told me to write a story about the burn. I then saw him a couple of times by his car before he left; he commented "you look like a gypsy," and I said I wasn't happy enough to write, as I lacked "the inner connectedness" he used to give me. He said "don't look at me like that," and I replied "I can't help what my eyes are saying." I begged him to come and see me somewhere in the middle of the three weeks, and he said "I might." When I saw him a second time I gave him a card with a poor sad blue teddy-bear on the front; "a teddy-bear out in the cold and sad, just like me!" He was amused, but still wouldn't say when he would come and see me.

I thought "why do I have to see so little of him!" I was grateful that he was no longer cold and rejecting, but I would never find fulfilment if the person I loved I could hardly ever see! It struck me it was a mistake to let my happiness depend on him; but I had to carry on, "to pick up the pain of loving, and walk with it long-distance." It would come alright in the end, I thought, echoing the words of Dame Julian; "All shall be well." It struck me "love is kept; with far fonder a care kept." He was still in existence, for me to love.

I wished I could have told him before he drove away; "I'm having powerful dreams about you; my yearning for you has no outlet." I remembered how I had known real happiness for a while, when he filled me with that "Deep Peace"; now I was yearning, and it was like the "loss of heaven." I certainly hadn't got that heaven back; though I was no longer in hell, I was continually aware of the heaven I'd lost; it was like being "in a limbo-land." *I prayed that I should be able to "hold onto a belief in that love," as I said I would on my Iona trip, but the reality of my loss began to overwhelm me. I saw how everybody builds ties of love that last through their self-giving; but a two-fold loss had greeted my self-giving; both my son and this man had absorbed me and left me with nothing. I had nothing at the end of the day.*

I felt I would be at the end of the day like Ms.Havisham in "Great Expectations," never going out of myself, but mourning forever over a happiness lost. I wrote letters to everybody on the last day of July, in particular one to Prof.Gray, saying "we were able to forgive each other, however"- - The "however" encompassed all this sad feeling that I was only aware of what I had lost, that I was perpetually looking back at a heaven lost. "My anguished sense of loss disables me; I'm not able to walk on."

One thought rose from the mind's abyss; "it was the only understanding of love I would ever really have, and if I didn't hold onto it, there would be a non-meaning in my life forever." How could he think that I had loved many times like that! It had to be really special before I could give myself to human love; I had to see divine love through it. I gave him my virgin soul-life, though it made me now "blush before God" because it robbed me of my aloneness before Him. After total self-giving and being left with nothing, that's the end of life,- "life as we know it."

I fleetingly thought of taking solace in other human love, as with Jim or Gavin, but I quickly realised no good could come out of such attempts; "it cheapens what we have valued, cheapens love, cheapens pain." It wasn't valid to seek "another You" to replace the You I had lost. I felt I'd rather go through pain for love, than get cheap happiness without it; *"real Love, an understanding of real love, is got through pain."*

What I wanted, what I really wanted and needed, was that he should "walk with me in my guilt"; because it seemed to me unless he walked on sharing the guilt with me, I couldn't walk on at all. "We must bear responsibility for each other, because we owe each other; we must bear one another's burdens like Abelard and Eloise."

I realised I must stop "dreaming" about it, and find "a new life for myself," some other way of self-giving. If I was going to renounce such love for a particular person and seek to give myself to something else, such as this ideal of "caritas," I had to be courageous and clear what it was. I had been trying to contact the Salvation Army, to follow this "path of giving myself to the poor," for which Pater Leo so praised me, only to find it all came to nought because they didn't operate in

Kirkshire or Invertay. I had to stop dreaming about him, or I couldn't healthily give myself to anything else.

I wrote a letter to Pater Leo, answering his in which he said it wasn't "wise" to commit myself in such total self-giving to the one man. I said it was true, as in Shakespeare that love is never "reasonable, rational, wise," a matter of choice and of the will; it can't be helped, in that it seizes us. But I told him earnestly that I was now "giving up human love" to choose a different way, and that I discerned God's purpose in this. *"I have to walk on with the guilt, with the knowledge of all love and happiness lost to me. Any escape from bearing that pain is an escape from the scrutiny of God's love. I must bear this wound in my flesh, of having given my All to human love, and having been stripped of all my happiness and all that I gave. It is the wounds that will get me to heaven, or nothing."* I flooded with tears, as I wrote *"I wish I hadn't given myself to these experiences of human love!"*

Then one day, on my way to the "Summer school" event in Kirksferry I opened and read an unkind reply in the form of a letter from Prof.Gray; it said "you fill the void by investing passionate emotion in a relationship." I felt that wasn't fair, and was hurt that he had a sad opinion of me. I wasn't just relating to Dr.James in order to "fill my own void", and I felt it an insult to imply that I filled my own void with my son, after all my selfless efforts to "pick up that burden and walk with it." That day I looked out to sea in Kirksferry and wished I could drown myself! *I had a sense of my life closing down, and having nothing. I felt how people compromised and made do the best they could to find relationships of love and self-giving, rather than living in the realm of absolutes as I had been doing. But my idealism had left me with nothing, and in reality my happiness was over.*

I remembered that bliss of "Deep Peace" in which I felt I "touched the finger of God"; if I had not known that bliss I could have found happiness in other ways, but having known it, there could be no happiness for me. *This is what I blamed him for; he had made me need something, which before I had I didn't need. "You have left me with the need." I came to depend on the bliss of that "Deep Peace"; and now that happiness was no longer before me, but behind me. And I blamed him for something more. For a while he had diverted me from my pain, and buoyed me up, when I lost my son; when I was vulnerable he took me up. But he only did so to now throw me down upon the thorns! And that was unforgivable! By diverting me from pain by something that didn't last, I felt he had done me the power of harm.*

My sea of pain in that loneliness seemed to go on ad infinitum. I felt that he had effectively "crippled me"; and I began to think again, in terms of that letter, that he was "the bastard who had destroyed my capabilities of loving," because he had secretly destroyed my heart. And so I went through my long aridity of pain, feeling "you can die of pain like this!" At the time I was writing a tragic story about a young prophetic girl who drowned her baby in the burn; *in the same way for those three weeks I was walking though "the long loneliness of pain," which "cracked the bonds of reality!"*

The reason I ended up suicidal, then manic, then hospitalised soon afterwards, was that after my walking alone for so long, when he returned he didn't help! The sadness of it is, that after feeling we owed each other that forgiveness, he seemed to spend the rest of the summer offering a friendship of such "aloof coldness" that it plunged me into a solitariness of pain, a mood of mind which left me"walking on the edge!"

Chapter 94
On the Edge.

Finally, on 15th August, he returned, and after a bright and sunny moment of seeing him by his car, he came round. After that "ache of the long loneliness" I'd been through, so disabled by my anguished sense of loss that I couldn't walk on, I needed his kindness, his warmth, his listening heart. I needed us "to bear one another's burdens like Abelard and Eloise." But he was cold, and wouldn't listen to me, and I felt "he really doesn't care."

I was hurt and wounded beyond measure that night; he said something about Gabriel, read my story, then his attitude was "right we have shared thoughts, now I'll walk straight out." I tried to say "give me a chance to say what is in my heart, listen to me for a bit," but he walked out. All I said at the door was "you can die of a broken heart you know." *The moment carried pain for me because it curtailed all my natural warmth and affection. I felt how I'd rather not see him at all than go through this kind of pain; however "real love is got through pain; does it need to be etched upon my forehead!"*

I became totally suicidal overnight! I was thinking of a quick way to die; I was walking on the edge of sanity and the edge of life; my grip on reality was slipping away from me. I felt like the girl of my story, in that I had known "the long loneliness of pain that cracks the bonds of reality." I wrote him a note which was a plea for help, giving it to him in his car; it said "there is a limit to the amount of pain that in my loneliness I can endure." The greatest grief to me, which was pushing me over the edge, was that I felt like saying "don't bother then, I don't want to see you again; I'd rather not see you at all than suffer this cold dying." But he never came. And it showed to me how little he cared. *A great outcry came out of me; like a wail, existing on the edge of life!*

I was going to say to him if he had come, that there was the chill of death in me, killing me from the inside out; *"I'd rather die a quicker way than to be slowly crucified in the cold climate of your platonic friendship."* I remembered how, out in the cold North sea that time, there was some faint hope that kept me from dying, but I didn't have it any more; "I had some kind of wholeness, some capabilities of loving, some reason for being alive, before I got involved with you; now I'm not fit for either life or death, either human love or God, but am suspended in a limbo of pain without end." I reflected how the only prayer I could offer before committing self-murder was "Lord have mercy on my soul."

Then I wrote my suicide letter; - *"You might think you can handle it this way, with your cold platonic aloofness, but it adds to my burden of pain already too much to endure, too great to walk with. You might think you can "walk on," but I am not walking on with you; I gave too much of myself to be able to walk on. I am sure Abelard and Eloise in the tragedy of their lives found some better way. But I forget, you never gave me yourself, and you take no responsibility. I really love you, you know. But I cannot endure the pain of loving you, and hating you for what you have done to me at the same time. It is like being suspended on a crucifixion. And I will always be locked in this agony of love, and you won't let me know its bliss any more by caring for me. I loved you too much; I loved you too much to be able to stay alive after the bliss of it was past. I go to seek the embrace of another Love, which is never past. I might have endured this pain, if you had helped; but never mind. - - I commend you as well as myself to God's love; it was my sharing in God's love that I shared with you; and in that love, I'll love you forever."*

But I never carried out that act of suicide, as I had in November of '92, because I was stopped from doing so by a vivid dream in which I was speaking to an Abbess. *And I said on waking "I will bury myself into death, it's what I really want; I will offer myself in a hard cold slow dying to the divine caritas."* And so I made my decision; I would take one step less, though a harder way than killing myself; I would renounce the world, bury myself in death, leave everything behind, as if I were dead, by entering a convent in Austria. Thus going back to my roots of monasteries in Austria, because it was what I had wanted first, was to me like going "back to the original."

With this intention, the next day I changed my will at the solicitors; in order to leave all I had written to Dr.James, and to make him guardian and trustee of Gabriel; I thought this was a way of "giving them to each other." I would say of the writings, "consider yourself as a repository for a life and a knowledge that was and always is beyond you." When I went round to the surgery to give him this will, I was twice deeply rejected; he accused me of being "inhumane" because he had flu. I went to his house; he had said "be humane, other people can be unwell." I was going to say "and other people can walk on the edge that exists between life and death." My doubt of him was utter as I waited for him in his room, and when he came in I said "don't be angry with me; I can't go anywhere without making sure I can trust you to receive this and can trust your response." He told me to give him time, a few days, to read and consider it; "I'll wait" I said. I tried to say "I came back this side of the edge, because I am attached to you." I reflected to myself that I shouldn't expect him to save me from the way I had chosen.

So I then wrote to him a nice kind letter, saying I was sorry for not being "humane" toward him when he was really ill. *"Can't you be more humane toward me? You've let me walk on in the loneliness of my anguish so far, that I am poised on the edge, the Edge that exists beyond life, the edge of sanity."* I told him how I had a lot of health-problems; "I lost my health when I lost you." But I said I could be "trusted to wait." I gave him a copy of one of my favourite books with this letter, to read in bed. Actually it was good that in trying to be "humane" to him, it forced me to be humane to myself.

I decided to find somewhere to stay in the East Holme, whilst I had to "wait on his understanding." I couldn't abide my own house, because it felt like a morgue. I wasn't able to sleep, which was a bad sign for me; the Lithium was no help in this situation, as it used to keep me awake with itchiness. I applied to other doctors for some of my minor ailments, but when Dr.Hughes implied that they were all "psychosmatic" I decided not to go near the Health Centre again. I stayed in KirkOswald for a few days, then found a B&B in Kirksferry; I had to attend a case conference about Gabriel, and I had to have a lot of treatment at the dentist. I became convinced that I had "wait in transit" in the East Holme for a couple of months before setting off to Austria, for two reasons; firstly to gain some understanding with Dr.James before I went, and secondly to "save" whatever I could for my son.

I left him a message to say that I'd wait on his understanding as long as he needed, and that I would be sleeping and writing in the East Holme. Twice he got out of his sick-bed to leave notes at my door; saying he was still fluish and back to bed again; they gave me the sense that he really "cared." *Those notes showed he cared, and I think we were indeed "bearing each others burdens like Abelard and Eloise." I think he tried "to walk on with me," he just didn't realise the long loneliness of the pain I was going through, and how it was driving me "to the Edge."*

My journal writing ended, because I had run out of ink, with the words "I think I have transcended my own pain." I had kept myself "sane" thus far, but then I was spooked by the fact that police cars were looking for me, and not being able to refresh my mind with sleep caught up with me. So finally, because I knew I was becoming manic, I hastily got travellers cheques, and went off on the train down south, with the aim of getting to that convent in Austria! *I was being driven over that edge of sanity!*

Chapter 95
An Ignominious Return from England.

After a few days of thus "walking on the edge," having left my house and endeavouring to write and sleep in the East Holme, on my way to an Austrian convent to "bury myself in death" there, but waiting around to gain an understanding with Dr.James and save what I could for Gabriel, I knew I was in danger of becoming manic.

Then an incident really "spooked me." When walking somewhere between KirkOswald and Kirksferry, a police car drove opposite me, and the policeman said "Get in Mairi." I was astonished, wondering how he knew who I was. "You're Mairi Colme, aren't you?" he asked. I got in the car, fearful that I was going to be taken back to Craigdene, thinking some doctor at the health Centre had ratted on me. "Are you arresting me?" I asked. "No, we just want to know where you are staying," he said. He took me to the B&B where I was staying, telling me I had to call in at the local police station next morning.

After this I was "running scared." I always had a touch of paranoia when manic, but it seemed to me true that "they were after me." I had finally got out of the Psychiatric System by that month's escape to Lytham-St.Annes; I didn't want to get into it again; at all costs I had to maintain my freedom. And so the next day, after going through a gruelling tooth-operation, in which I had all my fillings at one side removed, in an effort to find the cause of my toothache, and after obtaining as many £100 travellers cheques as I could from my Building Society, depleting all my savings, I got a taxi to take me to Edinburgh. I felt I had to get away from the area as fast as I could.

When you are manic you throw your money around. I gave this dentist, though I owed him nothing, a £100 travellers cheque, and I gave the taxi-driver another one. I was in an Edinburgh bank, trying unsuccessfully to change another cheque into cash, when the taxi-driver drove off, with my handbag and some luggage in his back seat. I was glad that fortunately I still had possession of my small backpack containing my prayer-books and journals. As I pursued my way through Edinburgh I came upon a shop which sold the candles which I desired for my prayer-time; I paid a £100 traveller's cheque for a £2 candle!

I hastened through Edinburgh to the railway station, and there got on a train bound for London, but without getting a ticket; I thought I could get one on the train. My aim was still to reach that Austrian convent. I very stupidly, manically, left another £100 travellers cheque on the seat under my backpack, and went to get something to eat in the diners car. I was talking to a nice young man there, who was buying me a drink, when the furore erupted about the ticket. The guard told me the £100 travellers cheque wasn't acceptable for the fare; we shouted at each other, and he said I had to get off the train when it went through Newcastle, where the police would be waiting to arrest me.

They did arrest me at Newcastle. They bundled me off to their police station, looked through my backpack, though I told them there was only books and writings in there. And realising I was obviously mentally unwell they took me to the large local general hospital; it was a very modern and impressive place, and I remember waiting there in the middle of the night with a policeman, waiting to be examined and admitted by a doctor. All I wanted to do, desperately, was to rest and find a bed, and get the cooling balm of sleep; I didn't care where it was.

I liked that hospital ward in Newcastle; it was the psychiatric wing of a large modern hospital, and they were very enlightened in the way they treated us. I was given that "Acuphase" again, designed to facilitate large shocks to the brain, and was introduced to Sodium Valpurate as an alternative to the dreadful Lithium, which had blighted my life for years. The meals were wonderful, the bathroom was wonderful, the nurses were kind, and I made a number of friends among the young men there, in particular one called Daniel. *It was a wonderfully sane, kind, fair, open place compared with the "psychiatric concentration of minds" that went on in Craigdene.*

They found out who I was and where I came from by the medical records on the computers; and to my great chagrin they said after a week that they were returning me to Craigdene. I didn't want to go. At least they took me on the journey north in a car rather than an ambulance; I remember how on the way when we stopped at a restaurant and shop, I spent another £100 travellers cheque on new clothes. *And so I arrived back in Craigdene, transferred there by an act of the Secretary of State no less! I remember how, after the nurses were nice to me on the journey, I was ignominiously bundled in the door of Morlond Ward.*

One of the first things that happened was that Dr.McNeill, now I was in his grasp again, changed and increased my medication. I had been feeling well on the Sodium Valpurate, which is a mood stabiliser equivalent to Lithium, the dreadful Lithium which had cause me nausea and itchiness of the skin for the past 7 years; Dr.McNeill changed it back to Lithium. And he put me on a dose of 200mg of Largactil 4 times a day, which was 8 times the dosage they were giving me in Newcastle; and he put me on the dreadful Haloperidol as well. I groaned with the thought of how I would be a "zombie" under the weight of all these drugs! (I didn't take them of course, but spent months spiting them down the loo, but I remember the oppression of perpetually being administrated them.)

I remember him well in his arrogance, sitting there with his drug-chart, changing it all, and myself groaning with the realisation that I was in his power again. I remember how I talked of "Donald Duck"and "Thomas the Tank Engine," which were my fond pet names for two of the nurses; and he thought I meant it and was living in a fantasy land peopled by these characters! And Steven Peterson my social worker spoke up, saying "she means Finlay and Alex McDougal". Then I said "there's always three nurses on at night, and one of them is always a mean little bitch." "She's right you know," commented Steven with amusement.

Steven Peterson was very amused at the time by my mood and insightful sense of humour. When he was dealing with the legal hassle of my transfer to Scotland by an act of the Secretary of State, I commented to him "those who live in England would do best moving to Scotland." "Why is that?" he asked; to which I replied "England is sinking!" He thought that funny. Upon him fell the onus of rectifying the mistakes I'd made when manic, such as getting back the £100 travellers cheques, and getting my handbag returned from Edinburgh where it had been handed in. It was because he didn't succeed in doing this for ages, that during one clinical meeting I called him a "fucking idiot." He was upset by this, but really it was at the time for me a term of affection. I liked Steven enormously, and I used to perch myself on the top of the table outside the office, waiting for him to come out, so I could talk effusively to him. He said on one such occasion, "if only you could see yourself when manic, if only you could see a tape of yourself!"

I talked with Steven about Dr.James at that time, telling him that both of us were struggling to come to terms with things; I remember Steven telling me, when I was talking to the chaplain, that I would regret talking thus openly; but I suspect they viewed it as "the rantings of a lunatic." The chaplain was a wonderfully kind and supportive man all those months, and he took messages to Dr.James for me, after I explained that he needed some help to "forgive himself." It was he who told me that Dr.James had fallen and hurt his back, cracking some vertebrae. I wrote some touching letters, saying how I loved him "more than life," saying how heavily I had "lost" because of him, how I had lost everything by "waiting on his understanding" instead of setting off earlier to Austria. I wrote that I was suffering in such an evil place, but *"I believe in Christ, the white light and the angels!"*

And so I dwelt for long months in Morlond Ward, remaining "manic" in a sense, but going around, my backpack of writings always with me, self-contained and "neat."

"Is there anybody there? - said the traveller knocking on the moonlit door, and his horse in the silence champed the grasses of the forest ferny floor, and the slippery snake slithered through the long green grass." Everyone has disappeared. I said to Petal "Actually I'm in agony, but I'm happy." - - Those wash -days when I was in hell; I'm nearer to heaven than I was then; I have angel-wings behind my shoulder blades. Petal laughed; "That's what they need these days,- peace talks - our lady- intermediaries."

Saturday a.m.: Lemon verbena yellow primrose room; at last the cure for all of me,- Colour. I remember Uncle Harold and Aunty Gladys. The light has altered. "Is it morning-time yet? Am I alive? Where am I? I hear voices."

Superman /Adrian Barton has lost his bottle, has become mortal since having a baby. It was a blue baby-boy; I well remember his entrance to this world; since then Superman has become peremptory. I said to Neil, "My Grandad always said, never eat with your mouth full; don't speak whilst you're eating."

Saturday 4am: "You're not doing your knitting at this time in the morning"; green on the lemon bedspread. "And who is going to stop me?" Orange street light shining under the high heavens. Monks always get up and pray before daylight; by now they will be going to the fields; my soul is in tune to Austrian-Benedictine-mountain-tops.
To Petal, "Help to neatify my bed." (Glossary; neatify = to make neat) Laughter about "snuggles", "fiver" and the rabbits breeding; a baby rabbit in the bed. My son will kill me if anything happens to "the Prophet". Washing accurately folded.

Saturday 6am: Father Tweedy said "you are the most selfish person I ever met", because I tried to give my life meaning. To Superman: "I'm recording these conversations, then you'll look a fool." He replied "you don't need help to get washed; there's nothing wrong with your foot." I had been told by the chiropodist yesterday to keep the right foot dry for at least a week, the dressing on my toe for at least a week. Elspeth was supposed to report this, but she gave me rabbit slippers instead.

Weather forecast freakish; frost and snow after a summer heat wave; Earth's climate changing. Superman was trying to maximise my sleep. "Ah I see!" Susan said "You just Awol." I replied "But I didn't awol; I came back." (Glossary; to awol= absent without leave and crazy and brought back). She replies "I'll give you a form and you can discharge yourself".

I come from an ingrown family. I was born Spastic, with a speech impediment. But my feet were never healed. I'll get surgical boots out of this. The chiropodist has reconstructed my fourth toe! I am rapidly losing teeth and digits as I hasten toward my end! - - Grandad's wisdom; "Pay no heed to what children say; watch what they do." Superman has learned that; from his baby boy!

Saturday: Breakfast was nice,- warm coffee and bread and butter with a little blackcurrant jam. Kim is climbing tables, throwing milk around. "Oh Kim - you ought to be incapaxed." (Glossary; to incapax = to render incapable of spending money). - - They believed I was psychotic and raving about elephantitis!

9.30 Saturday morning: Sabbath day, day of mourning and death,- now used by
fallible-multi-copied-humans to celebrate the release from the world of their work. (Glossary: fallible-multi-copied-humans - 9 syllables, how many letters? - Count and whilst you are counting, the world population is increasable and increased.)

Superman was trying to make sure last night that I had the maximum of sleep. His aim of kindness, not seen or perceived by me at the time, was to maximise my sleeping -time, for my healing, and for the sleep-chart. (Glossary: to sleep-chart.) He was sleep-charting.

Saturday High Noon: I've paid for the suppleness of my fingers by the breaking down of my feet. Metadental arches mal-formed. I was born a Spastic; I have transcended my limitations; my speech-therapy worked, was effective. - - Spasticified.- - Limitation-transcending.- - (Glossary: to spasticify, to limitation-transcend). - - "Jonathan livingston Seagull" - - Transcend.- - Dream.

I had a certain "neatness" about me during those long months in Morlond Ward; Petal the nursing assistant said years later, "I admired you, the way you kept yourself neat." I kept my writings in a backpack on me at all times, and tucked visibly in the back of it was a toy rabbit that I had meant to give to Gabriel and now carried continually as a "sign" of my love of him. I was self-contained, kept a certain space around me, and was ready for anything that the place had to throw at me. The dentist, the phone, and the washing were my preoccupations.

The hospital dentist was a wonderfully kind man, and I had to go see him weekly for months on end, whilst he tried to solve the pain in my right upper teeth that had been raging for years. My own dentist for years had refused treat this saying it was imaginary because I was a "psychiatric case," and I had to go to the dental hospital for X-rays and then, finding another dentist, had a large tooth out with pliars, then suffering the pain of an inflamed "dry socket." But that tooth apparently hadn't been the problem; the day before I left on the train I therefore had all my fillings removed on the right hand side to try and find the cause, but in vain; it was now left to the hospital dentist to patch me up. He found there was an abcess behind a nerve; he took the nerve out, and I waited weeks for him to drain the puss and apply temporary fillings. The nurses in Morlond always refused to let me attend these sessions, saying they didn't have the nurses to escort me; but every Wednesday I used to "escape" out of the back patio, and then when they found me at the dentist, in the dentist chair, it was too late and they had to wait for my treatment.

I remember clearly the day the dentist finally decided it was time to apply a proper filling. When he tried to do this, I went through the roof with pain. There was apparently a second nerve in there which he hadn't taken out. The kind nurse called Tim had come to get me, and I returned back with him absolutely hysterical; and on my return I sat hysterically by the phone at the entrance howling and sobbing. Finally when the task was all done, I remember phoning Pater Leo telling him it was like a "miracle" that it seemed that I had gained an extra wisdom-tooth.

The phone in the entrance hall was more a torment than a blessing. Every time I went to use it, needing the space around me, and having gone through hell to obtain the money, someone always came, and started ranting at me, and yelling that I wasn't speaking to anybody when I was talking to Pater Leo in German, getting me into trouble, bringing nurses to cut me off. It was a very dangerous and emotion-laden place was that pay-phone; several times I got beaten up there. And then because I was making what was termed "abusive phone-calls" to my family I was frequently forbidden to use it. For I was shouting to my Dad that he was a "bloody bastard."

There was a reason for this. Nobody can possibly imagine unless they had been locked up in the place, what I had to go through to obtain "money that went down the phone;" that is, 10ps and 50ps. Everybody who came into the place quickly ran out of phone-money, and as almost everybody had to stay in the building, there was no way of obtaining change. And therefore 10ps were more valuable than £1 coins, or even than the precious cigarettes which were used there as a kind of currency. When visitors came in the door I had to try and trick them, or beg them, to give me 10ps; I even remember stealing them from unwitting old ladies' purses. And as for 50ps, because they would allow you a longer conversation, they were like gold! Therefore, because my Dad had been refusing my "reverse-charge calls," and because of going though the long torment of obtaining a solitary 10p, imagine my chagrin when I got through, paid with my precious 10p, only for him to say "you are not to phone," and put the phone down! I desperately needed my Mum, I always needed my Mum; she was always there for me, though the long struggle of bringing up a baby, and I loved talking with her about Grandad; I can remember the ache of the need to speak to my Mum. And my Dad wouldn't let me. I gained a precious 50p at last, saying "I'll phone my Mum," I had to use endless wits to get to phone as I was forbidden to use it, and I got there, I put the money in, saying "let me speak to my Mum," and my Dad said "No you can't." So I yelled at him "you bloody bastard!"

(And that was what estranged me from my family, except for "my good old Mum," for years to come, and why my Dad disinherited me. This fact, after he died in '97 and my Mum a few years afterwards, left me struggling under the burden of a mortgage, whilst having to pay food for my son during access visits, for many years, in a real poverty. It is very ironic that the date he disinherited me was the Summer of '95, when I finally escaped for the grip of the Psychiatric System. He had no idea what suffering lay behind the emotion of my yelling "you bloody bastard" down the phone!)

The washing was another obsession. There were two machines in the kitchen, a washer and a drier, and because they had the glowing red lights which I regarded as a sign of "intelligent life," computer-life, I called them, after the names of twin robots in a film, "Huey and Dewy." I used to look after them, making sure they were carefully treated by the patients; I remember being very upset once on finding one was out of order because I patient had left a kipper in the pocket of a dressing-gown they had washed! I did lots of washing myself, but refused to let anybody else touch my washing, or transfer it from one machine to the other, or hang it out to dry on the washing line. I had to do the whole process myself, and my things had to remain "untouched by human hand." This was almost an impossible thing to accomplish, because the nurses and nursing assistants were constantly handling washing. That was why I frequently took bowls of washing along there late at night, or in the middle of the night when I couldn't sleep.

Another of my preoccupations was cleanliness. I showered frequently and washed my feet and underarms with creams. I was very aware of the "lameness" of my feet (I only walk on four toes and have a couple of painful foot conditions). I also had a problem with my right middle finger which had been hurt by a nurse. I had this strange surreal idea that I was "losing digits" as I got older. After the cleansing milk Patricia had brought in had run out, I had nothing with which cleanse or moisturise my face, seeing I was allergic to the carbolic soap that the hospital offered; and the only thing that would do which the hospital shop sold, was a combination of baby oil and baby soap. I remember secretly giving a young man a £20 note to go buy for me this baby oil and baby soap from the shop, saying he could keep the £18 change! This made sense to me in terms of how much I wanted it!

Sleeping was a problem; they mostly had me in the single side-wards rather than the dormitories, but they frequently kept moving me, without warning from one to another. But I didn't like anyone to so much as touch my things, so I had to keep on my toes. And every time they moved me, I found my bed in a different direction, and so they found me struggling to move it round in the dark in the middle of the night, because I felt I could only sleep with it in one particular direction. This occasioned nurses to threaten to inject me unless I kept quiet, or kept still. For the most part I hardly slept, but the nurses did "observations" all night, so I had to keep lying there pretending to be asleep!

Staying there for so long, I got the measure of the place, and began to see it as a kind of "home." I looked after some people, with a certain kindness; a certain old lady, whom I helped to shuffle along the corridor, and a young girl called Anne, as pretty as a princess with long golden hair, whom I took under my wing and did my utmost to help. (*I was really upset when years later I found out that, believing her only escape from the psychiatric system lay in suicide, she had hanged herself by the shoelaces in the bathroom.)* I also made friends with the ancillary staff, Katherine in the kitchen and the kind cleaner; and I made friends with a cat, who used to visit the patio, secretly feeding it, for which I frequently got into trouble. I got to know all the nurses well, working out their strengths and weaknesses, and had good friendships with all of the nursing assistants. I had a scheme of offering to everyone who was my friend or to whom I wanted to return kindness a chit of coloured cardboard out of an autograph book, on which I offered them a holiday on "Austrian-Benedictine-mountain-tops;" I believed this was a way I could repay them all someday.

And so, patiently settled there, the time passed. It is the one time I settled into Craigdene without perpetually planning to escape!

Chapter 98
Craigdene Madness: Part 2.

Character Profiles: -
Elspeth: bossy busy middle-aged woman with hair curly with large curly couplers; typical statement - "If we had been born in the Renaissance we would have been painted beautiful by Botticelli, but our bodies are now supposed to be thin." - - Article 39 called "lapsing out".

Superman: alias Adrian Barton; OK, in the end will still accept truth when he sees it; "Elephantitis is a real disease; look at my foot - the chiropodist has operated and reconstructed my fourth toe". - Accepted as Truth.

Denise: kind and thoughtful; a genuine help with the washing; treats like a general, rather than a psychiatric nurse; an early-thirties-mother.

Susan: an early-thirties-mother learning fast; like her now likeable memories; slapped her face for calling me Mairi; - Forgiven.

Geoffrey: crisp clean young man in pinstripe red shirt, born in the sixties; likings-   mint humbugs, nice sweets, red pinstripe shirts, fresh clean appearances; favourite sayings- "no probs" and "lovely"; designation- a war baby (the Vietnam war); relationship with filial love.

May: short black flat cropped hair, an early-thirties-mother.

(Glossary: "an early-thirties mother" = a mother who has had her first baby in her early thirties. i.e. a prima-gravida-geriatrix. Glossary: "a war-baby" = someone whose parents came through the war and was conceived during the war-time. - Why War?)

June: War-baby (here as applicable to World War 2); grandma-type, pink glasses, grey wavy hair, no make-up for work.

Linda: auburn full-curled-shortish-hair; one child- Darren, 8-month-baby.

Freda: lovely, bubbly, straight-black-haired; typical jokes - "Mary had a little lamb and the midwife fainted", "Have you heard about the man who died drinking milk? The cow fell on top of him"; full of witty jibes; expert-extraordinaire within the field of nursing; designation - an early-thirties-mother; one child- Rachel, 15-month-baby,

Conclusion: - Motherhood matures you; makes you compassionate, healthy, wealthy and wise.

On my Madness:
I had/have a Schizo-affective Disorder.
a) Psychotic = mad   b)Manic = creative.
The zuchlopenthixol-decanoate saves me from a).And the mood-stabilizer cures me of b). And I am well.

If my son suffers from the same illness as me, and apparently he does, he will probably benefit from the same treatment!- Sodium Valpurate (purple hearts)!

To Alfred, retired university tutor; "We want to stay here and get it right this time; we want to be A1 when we go out, squeaky-clean! (Glossary: A1-squeaky-clean)

Please check; SodiumValpurate levels, Clopixol levels, new glasses, new dentures, curing of my ears and teeth, curing of my lame foot so I can walk, that I'm sleepy; give me Disprin and Largactil please on regular prescription.- I have loads of both back at home; I'm self-medicating. I need at least one month.

I'm in too much pain and intensity to sleep. - - Make me sleep. - - Pain in my head, and eyes and ears and toes and feet. Give me a stronger painkiller please.- - Same old dream. I sleep-walk and I sleep-talk. I wake out of nightmare at 6o'clock with Lorenzo staring at me; - - I can't wake up you see; - - sleep so deep that it's frightening.

Nightmare: - Having eyes bitten out by wolves, having digits/toes broken off, and digits eaten by lions, people, evil figures from my past; evil stalking me. - - Nightmares because my sleep is too deep.

When I dream/sleep I go to the land of myth, i.e. Mythology, where there's dragons; - -"here be dragons" said Patrick Bellamy. Grimm collected them. E.g. a girl cuts off her little finger as key to get her nine brothers back, changed into swans by the nettle shirts woven for them and thrown over them by an evil snow-queen witch! - - Archetypal. Grimm's law about language declension; the same Brothers Grimm. Compare my sitting as an 18-year-old schoolgirl looking after kids on the doorstep of the Sudtiroler kinderdorf south of Innsbruck; the other aunty drunk with too much egg-flip. - - My youth spent mountain-climbing, romancing with soldiers. My pretty young life 14-21 ended up in a Benedictine monastery. I'm now 42; had to experience the world first. Needed freedom from my dad; threatened to drown myself; he was having a heart-attack; I made him leave the island! - - I like islands. Mountains 10,000- feet-high looked like islands in a sea; mountain-tops above the cloud-level! I saw sunrise and sunset on top there; and went to a hut for Bauerbrot and hot milk.- - My own mountain-top.

Rest your eyes; shut them; sleep - - I am one-eyed. (My right side no good.)

Question: "What do you call a one-eyed deer?" Answer: "No idea!"

Question: "With no legs?" - "Still no idea."

I am Insane with Pain.

TO HEAL
=Healing, whole, holy, to make well, to make whole, to make tranquil.
=Heil, haelan, Heil Hitler, in the mid 20th century.
=To tranquillize, to make the mind dead, in the 21st century.

Regress to McNeill, the Asylum-doctor:
I said to him, "We'll get all the monks to pray, to get the fingers off nuclear power-buttons." McNeill; "Sounds a good idea."

Austrian-Benedictine-mountain-tops; where I come from; - - like the "Sound of Music"; - - "How do you solve a problem like Maria?"- Let her be Schizoid! - - I suffer from a "Schizo-affective disorder".- - I had adventures in St.Peterskirche. But I wrote "the Book of the Beloved".

Who is the Beloved? Our Lady- Maria; not me!

Stop! I need a computer; - to be my friend.

Chapter 99
A Near-Death Shock.

I had been patiently settled in Morlond Ward for many months, before the beginning of December, when the event happened that lost me many more months. *For the "bathroom incident" which brought me near-death was also the occasion of the starting of me on the dreadful depot injection called "Clopixol," which then, although I was told it made me "normal," left me as "dead as a doornail" until the following May. So many months of my life I lost due to Craigdene!*

The bathroom incident happened due to the animosity of a certain nurse called Vera toward me. I had been running about as usual, in my "neatness," carrying with me all the time all the manuscripts I was writing and my few valuables in my backpack, the one with the rabbit sticking out of the back, when she accosted me one morning saying I had to have a bath. I naturally refused, as I had already been washed and dressed; but she forced me into steam-filled bathroom, together with a nice nursing assistant called Debbie, and they attacked me, forcibly taking off my backpack and trying to take off my clothes. I went bananas; "water and manuscripts don't mix!" There was all this water and steam, and I didn't want my backpack in there! I threw a kind of fit; wedging Vera there in the corner of the room, I just thrashed my arms and legs back and forth; I beat her up.

It caused an extreme and immediate reaction. I had run back to the safety of my room with the back-pack, when the three nurses, the charge-nurse Rob, Vera and the Tim that I liked, forced their way in. They held me down on the bed, and started giving me an injection of Largactil, but I thrashed about so they couldn't keep the needle in. "Hold her down" came the cry. So they threw me down on the dirty and smelly carpet, all sitting on top of me, with Vera giving me injections over and over again. This was Vera getting her own back because I had punched her. I remember the stench of the dirty carpet, I remember the sense of being "raped." *My neatness and my self-containment had been violated!*

The next thing I knew I was being carried or dragged along the corridor to the observation room. And Rob shouted out "Quickly, she's stopped breathing, she's stopped breathing." I remember being thrown on the bed, and everything going round me like slow motion. I realised I had stopped breathing; I remember realising I wasn't breathing. Rob tried unblocking the airway and giving me mouth to mouth; and he was yelling for someone to bring injections of Procyclidine, which is the antidote for side-effects. I was always grateful to Rob ever after, feeling that by his quickness he saved my life. The next thing I was aware of, the doctor who had been called was running his key along the souls of my feet, to check my responses; "she'll live, she'll be alright now."

But I wasn't alright. This near-death experience was a shock to my brain; I always believed this; for months after I dreaded that this was the fact, because it was a long time before I became "normal" again. I lay on that bed, as pale as death, having endless injections for days, - 13 in all I think I counted. There was the ones that nearly killed me, then the ones that saved my life, then more "Acuphase" to help me get over the shock, then more of the "Clopixol" they wanted to establish me on. (I noticed that the Acuphase was ZuChlopenthixol Acetate, and the Clopixol was ZuChlopenthixol Decanoate, so they were the same family.) The nurse I called Superman kept coming in a kindly enough fashion explaining to me what the injections were for; he said the "Clopixol" was a modern anti-psychotic drug, recently created especially for females, and I would be stabilised on it and it would keep me well. My friends who were on the kitchen staff said that in those few days I looked ghastly, as white and stony and deathly as concrete!

It had apparently been Steven Peterson's idea that I have the depot injection, instead of the dreadful Lithium which never worked on me, which Dr.McNeill had forced me to take for 7 years, since he had first sectioned me in '88. The Lithium had caused me problems with nausea and itchiness, but I least I could have some kind of meaningful and creative life on it. The new "Clopixol" deadened me entirely, making me feel I had concrete instead of living tissue in my brain! They partly forced me to have it, I believe, in order to force what they term "compliance," for when they had ransacked the room I had been in, they found a lot of tablets hidden away. And Vera had come away triumphant, shouting "she hadn't been taking her tablets; that's why she wasn't getting well!" *I ask you, what did "well" in this situation mean! It certainly meant, rather going around creative in my "neatness," than existing without any capabilities of thought or feeling, in a state of being "brain-dead"!*

But they insisted that they had made me "normal!" And they gradually let me out, more from week to week, over a long agony in December, going back and forth daily on buses, till finally it was called "trial leave." I remember seeing Dr.James over Christmas, and he drew his finger over my forehead to see how much make-up I was wearing, and I knew he saw the deadness of my face and my eyes!

401

I didn't recover; I went on "living in concrete" for many months, until in May I became manic despite the injection; then I was back in the hospital, from which I made many and persistent escape attempts, until I succeeded, so that at the end of the day I could carry on under Dr.James' care on a "minimal dose" of the Clopixol. For the cruel Dr.McNeill had refused to reduce the dose, despite all my desperate appeals, and it kept me "brain-dead" in a way I couldn't endure. Finally free of my section in September of '95, able to choose and no longer forced to take anything, I worked out a medication regime together with Dr.James. *The irony of it is, I was indeed kept well on this Clopixol for the next 7 years, but on one sixth of the dose!*

Chapter 100
In Concrete.

Thus I was thrown out of hospital back into the community, around the time of the New Year '95. They thought they had made me "better" and "normal" by establishing me on a depot injection of "Clopixol," but in reality I was "as dead as a doornail," incapable of thinking, feeling, writing. *I continued in this dreadful "living death" for the next four months, unable to function; it was as if the living tissue of my brain had turned to concrete.* I remember saying to the kind and sympathetic Gail Bryans when I one day met her in the Baptist church, "But it's like going through concrete." And she replied, trying to restore in me some hope and faith; *"you've got to go through the concrete in order to get onto the grass." But I never found that grass at the time!*

I could hardly get out of bed every morning and hardly function; I was suffering "tardiv diskinesia," my legs shuffling and twitching and my speech slurred. I remember going every Wednesday night to a bible study meeting, striving only to stay awake, and striving to restrain myself from saying in the car "I want to die." I begged Dr.McNeill to take me off the horrid injection that was doing this to me, and to return me to a regime of tablets; but he commented that I was "very well," and that I was comparing it to "the whiz I got when manic." I begged him every time I had these appointments with him at the local hospital to at least reduce the dose of this injection, but he would never listen to me, and I felt he only wanted to keep me "under his thumb." *I was forced to take this medication, entirely against my will; once a week a psychiatric nurse would come to give me it, and the threat was perpetually there, that if I refused it, I would be sent back to Craigdene. Thus the regime of fear and coercion under which I lived!*

I wanted Dr.James to support and help me; but the ten-minute slot on a Friday morning in his surgery didn't solve my loneliness. I was trying to come to terms with "the fact that the friendship was over." I said to him once "thankyou for the happiest year of my entire existence," meaning the year of '93; but he wasn't really in my life any more, and I had to get used to the fact that the Friday slot in his surgery was all I was going to have. He kept saying I was "normal" now; he said "when you are not mad, I like you."

But it was because he wasn't supporting me at all that I turned for comfort and support to Walter. He gave me affection and showed me kindness. I kept saying to him "thankyou for being so kind to me." Every Saturday in particular we spent the whole day together, going out with

Gabriel, returning to a roast chicken dinner, and then I would help Gabriel with his bath and putting him to bed. I needed the affection.

Often there were squabbles of bad-temper between Walter and Gabriel, and I did my best to keep out of them. I kept saying to Gabriel "mummy always loves you, mummy is never angry with you." Gabriel sometimes said very sad and plaintive things to me, because he could tell I wasn't well. He kept saying "you are different than you were before; when will you be well?" or "Why are you so different than when I was a baby?" These things pained me so much. I managed to get unsupervised access again, and took him out to places in KirkMichaels, but was disheartened by how naughty and undisciplined he was. But, as opposed to Walter's bad-temper, I was trying to show him "an alternative way of life, which has real freedom and love in it."

My real struggle at the time was with Dr.McNeill. He had sworn to me that when I would see him on the 3rd March he would reduce the medication. Steven Peterson had been to see me, and when he had said the injection was "keeping me well," I had replied that I wasn't able to think and feel and write; "I don't have a soul any more." I said it was as if, "to stop me from swimming too fast, they had fastened me to the ocean floor with concrete, and now I couldn't even surface to my normal self." Steven agreed with me that it was "a matter of getting the balance," and he would ask for a reduction for me.

On 3rd March Dr.James filled me with hope when I saw him, because he said he would come and visit me on his return in three weeks. I had said to him earnestly; "I need you with my whole soul and my whole personality; I've been masterless so long; come back into my life again; you are like an umbilical cord, connecting me with everlasting life." And he gazed at me with his grave grey eyes. And I went away jubilant, feeling his presence, so prized and so valued, "graced like an angels tear!"

But the same day I felt complete despair by my encounter with Dr.McNeill. For after he had promised he would reduce the injection by half, he refused to do so, and when I pleaded, he said in a denigrating fashion, "you are an actress; next month you will be pleading for something else." He said he wouldn't consider it for a further 3 months. Then he said insultingly "your lack of well-being is in yourself, not in your medication; you've been ill so long you can't tell when you're well." I was outraged, and I was upset that he condemned me to live like that for a further 3 months! "I'll have to escape" I said to myself.

I did run away, to Edinburgh a few days later, in a bid to crack my section again, so I could get out of this coercion. I found an old cold bedsit, but when tracking into the town in order to find something hot to eat, I realised I couldn't go through with it. I had visions of becoming gradually psychotic in the cold bedsit, and it would take me back to square one in Craigdene. I had left a note saying I was absconding, but I phoned from a public phonebox, to say I had realised how stupid I'd been. I realised when I came back from that trip, "It's a mentality; I'm always escaping." Walter said "it is like running away from yourself." I realised "it's a mentality I must transcend."

I began to realise I would have to stay on the injection, as it was my only chance of staying well. I wrote about the pros and cons of it. *On the one hand I felt so trapped; I'd rather have a short high quality of life, with the possibility of being manic, than this flat deadness for ages; "I can't be myself unless I'm capable of being manic." I said to myself "this isn't the answer," this mind-deadening medication wasn't the answer! However, realising that I had been more mad than sane for years, I could see the argument that "any medication which gives me a chance of maintaining a life better than that, is sure to be worth its salt." I felt if I persevered with it, pressed ahead and went through with it, perhaps it would give me a chance in the face of my own illness. Going though this "therapy" was perhaps the only way I would ever get free. I meant it when I said "I want to stay sane."*

So having returned from my failed attempt, I decided the only thing to do was to plead with Dr.McNeill to reduce the injection. I wrote a letter to him, pleading that I was so deadened in my responses, and so incapable of living a meaningful life, that I would be driven to do something desperate, though I knew absconding was not the answer; could he please put me "on a minimal dose"? Could he do this to give me a chance? "I have to have some hope." I went to see him, begged to be put back on Sulpiride; he recognised I might be what he called "depressed." Then I voluntarily put myself back in Craigdene for twenty-four hours, and he finally agreed to put me on anti-depressants.

Steven Peterson came around again, and insisted that I was "normal," and that "this is reality." He said "God isn't up there with the manics, He is down here with the rest of us." Dr.James also was telling me that I was "normal," saying, showing me myself in the mirror, "Look at your eyes; I don't like you when your eyes are mad, but now you've got normal eyes." He said it would do no good living in the creative stage of hypermania "because it is only one step away from that precipice."

But I still averred "I refuse to accept that this is my normality." I averred "I am only myself when I'm capable of being manic."

Then the last few days of April I found myself getting to feel well, and told myself "I've come through." But I soon realised I was getting into a euphoric state, and I asked for an extra injection at the local hospital. Then on the Monday I went to Dr.James saying "I'm too high," asking if he could help my precarious mental state; "can I please have some care!" I appealed to him in the privacy of his car, when he was giving my son and myself a lift, "can't we work this out between us without the psychiatric service knowing?" I found it very hard trusting him, remembering how he had been instrumental in putting me into hospital in the past; but "I know he cares about me, though trust between us is sometimes thin."

In those last few days I got myself a boyfriend called Ernie, and I found him fun to be with; we were both trying to get healthier with good food and exercise. I was delighted when he took me out every evening; and I decided I was going to make a stand against the sexual harassment from Walter. I was determined to tell him "go take a hike." Walter became jealous, and shouted in the back garden "Is Ernie your boyfriend?" Meantime I was astonished when I talked with Isabel and the psychiatric nurse in the back garden and they couldn't tell that I was manic!

By 3rd May I was properly manic, though I still had insight into it. In a sense you can't be properly manic if you know that you're manic! I wrote a note that morning to Dr.James, saying, "I'm having a whale of a time, but I don't think I should be, because it's dangerous; it's like balancing on a knife-edge, or balancing on a wall when down one side is a cliff." I asked if he could get me down from this condition without telling Dr.McNeill. He gave me a further injection that morning, and whilst he was giving me this oil in my backside, he said to me earnestly, "Don't go mad on me Mairi!"

The next day I felt "saved by my friends," in that Patricia and Elizabeth were trying to look after me, like a real mother and a sister in Christ. And I felt Dr.McNeill's poison was pitted against Dr.James' remedy, in that, against the rules, Dr.James provided me with Sodium Valpurate, in a last ditch attempt to save me from "going over edge." I was in his surgery, feeling it a sanctuary, knowing I had gone manic, bouncing a tennis ball that I had got for Gabriel. I can remember this was a day of great national celebration; the 50th anniversary of the VE day which had ended the war. *Thus I went from having a deadened mind to having a manic one in just the space of a few days!*

I ended up in Craigdene of course; I went there on the bus, thinking I could ward off the evil of the ambulances coming after me. I knew they were coming after me, because in walking past my friend Vivien's house, she came to the gate, and noticing I looked "peculiar," with my hair down and my glasses on, she said "just wait here whilst I call the ambulance!" *I thought that by making my own way there, and "giving myself in" as it were, I could win some vestige of freedom, of being able to walk around the grounds. I told them I couldn't tolerate living at my home any longer because the whole experience since the New Year had been like "living in concrete!"*

Lorenzo: "I'd be offended if they put a picture of my head, and put "Missing"!
- - Green for Laughter. - - Laughter about woollen mills and smog; mills and dirt led to escape from industrialization. - - That was in the bad old days,- of time-out rooms, before the 1984 Mental Health Act.- - I said to Lorenzo, "I had to go to school in a smog-mask and they all laughed at me because I looked like a Martian." Why did they laugh? - - Fact of Smog.

Character-profiles: Lorenzo: tall, distinguished, a character of wit, grandfather of many children, and father to all. Neil: decent guy. "I love you," I said to Neil, after talking excitedly, and showing him my lame foot mended; "I love you too," he replied.

Laughing and hitting Lorenzo at midnight, after my washing seen to, and everyone else put to bed. With Neil: spirits, ghosts, poltergeists haunt this place. Back to Lorenzo: "Walk on your heels, and save your soul/sole." - Laughter.- -

With Neil: "Ee by gum!" - A yorkshire saying; - like the stamp saying "Ee by gum I'm stuck." With Janet, saw to my washing. With Neil: "That little mermaid story, is the story of me. I see you in the dark; my eyes were burnt out on mountain-tops as a schoolgirl."

With Lorenzo, must be sober to take my medication. - - "Be sober, be vigilant, for the devil goeth around like a roaring lion, seeking whom he may devour, whom resist, steadfast in the faith." Lorenzo: "He will be after your rabbits then." (rabbit slippers on my feet.) Back with Neil: " a friseur means to shiver." Finally back, Lorenzo says: "What is verba-bit? That's what we've been playing all this time,- (all these years). It means verbal diarrhoia." Hit him!

I came back out from medication; Lorenzo: "I have a flair for dancing." Beat him up: "I'm going to beat you up. You make a good father don't you?" He held my wrists,- like a father. "You make a good father don't you?" That's been the most enjoyable part of my life!" "What? Being a father?" "No; making bairns!" Laughter.- -Lorenzo's rhyme (to teach his children): "I'm not a pheasant-plucker, I'm a pheasant-pluckers son, I'm only plucking pheasants, till the pheasant-plucker comes."

About my Grandad:

"Brothers and sisters have I none, but that man's father is my father's son."- Grandad would never tell me the answer; not allowed to guess. - - First epileptic fits and first poem about his death. - - "And my very soul is crying out for love and understanding, for he is dead."- - Guardian Angel.- - Combination of two ingrown families produces spasticity; a very potent combination of two families, which left me as the weak link. - - Lesson on the photos; we are the love-babies born after the war; I was an unwanted child and had to be a boy! - - Grandad chose me!

Struggle with friends Neil and Kim over footwear and money and washing-computers. And I said, "All things are possible; God's not God of the possible, but of the impossible."

People break things (i.e. inanimate objects) because they don't know how they work. - - Symptom of Violence in our society. - - But irons, washing -machines and tumble-dryers are now living inanimate objects, because they think.(Everything with a red light on is alive.) "Anima" = soul, psyche. - - Title, "Her Psyche danced with God".- -Dancing!

My personal tragedy: That the man who raped me took custody of my kid off me when I was in Austria writing a book. - - It's behind the scenes, it's evil, it's the freemasons.

Ernie offers to get shoes. - - God sending you what you need. - - "There is a special providence in the fall of a sparrow." - - "Deus providebit."
To Freda and Janet at the nursing station; "Is he a neighbour?" - - "Who is my neighbour?"- Christ answered. And so my kindness is being repaid. You can say "Everything is working out wonderfully for her!"

Character Profile: Ian: "A gentleman in whom there is no guile"; like Superman, kept tucking me in; boyish, same age as Superman; supreme gentlemanly care of a lady, a woman in distress. - - How the age of Chivalry is not dead. - - "Sir Gawain and the Green Knight".- - Chastity, Integrity, 5-fold Pentangle.- - I wrote a story about Medieval romance. - - Courtesy; Dame Julian.

We're middle-aged (Elspeth, Petal, myself); we came through the War; we were in our mothers' tummys 1939-54, and in the intention of our fathers'eyes.

My mother called me Maureen; -"little Mo", after the tennis champion of that era. My mother says she should have called me "Kelly", "because

I always bounce back up again!" - - Identity is through the meaning of words, the meaning of names; self-identity through the passage of time and unique experience.- - I wrote an Anglo-Saxon short story. It explained the meaning of Rape.

Meaning of Rape can only be seen in light of the meaning of Freedom.- "Free choice, free doom". - - Iona, the Island of Doves. - - My meeting with the Iona Peter; loss of him; "ships that pass in the night." - - Living earth theory; "Gaia hypothesis".- - Dance of atoms, Einstein, the Zen of Physics. - - Elderly wise men; my Grandad, Prof.Robinson.

Chapter 102
The Horrific Punishment.

The reason I was always acutely anxious about being "caught" during one of my great escapes lay in what happened to me after I was caught on Iona, years earlier in 1982. On that occasion my punishment was severe.

I escaped from Ward 6, the lock-up ward, which was quite an achievement in itself. I had been put there in March of 82, transferred from the old Ward 19, because of my frequent escape attempts, usually across the grass in my nightdress, with the wind billowing through me. I felt I had to get out of a building of such torture, even if it were only a short while in the gales and the rain, felling the rush of the air and the sporting of the seagulls. I remember feeling there was nothing wrong with me at the time, not convinced at that time that I had an illness, but was viewed by others as manic. I remember trying to convince a darling old nurse called Nurse Hopkins that the fact that I could balance a cup of tea on a chair-arm proved the fact that I was well. I remember climbing out of a high window when only half dressed, running fast across the dewy grass, and when I was caught yet again, saying I'd just "gone for a morning jog."

They finally put a stop to this behaviour by locking me up in Ward 6, where, as well as greater security, there was one nurse to every patient. It was a "behaviour modification" ward, and if you did not do as you were told you were relegated to pyjamas and plastic eating utensils. Everything was controlled by keys and locks, even the toilets being locked up, and the upstairs dormitories being closed off by a heavy-duty gate. I made the mistake, the first night I was there, tired of being herded around like a prisoner, of saying "I want to be alone." The result was that the unintelligent night-nurse said "come with me then", showed me into the time-out room, and shut the door on me. This was my first introduction to the "time-out room."

It was a dreadful and dreaded place. There were just four plain white walls, and bare lino floor, and in the opposite corner from the door a huge mirror covered by a wire mesh, so that it couldn't be broken. The only window was a small one on the door itself, which was covered on the outside by a wooden slat. And the only light was controlled on the outside by a dimmer switch, which put it on or off. I quickly turned round when the nurse closed the door, realising this was not what I wanted when I said I wanted to be alone; it was for "solitary confinement." But I got a shock when I found no handle on the door. It couldn't be opened from the inside; everything was controlled from the outside, and the mirror was so angled that a nurse peeping in could see every corner of the room. *(NB. This was the room which later proved my bane, was I was locked in there for long periods during my pregnancy.)*

I was alarmed and banged violently on the door; the nurse came back and shooted back the slat; "What's the matter?" she asked. "Let me out, I want to go to the toilet," I replied, thinking this a good excuse. The next thing I knew, the nurse threw in the door a small cardboard potty!

I can't recall how long I had to stay in the time-out room on that occasion; I think it was several hours; there was no way of telling the passage of time in that room; it was a dreadful place. The following evening I watched a similar performance with a very young girl called Lynn; she was put in there for misbehaviour; again she was thrown a cardboard potty. This time I noticed the nurse came back saying "oh I've forgotten to lock it!" *I was appalled by the realisation that this nurse didn't seem to know that once in there it was impossible to get out again, there being no inside handle; it seemed she thought the poor inmate could get out again when they wanted. I was so appalled by watching this young Lynn suffering that I decided I would "strike a blow for freedom" on behalf of everyone in the place!* They all shuffled along like lost souls; they were herded into and through locked doors as if sub-human. I watched Danny McAlpine being punished for drinking water, reduced to pyjamas, and stuffed full of injections in the time-out room until his blood ran down the walls. I was determined to escape from the place, though such a thing was deemed impossible.

I planned it for ages. I asked the inmates when the times of change-over were, I found out when the nurses were at their most vulnerable; I asked about all the exits, and especially about the fire escapes and were they were situated. I found out what was on the outside of the fire-escapes. I was told that once the fire escapes were open, all the fire alarms would go off, and the relevant breach would be shown by a red light in the office. I watched again and again where the nurses would be at any particular time. And so one night I found myself ready and poised for this act of daring. Realising I had to travel light, I had put layers of clothes on, and I had put that morning, ready packed, my rucksack on the bed. We were ushered up the stairs to the dormitories, the female nurse coming up the stairs behind us; I realised this was the moment of her least attention, the best moment to seize. I rushed into the dormitory, ahead of the others, put on my anorak, slung my rucksack on my back, and launched myself through the fire-escape door.

I was instantly terrified by the noise; the loud fire-alarm sounded in my ears as I ran fast down the narrow fire-escape steps. I was down! I knew the way out of the grounds, the quickest and best way; down the path and through the gate I ran, not looking back to see if I was being pursued. Then I was on the main road, and a new fear struck me, - soon police would be searching along that road. "I must get off the road" I told myself, and seeing a wooden gate through to a copse between farmers fields, I climbed over it and hurried on. Quickly the darkness closed around me in that little wood; it was very dark away from the lights, and I couldn't see anything ahead, except incessant trees and briars which clawed at my legs. I began to regret this; I didn't know where I was going; I hadn't planned anything; I knew I had to be absent for a whole month for my section to lapse; how on earth could I manage that? I had wellingtons on, but the bushes and briars were becoming a nightmare; I felt I was stuck and lost.

I went on and on, until finally I hit another road. I breathed a sigh of relief; at least this was a different road, so hopefully the police wouldn't be searching down it. I saw a car coming with its headlights; it could be a police car; I hid in the roadside ditch. I was thankful when it passed. I walked on. It struck me I could try going to Iona, because I knew the place, and I would feel safe there. I walked on and on in the darkness, throwing myself in the ditch every time I saw a car coming, fuelled inwardly by the fierce hope that I could get to Iona, and also chased by the dread of what would happen to me if I were caught. I walked about fifteen miles that night!

I arrived at Kirksclare railway station in the early morning light, having come upon the railway tracks and walked upon them for some distance. I knew there would be an early morning train through that station, going to Edinburgh, carrying me yet further away from the dreaded hospital. My instinct was to get as far away as possible from the hospital as quickly as possible. I can remember the station-master gave me a shock by shouting at me from the opposite platform, "How did you get in here?" But I just ignored him and sat on a seat trying to look small. A few other people arrived for that train, and then finally it came wooshing along. I didn't have a ticket or any money to get a ticket, but I just thought I'd use the ruse of hiding in the toilets until the guard went by; and it worked, and I spilled out onto the platform at Edinburgh. Then I pursued my way via ticket-less train journeys to Oban, which is on the West coast and the main port for ferries to Mull

413

and Iona. I realised that there I would have to get hold of money, so I went to my own bank, the Bank of Scotland, spun a yarn about being stranded, producing a bus-pass with a photo and the number of my bank-account, and pleaded with them for cash. I can remember standing there petrified whilst the girl went through the back to ask the manager, thinking the police would have alerted the banking system and I would be caught. However I obtained the money, and then went on a spending spree in Oban, buying toiletries and extra clothes, and a camping knife attached to a belt, before I boarded the ferry.

Soon, after two ferry journeys and a bus journey in between, I arrived on my beloved Iona, and felt safe. I can remember laying myself down on the grass in the nunnery ruins for a while, enjoying the sunshine; I heard a couple of girls passing and I was sure I heard them talking about KirkMichaels university, my home-town. However I told myself not to be alarmed, because I had escaped to Iona several years ago, when I was fleeing from another psychiatric hospital in Aberdeen, and I had managed to stay safe; and I had also camped in my tent there the previous summer. I knew people on the island, and also I had used a different surname here; so there was safety in that. Somehow or other that day I managed to obtain a tent from someone I knew there, carry it to a far corner of the island, in the hills beyond Sandeels Bay, and set it up. And I slept there, jubilant that my escape from Craigdene was a success.

Something dreadful happened the next morning. I was walking over the brow of the hill, toward the village, when I saw two policeman talking with the farmer on whose land I had camped, and then coming toward me. *Adrenalin rushed through and through me; I knew they were coming for me! I didn't know how they could have found me there, but they were coming for me!* I later discovered that the local policeman, who had been alerted by the force, had happened to see me getting off the ferry; and then it just took some phone-calls round the island to locate someone of my description. As the police came up the hill, I fled the other direction, but there were cliffs, so the only thing I could do was to climb a little down one of these cliffs which went beetling down to the rocks and sea-surge below, hoping I could hide there.

No such luck! A policeman peered over the cliff-edge and shouted. "Mairi? Is that you Mairi?" I can remember how I was petrified in that awful moment, the fear of being punished and taken all the way back to Craigdene's time-out room on the one hand, and the terrible attraction of throwing myself into the sea, and maybe finding a tragic ending to my life, on the other hand; it was like a terrifying endless conundrum. I

414

realised in that moment what a terrible mistake it was to flee to a sea-surrounded island; I was trapped.

So I gave myself up. I insisted that the police helped me to take down the tent , in order to return it to its owner. They put me in a police car and drove me across Mull, letting me out on the big ferry with handcuffs on. I can remember asking why the handcuffs were necessary, and I was told it was "in case I jumped into the sea." I was taken to Oban police-station, having first my belt, knife and shoe-laces confiscated; they showed a lot of concern about my having a camping-knife. And then I was shoved into a cell, with merely a bench and foul-smelling blankets. They were going to shut the slat on the door when I asked "But how do I contact you?" I was answered with a broad Glaswegian accent, "You don't contact us, we'll contact you!"

After being left in misery there for a while, an ambulance came and took me to the nearest psychiatric hospital, - a dreadful place in Lochmaben. Here I was put in a room, which smelt strongly of Largactil, with loads of aimless zombified people milling around. I was made to drink liquid Largactil and mill around with them. Shortly an ambulance from Craigdene came to collect me from there. I was dreading the punishment which I knew awaited me, though I couldn't know what dreadful form it was going to take.

I had everything taken off me, including my comforting small gold cross, and was left in the time-out room in a nightdress, by the time Dr.McFannen made his rounds. I was led out to see him. *"You are costing the health-service a fortune Mairi; we must stop you from escaping. So we have decided to give you ECT, as maybe that will calm you down."* (ECT stands for Electroconvulsive therapy, and is a severe method of applying electrodes and sending electricity through the brain; it is supposedly used to cure depression.) I panicked "You can't do that" I screamed, "I haven't signed a consent form! It's against the law to do that; you can't do that to me." I shall never in my entire life forget his awesome and evil reply: *"You are a sectioned patient, and therefore I can do anything I like to you!"*

I fled. I was wearing a nightdress and barefooted, and there was a cold flurry of snow outside, but I rushed straight through a fire-escape. I ran down the path and through the gate which I knew led to the main road. But I didn't get far; a car pulled up in front of me, blocking my way; I sat down in front of it, feeling that escape was now hopeless. Dr. McFadden got out of the car; he and other orderlies took hold of me and took me straight to the building where the ECT was taking place.

When I came out of there I can remember saying "Who am I ?Where am I ?What's my name?" The reply came unsympathetically and matter of fact. I had a course of the treatment. I felt terrible; I felt lost, dead; I couldn't think, I couldn't feel. They had done something terrible to me; it made me brain-dead. This is what I kept saying to my Mum and Dad when I went down to their home in Yorkshire for comfort and the care I needed; *I kept saying "I'm brain-dead aren't I? Will I be like this forever?" They did their best with me, whilst I shuffled along the streets, feeling incapable of thought or feeling, unable to write or converse, for the good part of a year.*

Finally, and most thankfully, my brain then gradually came back to normal functioning, and I returned to Iona and then my beloved KirkMichaels in the following spring. It was the most horrific mental experience of my life, *and I never forgot it as the "punishment" meted out to me for an "escape" from Craigdene!*

Chapter 103
Craigdene Madness: Part 4.

History of my Late Childhood:
From Austria came back for a university education, longing to escape from my roots; from dirty snow, fog-pollution, of Yorkshire woollen mills. - - Grandad the Master of the last decade.- - Love of Mum.- - Bust-up with my Dad. - -"God forgive this man, I cannot."- - Called him my step-Dad; can't accept as my Father. - - Search for a father-figure; my platonic relationship with Dr.James; Austrian letters to him. - - Sexuality is spirituality at the point of self-yielding; St.Theresa's ecstasy sounds sexual. - - The Beloved, heroine of my novel, is capable of ecstasy.- -A capability, not a disability; my condition is gifting. - - I am a poet.

I am a single-parent family, and proud of it; I have Gabriel and "Annatina"; both I baptised, and have been given me to look after. ("Annatina" I've just baptised with lemonade when drugged and asleep.) - - Politics and the Evil of the social-security Welfare State to young mothers. - - Key-cupboard keys; everything is locked up to keep it safe,- all except people. Annatina on special obs, - watched all of the time.- - Einstein's theory of relativity.

Violence at the tea-table is beyond the tolerable; two nurses jabberwocking and pointing their fingers at me,- wagging jabbing fingers.- - Character profiles; bullies Gillian and Spotty-Dick Alistair. - - Nurses join the psychiatric profession, either to care and heal, or, to pontificate, dominate, bully, terrorise, oppress. - - Like "One Flew Over the Cuckoo's Nest." - - The victims are generally prone; the patients are the ones who are ultimately put down, sent to sleep, like animals.

Count digits, teeth, toes, fingers, hands, feet, as we lose the youth we had,- as you lose them to old age, to senility. - - Shakespeare's 7 golden ages; I am 42-56; compare "boy with shining morning face".- - Wordsworth's vision of boyhood; Blake's 4-fold vision; our spirits get too heavy and earthified. - - All my knowledge is contained in my MA English literature degree.

The Pathos continues; Sunday first light: "I danced in the morning when the world was begun, and I danced for the moon and the stars and the sun, - it's hard to dance with the devil on your back." - - The song-writer didn't write it, he discovered it.- - "The Singer and the Song." - - Songs are/exist in the ether. - - The Beatles songs, popularity of Elvis, Mozarts songs and melodies, Handel, Bach,- they catch the rhythm of the ether. - - Poems about the sea in Lytham; "The myriad murmuring waves of rhythm surrounding Thy throne;" Tagore is a poet. - -CS Lewis; "All things wind in" to the magic centre, the mystic spiral". - - "If a man should find this place two times in time, his eyes are changed." - - Grandad read Wordsworth, couldn't put down "The Count of Monte Christo."- - My poetry -"Fallen in love, I sing;" "with dark eyes dying in the dawn."- - My theory of Rhythm; all poetry is based, not on the counting of Latin metre, but on Anglo-Saxon rhythm; - - "Beowulf" and Gerard Manley Hopkins.

I'm not a sensitive Artist; where my sensitivity once was, I now have strength.

About Health and Healing: think about our bodies; get well; think in pastel pink and blue. About Kim's desire to escape; staying, for our health and families' happiness. Kim and me: "you get the tar out of your lungs, and I'll heal my feet; we stay and do the impossible,- we get healed. What you do for my feet I'll do for your lungs; and we are doing."

Lemon and green; Jed taken in hand; "your data needs controlling;" "I'm concerned about your physical body;" causes overload. Definition of "control": a) Dominate, use as an "It"; eg. kipper in the dressing gown gone through the machine; b) like plaiting of hair, co-operation between computers, the calming of Kim's behaviour.

"Have you obbed me?" (Glossary: to obb = to check that present in time on observational status.)

Character profiles:
Michelle (first prize): star-sign, Leo, golden-maned;   shows much promise; as yet unwed and un-birthed; 21, Age/prime of life; one who will belong to the New Age, and will travel to the stars.
Debbie (3rd and 4th prize): on her way up; will be a brilliant social worker; cares; good at washing hair, for she was a mother; had a baby in her youth, now aged 5, and in maturity, with surety, marries the man; and she is very happy, because she is relaxed, and consequently looks like a boy; designation, prime of life; star-sign, Cancer; age 27; will travel to the stars.
Gillian and Shiona: the bitches throw their weight around; they throw their weight around because they have no real power.
Jed: my favourite Minder; likings,- crisp white shirts, blueness; star-sign Taurus,- mixes well with Saggitarius; Aldebran is orange-red and the star-sign opposite to mine; lovers of food and drink, stubborn and obstinate; both before the Winter or Summer solstice;

There's no difference between legitimate drugs and illegitimate; the first are described by a Doctor for our health (like Elvis Presley); the second are taken for their surrepticious delectification. - - Bubble, bubble. - - "Immortal, invisible-bubble, God only wise."- - Delectebubble, Indescribabubble.

Chapter 104
A Failed Escape-Attempt.

Three times I escaped from Craigdene in the summer of '95. My intention was to escape again from the Psychiatric System and the grip of the power Dr.McNeill had over me, and in particular to get the dreaded Clopixol injection stopped. It was a month I had to stay away, to break the section; the first two times I didn't make it, due to my need of medication.

I didn't much mind being in Craigdene at the beginning of May, because I had found living in my own house, solitary and without Dr.James' visits, suffering the terrible side-effects of the Clopixol, like living in a morgue. And so I welcomed the company of people, and seeing I had entered there of my own accord, I was allowed to be "on green," free to go outside and wander round the grounds.

However after a couple of weeks there was a summer fete, and my two acquaintances Jack and Gavin happened to come into the ward to see me; they caused a loud fuss in the usually quiet place, with their laughing and joking; and Alistair, the nurse in charge, took umbrage and said I wasn't allowed back out with them. I disobeyed, and went out with them to talk in the sunshine; he was angry, and dragged me back in, telling me he had put me "on amber." Amber is based on staying indoors and being "observed" every five minutes. I felt this as an acute blow. And then this Alistair insisted on giving me an increased amount of "Clopixol" injection, telling me Dr.McNeill had increased the dosage. I remember having this needle in my backside in the treatment room, saying to myself, "I'm not standing for this; I'm going to escape."

And so I did. I ended up walking for miles across muddy fields in my shoes! I think this was because I didn't dare stay on the bus as it was passing the police station, and I thought I would be able to get to another road further away if I went through some fields. I remember my despair, when I was stuck in the corner of a field in a mud-bath, wondering which way to go to get out of it; it was dark and I couldn't see my way. Finally I came back into Kirkcraig and, afraid the police would be looking for me, I hopped into a taxi at a taxi-rank and asked to be taken to the nearby station at Langport. I had some money, hidden in the secret compartment of my handbag; it was worth spending it to get away from the area.

When I was crossing the Strath Bridge on the way to Invertay I had a great terror of the water. I often had a fear of water when I was manic, partly due to my memory of my near-drowning in my suicide attempt in November '92. I swore to myself that I wouldn't cross any more water, on my way to Dumfries and Hawkeshill to stay with my friend Maggie, for that was where I intended going. I remember when I told Dr.James of this, he commented "it's witches who won't cross water!"

Something horrible happened in Invertay. I had to wait there overnight, before the buses started running in the morning; then I could use my free travel pass to go anywhere in Kirkshire, or as far as Glasgow. It was very cold; though it was May, there were flurries of snow in the air. There were lots of very shifty, shady characters hanging about the bus-station; there was drug-dealing and prostitution going on. *I always myself aimed for the "prostitution-principle" during my escapes; it ran like this; "to gain the freedom of your soul it is worth the selling of your body." I often found myself in such extreme circumstances, of cold or hunger or tiredness, that this principle made sense*; I felt my body was only physical and could be used as payment when I didn't have the money. This would be seen by doctors as part of the "disinhibited" nature of my illness, which meant I needed to be sectioned; but ironically to me, it seemed worth being disinhibited in order to gain my freedom from such a section; for the section "imprisoned me in other people's minds," and in places which were like prisons to me.

So I was cold, hungry, tired, in Invertay with no money left and nowhere to sleep; and the snow flurries were falling from the skies. A nice young man seemed interested in me, so I walked along with him, appealing to him to "spend the night with me;" I said he could spend the night with me if we could check into a hotel, and get a nice warm clean bed. The "nice warm clean bed" appealed to me so acheingly. But he led me into some bushes, saying it was a short-cut to the hotel we could see, and effectually raped me. I was saying "No, No, let's find a nice clean bed." Imagine my horror when he just left me there, saying "here's some money," and throwing me a 50p piece! I felt grotty, but I went into a garage, and bought for myself a Marsbar with that 50p piece, and my slow eating of it was some kind of comfort through the long hours of cold darkness.

I got to Invermor the next morning, with my Bus Pass. And there I promised to pay a taxi driver a lot of money for driving me to the local branch of the Dunfermline Building Society, which housed my savings. I leapt in, said "I want you to speak to my bank manager to let loose some savings to me, and I have for proof of identity this bus-pass." I was very scared whilst waiting for the phone-call; I thought they might be contacting the police. But the ruse worked! I got some money, paid the taxi-driver. And then I got out of Invermor as quickly as possible; I thought they might be looking for me there, and I could never rest where I couldn't feel safe.

I got to Dumfries on the buses; I intended going to stay with Maggie, who stayed in a place called Hawkeshill in Whitmore, which is beyond Dumfries, because I'd stayed there the year before, and I couldn't think of anywhere else that I could go to remain hidden for a month; I couldn't even return to my beloved Lytham-St.Annes where I'd stayed in '94 because the police would look for me there. Pater Leo had told me that they had even sent Interpol to his monastery in Austria when I was last missing. I had to find somewhere new where I hadn't been before. However on the way to Maggie's, a dreadful doubt overcame me, in that I knew Dr.James at least knew of her address, and I would be found there too. So I got off the bus at a village before Whitmore, and checked in at a B&B thinking that the next day I would make a bid to get to Ireland on the ferry from Stranraer. But Maggie came and found me at this B&B and insisted she take me back to her house.

By this time the Clopixol injection, which had been heavier than usual, was having a dreadful effect upon me. For the 6 months that I had been having this injection I had always take Procyclidine for the side-effects; Proclyclidine is the "antidote" to all the anti-psychotic medications, and without it, especially when you were used to it and dependant on it, the effects of Clopixol were dire. It feels as if your mind has been twisted, round and round, and you only desire to untwist it; your tongue is so dry and thick that you can hardly speak, all your limbs are stiff and twitchy, even you eyes are stiff and unmoving, you get a sense of enormous pressure built into your head, and all you want to do is release it in some way, untwist yourself in some way, but there is no way to do it; you can't find a relief, except in this little white tablet, which I was lacking.

I felt dire, as Maggie settled me into her son's room. I told her "I've got to get some Procyclidine." But she insisted "you've got to go cold turkey." I couldn't, I couldn't! I felt so ill that night I thought I was going to die! I remember I went into Maggie's bedroom, really "twisted" carrying my shoes, saying "tell Gabriel the last thing I did was to tie my shoe-laces together." She laughed her head off at this, but it wasn't funny! I didn't die that night, but there was no relief for me. I was horrified the next morning to find that Maggie had phoned a few people in the Kirkshire area, telling them I was there and that I was "safe." But I didn't feel safe! I felt I couldn't stay there, because I wasn't safe.

But I think I didn't care any more; I felt so "ill" that all I wanted was the Procyclidine. Maggie had washed all my clothes, so I put some of her clothes on. And I went out onto the main road nearby to try and attract some attention in order to get some help.   Maggie insisted that I mustn't attract attention to myself, because there was a man who was a psychiatric nurse a few doors away; she insisted that I would be OK if I stayed there "cold turkey" for a month.   But I felt I needed to get help to rescue me from Maggie! I tried to attract attention; I was walking on the green grass barefooted. I felt I'd get some relief from the "twistedness" and pressure in my head by going to the toilet or walking barefoot; but nothing helped. *I thought I'd go through anything to get some Procyclidine!*

From that point, events went fast. I managed to attract the attention of an orange-suited engineer, and he went and fetched this psychiatric nurse Maggie had spoken of; he fetched the local doctor, and this doctor phoned Dr.McNeill. When I found out Dr.Black's plan was to admit me to the local hospital and sedate me, I ran away, back to the house. I was in the room, carefully trying to pack and preserve my things, for I had stored everything carefully away in the bureau in the bedroom, locked with a key. I had carried all my writings there carefully bound up in a shoebox with green wool, and had a black handbag too. I was in this room when Maggie and the nurse and the doctor came upon me. I yelled that they had to give me time to pack, because all my things were locked away carefully in this bureau. But they wouldn't wait; they pulled me backward, hurting my feet, and carried me down the stairs headfirst. When this Dr.Black tried to get me in his car, I wouldn't let him push my head down, and so it was agreed that Maggie should take me in her car. I was feeling very hurt.

The whole point of my giving myself up was to get some Procyclidine. Imagine my horror when, once in the local hospital this Dr.Black came at me with an injection! He told me Dr.McNeill had said I should have it; I didn't need yet more tranquilliser! So I thrashed my arms and legs about, attacking him with enormous energy; I think the injection went into himself. Then I lay in the corner of the floor, and none of the nurses dared come near me. I think it was because I'd been violent that they fetched the police.   The young nurse whose name was Alan volunteered to go in the police-van with me; he kindly said he would "stay with me" through the whole trauma. They locked us up in a police-cell; Alan remarked that he has never been in a police -cell before. We must have stayed there for a whole day, not knowing what was going to happen. It was a memorable experience, though I felt very ill, being locked up in a cell with this nice young man; we talked a lot, and when we had to part, I asked for a something to remember him by, suggesting his wedding ring; he gave me some small thing, a button or a coin.

It came to an end when the "Craigdene squad" arrived; it was two nurses I liked, Gerry and Pam, and they took me back in an ambulance. I remember how, when I couldn't stand anymore the drone of the engine, they stopped for me to take a wee in a park in Glasgow, and Pam was kind to me, as she held me on the cold wet grass, whilst I entrusted to Gerry the holding of my precious wool-wrapped shoe-box. I believed that when I got back to Craigdene I would finally be able to have the Procyclidine I so needed; imagine my horror when Gerry and Pam, who had promised me it, disappeared straightaway, leaving me faced with unkind and unfriendly night-staff!

"Please, you've got to give me some Procyclidine," I begged, "I had a big depot injection just before I left, and I haven't had Procyclidine for days!" "You must know we don't give out Procyclidine for night-time medication," came the reply. I begged, but it was no good. I sat in my dark room, feeling far too ill to be able to sleep, and I dared to come out once again, only to be faced by the snippety female nurse who had once in Ward 6 dragged me upstairs by the hair in my underwear. "Get back in there," she yelled, "or it will be a jag in the backside!"

I sat in the dark, more miserable and more demoralised than ever in my life. I had given up my freedom, freedom I had struggled hard to attain, to get some Procyclidine, and look, I was again locked up in Craigdene, again treated like this, with no freedom and no Procyclidine either! I sat in the dark, suffering.

Chapter 105
A Second Brave Attempt.

June and half of July passed; a lot of my friends came to visit me, such as Elizabeth, Helen, Patricia, and Henry; they talked with me and took me out; I made friends and enjoyed myself with some of the nurses; I looked after the young "Annatina," and made friends with a manic girl called Kim, who was always setting off the fire-alarms. I was doing great, writing again, "getting my act together," having lots of home passes, seeing social workers about re-establishing access visits with my son; I decided I wasn't going to "abscond," but go out this way, the long hard way!

But then stupid little female locum doctors got involved and insisted that they increase my depot-injection. I knew I couldn't survive on a higher dose of Clopixol; it had been decreased under a nice doctor called Dr.Northgait, who had also introduced me to Carbamazepine to replace McNeill's Lithium. I had to go; I couldn't have people messing with my mind's health any longer. After my last failed attempt I knew of the importance of taking Procyclidine with me, but I had obtained a bottle of this from the house. As for money, I had been slowly saving it up, asking for a couple of £ a day from my funds, which was all the pocket-money that I was allowed; I stashed all these coins in a jar in the locked drawer by my bedside. One snippety nurse had said, laughing, "What is she doing with all these coins! She's saving them up for her next escape-attempt!" And I was!

I used to walk round in the car-park, balancing on the pavement edge like the cat did; when nurses saw me out there and told me to come in, I'd say "Rob says I'm allowed in the car-park;" it was my way of gaining a little more freedom every day, because of course the nurses didn't trust me after all the absconding I'd done! This time I was better prepared for a journey and better clad; I had obtained tracksuits from my house, and the small blue wellies that I always used to wear on Iona. And I also had got hold of the back-pack I had worn on my back for the whole of the previous year, - the one with the toy rabbit sticking out of the back-pocket with its arms outstretched. Apparently when I went missing and the police wanted a description, the nurse Alistair had told them I had this back-pack "with a rabbit sticking out of the back," and they had laughed and didn't believe him! And "went missing" is what I did, between one 5-minute observation and the next 5-minute observation! A car came up to the door, and there was a diversion as people moved and talked around it, and I was off!

Having made the mistake the last time of getting stuck in the mud in farmer's fields, I decided I must make straight for a speedy attempt to get out of the area, so I made for the train-station. I got a ticket and paid for it with my precious saved money, making my usual mistake of asking "where's your next train going to." When I was waiting there on the platform, imagine my horror when through the glass doors, I saw a police-car driving up! They came up to the ticket booth and asked the man, "Have you seen a woman that has absconded from Craigdene?" I was standing secretly just behind the door onto the platform. I was literally quaking in my boots! A painful flush of blood passed through me; I was so scared that I couldn't move; I was rooted to the spot.

Then the police said "she's wearing a blue denim jeans and jacket." And it was surreal, as I looked down at my own clothes, and realised that I was wearing a white tracksuit bottom and a green tracksuit top! "It isn't me, it isn't me!" And it dawned on me that it was the young Kim they were looking for, the Kim who was always escaping. And the next moment I was scared that the man was going to say, "No, but there is another wierd woman here, who doesn't know what direction she's going." I held my breath, but he said nothing and the police went away.

I was so scared afterwards that I went and hid in the toilets.   But I thought to myself, "No, I'm not going to hide on the toilets, I'm making a bid for freedom, to assert that I have rights over my own brain; I refuse to hide in the toilets."   So I sat on that same platform, where I had sat before, scared, afraid of what lay ahead of me, but above all frightened at the thought of a policeman's hand on my shoulder!

I travelled all round Scotland, reaching the Highlands on this occasion. I had nowhere to go; I could think of nowhere to go, where I hadn't been already or where the police wouldn't look for me. So I went round just trying to find "a safe Haven." Pater Leo had sent me a postcard, which said Christ had "opened for me a door," so I travelled round trying to keep the sense of this "open door" in front of me, a sense of freedom, a sense of possibilities and a future.

I stayed one night in Invermor, and bought clean socks and pants there, I travelled around on my bus-pass eating Mars-bars, and I ended up in Invermount, with no money left. My mind was set on the "prostitution principle" again; the idea that it was alright to sell your body for the sake of food and warmth for the body, when it was really for the sake of the soul's liberation. I was walking along a street, feeling desperate, and said to this guy, "Do you have anywhere to stay?" It initiated a conversation, and though he stayed in a house some way distant with his brother, he said he would take me there. We got to some green grass, sat for a while in the warm sunshine, then he said "Come into the woods with me." Like an idiot I did so; he just wanted cheap sex; I ended up with my white trousers stained with grass and dirt. He then said he would go to the local shop to get me something nice; I asked him to get me some Impulse deodorant, aware of my stinking feet inside my wellingtons. He told me to wait for him, on the green hillside; I waited for ages on the grass, watching the sunset, watching it grow dark; I finally had to accept the fact that he wasn't coming back!

So I was left in the council-house area of Invermount, with nowhere to sleep, nowhere to go, no money. At last I flagged down a passing taxi. The taxi-driver felt sorry for me; he asked me what I was "running away from." I could hardly tell him I had absconded from a mental hospital; so I told him I was escaping from my father. When he asked if this father abused me, I said Yes, and started crying, and wove a very credible story about it. I just wanted this taxi-driver to look after me. And he did, taking me to a B&B place, paying for it himself, telling me to knock the grass off my trousers before ringing the door-bell, and saying he would pick me up from there the next morning. I had a bath and good night's sleep in a clean comfy bed.

The next day we spent trying to find another B&B for me in the Invermount area; it was a problem because it was the height of the summer season; we found a farmhouse on the outskirts where I could stay for a few days. He took me out to a meal in Burger Bar. However, though he had shown me some kindness, I felt compelled to get out of his clutches; it bothered me that he had said, "I want you to be my lover." And so the next morning, instead of waiting for him, I got a lift into town in the farmer's wife's landrover. I'd decided I was going to make a bid to get money through the Dunfermline Building Society again, because it had worked the last time. So I went into the local branch, and wove this story about being stranded in Invermount, and desperately needing funds from my account. When they phoned up the KirkMichaels manager the answer came back "No." I asked to speak to her myself on the phone; I begged miserably; she said "Mairi we are not supposed to do this; this is the last time we will ever do it; how much do you need?" I asked for all my savings of £400. She said pointedly "and how much does it take to get from Invermount to KirkMichaels?" I couldn't tell her I was absconding in the other direction. She said "OK, we'll do it this once, but never again!"

So now I had money! At £20 a night for B&B it wouldn't last long enough though; I needed to find accommodation. I went to the local Information Centre, and asked about how to get up into the Highlands; I had my heart set on staying in Skye. I had a horrible experience in that information Centre. I couldn't stand the crowdedness of the place, and I said to this fair-haired young girl, clutching my back-pack, "Look I'm in a hurry, and I've got valuables in here, can you just give me these details." I suppose I seemed aggressive, as well as suspicious, because she went way for a minute, told me I had to wait, and then the next thing I knew the police had arrived. The policemen took me through to the back-room, and started quizzing me about where I was from, and what I had in my back-pack. I suppose they thought I had stolen loot in there; but they went through it and found it contained nothing but payer-books and writings. Now I had sat there exteriorly calm, but inwardly petrified; I kept saying to myself, "there is nothing, nothing, to identify who I am; there is no way they can know who I am." I think I had thrown the bus-pass away, to make sure that no-one for the next month could identify me. And so they then said "you are free to go."

I didn't quite get to Skye; I got to a place near it on the mainland, amongst the high mountains, but something happened there that gave me a fright, and sent me back southward again. The problem was finding anywhere to stay during the height of the Summer season. I had finally found a night's stay in a B&B; I had another of those frightening experiences when the local policeman came round to visit this landlady, though it had nothing to do with me. But I found a caravan just down the road, owned by a farm, who would let me stay for a fortnight at a much lower rate. Conditions in this caravan were rather primitive, but I paid to stay and was ready to move in there. At this point I did a very stupid thing. I didn't have things like towels, soap and toilet paper, so I pinched them from this landlady's house. I though they wouldn't be missed. Imagine my horror when early the next morning, after a night's sleep in this grotty caravan, I heard a commotion, after a car had driven up on the gravel; and I looked out of the window, and saw the landlady remonstrating with the farmer's wife, and then she came striding over. She said her towels were missing; I had stuffed them into my bag and thought I could lie about it, saying, "Oh look, I must have accidentally put them in my bag!" It didn't wash I'm afraid; a little later after I'd got dressed, the farmer himself came striding round, giving me my money back, and telling me, "Get out, we don't want your sort here!"

Distraught about what I could do next, I used the public phone-box at the corner of the road to phone Rachel in Cairndale, whom I had visited the summer before; her father answered, and when I asked if I could stay there for a bit, said "Oh Yes, come, because you can stay a while." I grasped at this, for it gave me the chance of lasting out the month. I went to the cafe on the corner of the road, whilst I waited for the bus to take me south. Whilst I was in that café having some breakfast, that policeman came round, whom I had accidentally encountered the day before. This time his coming did have something to do with me, and again I was frightened. He told me to get in his police-car and he would give me a lift to the point about ten miles south where I could find the main bus-route. I was scared as I sat in his car, but I chatted away merrily, in a bid to convince him that my state of mind was good; I didn't want him to suspect I was an "escaped patient." He was pleasant enough, and I finally said, as if jokingly, "you're not arresting me, are you?" He replied, "No, just escorting you off my patch!"

I was disappointed when I got to Cairndale to find that Rachel's mother was rather negative toward me. She was cross with me that I obtained a pair of old slippers from Rachel and a pair of clean trousers form someone else; and she told me that after one night's stay I had to leave. I was upset; I told her that I took "staying a while" to mean longer than that; I remember telling her that I had just started a heavy period, and for that reason I couldn't travel; but she wouldn't budge.

I phoned up Dr.James; I told him I had got to Ireland, though I hadn't; I asked him about the case-conference about Gabriel, which was due in just a few days; I told him to tell Steven Peterson that I would attend it. *For I had decided to return; to return to face the reality of my own life. For I needed to come back for an injection; I knew that if I didn't have the Clopixol in my system I would become really ill; and I needed to come back to fight for Gabriel. And I felt I could return, because I wasn't afraid anymore. I had been away for a week, but to me it had seemed a long time; I think I had gone through so many "frights" that I wasn't afraid any more!*

I hastened back to Kirkshire, stayed overnight in a hotel in Inverlang, and in the morning, believing I could have a swift entry and exit from KirkMichaels, got a taxi to take me from there to the KirkMichaels health centre. I went straight in, past Audrey the receptionist who protested "you can't go in Mairi," and landed myself into Dr.James' room. There were two elderly patients having a conversation with him; he looked up surprised. There was I wet from the rain, with my hair in wet curls over my forehead, holding my backpack and clutching a rosary of green-marbled semi-precious beads which a man had given me on my travels! He looked at me, urged the couple out, and I spilt out treasures from my bag, and told my tale; I remember I took out a picture of Christ, and he told me to take it off his desk saying it was "idolatrous." And so I snatched this short, beautiful time with him. I told him to phone to tell Steven Peterson that I was coming to the meeting; he said it wasn't safe, but I insisted. Steven Peterson gave the news that it was cancelled, but asked where I was; "she's here with me," said Dr.James. I said rather stupidly that he could tell him this; for I had fought with "fright" in the big wide world and I wasn't afraid any more. *I was upset that the meeting about my son had been cancelled; it seemed to me that "Gabriel falls like water through my fingers!"*

Dr.James showed me into another room, where I could wait until the Clopixol injection could be delivered from the chemist. He said I had arrived at a good time, because all of the town was bustling with golfers and visitors, it being "the Open," so hopefully "the police will be busy doing other things." However I soon saw from the window a couple of burly police-officers arriving in a van. I went straight to Dr.James' room; "I think they've come for me." He said with a groan, "I told you we shouldn't have let Steven Peterson know you are here; I should have used my better judgement!" There followed an altercation with the police-officers at the door-jamb of his room. *I fought it when they tried to lay hands on me; "Get off me! I am a free citizen of this country, and I have done nothing wrong; you have no grounds on which to arrest me!" Of course they replied "you are a sectioned patient, absconded from Craigdene."* Dr.James argued his best that I should be let free, and I said "I am waiting here to have an injection from my doctor; you will have to wait awhile." Their reply came, "you can have an injection at the hospital, once we get you there." There was no help for it but to accompany them to the van, but I said I wouldn't be manhandled; "Get your hands off me!" And as I went I looked back at Dr.James, and said "I love you." The policemen mocked me for it, "that's right, swear undying love to your doctor!" *They treated me like a piece of meat, swapping me over from the back of one van to another when halfway there, manhandling me despite my protestations; "we'll soon have you back in Craigdene!"*

And so I was back! Those stupid little female locum doctors were immediately all over me again; two of them came behind my bed-curtains saying I had to have an injection, before I had even managed to pull off my smelly wellingtons. "You could at least give me the space to take my boots off!" I yelled. When they asked how I was feeling, I said "just fine!" I looked at myself in the mirror, and saw this face looking back at me with its make-up worn off, and short wet curls hanging over the forehead. *"You look anguished"* said one of them. *I wasn't anguished, just angry.*

The next day I told Dr.McNeill "I went all the way to Ireland to get hold of this rosary made of semi-precious stone!" For he had said to me, "No wonder we have to section you when you go running off all over the country." *He scoffed, "It's just some cheap beads!" I came away with the triumphant sense that he could never break my spirit!*

Chapter 106
The Final Successful Escape.

It was practically only a weekend that I was kept in Craigdene this time; I was returned by the police on Thursday 20th July; on Tuesday 25th I absconded again. It was facilitated by the fact that I was let out on home pass, in the charge of my friend Patricia, to collect some clothes. I can remember the young "Annatina" bewailing, "Why should she be let out on home pass after just escaping? I never get very far when I escape!" (This was the young princess-like Anne, who at the end of the day hanged herself by the shoe-laces in the bathroom as her only way of escaping from the System.) *My own final escape, when I stayed for a month in Ruthwell, was successful, and I won for myself true freedom from the System, and with it mental health.*

I shamelessly deceived Patricia that day she brought me home for some clothes; I asked her to go to her house and leave me alone for a while, as I intended having a bath and getting changed. What I really intended to do was to get packed, stuffing a travel-bag with the clothes this time which I would need for a month, and absconding again. The money I had available to take was about £150, but I was taking my DSS Benefit book with me, with the hope that I would be able to cash it. *As for medication, I wasn't going to make a mistake this time; I wasn't going to be driven back by my need of medication; I had got a whole bottle of Procyclidine, and I had plans about the Clopixol injection.*

Having got packed and ready to set off, I went round to the health centre to see Dr.James. He said "Not now Mairi, I'm very busy; I'm in a rush to make a call at a public phone-box." I told him I was escaping again, and asked if he'd help me to stay away for the required month. "What do you want me to do?" he asked, willing to help. "I know Clopixol comes in tablet form, it is called Clopenthixol; I've seen them giving it to Anne, as lots of small tablets; could you give me a months supply?" He was hot and in a hurry and exasperated. But he looked it up in his medical book, and quickly made out a prescription. I took it and dashed out of there, whilst he shouted after me, "Look after yourself; be good!"

(NB. This seems to me the greatest single selfless act of love anyone has done for me in my lifetime. Its benefits to me have been enormous, for it served to crack the power the psychiatric System had over me; it set me on the road to true freedom and mental health. Though perhaps he shouldn't have done it, he did it to help me; because he

wanted me to escape from the System as much as I wanted to escape from it. He did it because he cared about me.)

I was now "running scared," aware that Patricia would be looking for me, and I was looking suspicious with the travel-bag; I didn't dare go to the local chemist and wait for that prescription, so I resolved to take it with me, and jumped on the next passing local bus. I can remember how petrified I was on finding this bus going past Patricia's house. But I got to the bus-station OK, and then used my money, passing through Glasgow, to travel as far as Greenock. I had a destination in mind this time; I was on my way to Ruthwell, because I found out on my last escape, from Rachel's mother, that the last Benedictine convent in Scotland, had been sited there, on the Ayrshire coast. So Ruthwell was where I was heading, with the hope that they would take me in.

Greenock was a bit grotty, both the place itself and my experience there. I ended up there late at night, on the last bus, and hung around by a row of shops, in what seemed a dying town. As per usual I got a young man to take me back to his place, willing to use my "prostitution principle" to find a place to sleep, but he was a decent guy and let me "crash" at his old flat without requiring sex of me. This flat was quite literally dilapidated, in that the roof had caved in; so it was very messy and full of plaster, and had no electricity or running water; and I found the next morning that the toilet was in a disgusting condition. He offered to let me stay there if I wanted, on my own; he gave me the number to get power-cards. I can remember sitting on the bed watching the arms of the great dock-cranes out of the window, wondering whether I could possibly manage to stay there on my own for month in such grotty conditions.

I was told there was a convent nearby; I went along there and pretended to be a bona fide seeker of the "religious life" rather than an escaped mental patient. The nun showed me into the house they ran for the elderly, and then showed me into the chapel, saying she would enquire of the mother superior; I had asked if I could stay and work for them for a month. I mustn't have looked "bona fide" to them, because the next thing I knew, they ushered me out into the porch, presented me with a meal on a table, and shut the doors against me; "Mother Superior told us to give you this meal, before seeing you on your way." I was horrified; they were treating me like a tramp! But I was grateful for the meal really, so I ate it and left without making a fuss.

I can remember returning to the grotty flat, watching the yellow cranes go up and down and back and forth. I decided I'd move on and try my luck in Ruthwell. It was a bright sunny day and the sea was sparkling, when I arrived in Ruthwell on the bus; a couple of children I had met volunteered to take me to this Benedictine convent, which had a lovely situation on the sea-front. I had no better luck at this place, though I put on my best act of being a religious seeker. It was a enclosed convent and you had to speak through a grill; I asked if I could stay for a while, as it had a guest-house attached, but it was full, as it was the height of the season. I went to the wee shop and tea-room that was attached; there I can remember pinching a wee purse for my rosary beads. The tea-room was pleasant enough, though run by some grumpy old ladies. I decided I could mange to stay there for month, because I could keep warm and dry in this tea-room, and attend all the services of the convent, if only I could find a place nearby to stay, to sleep. So I hunted around the area for B&B, and eventually was directed to the house of the local milkman, who I was told let out rooms very cheaply. He was a very nice man was this milkman, and always treated me very kindly. He showed me an upstairs attic room, a tiny room sloping under the eaves, saying I could have it for £50 a week; I agreed and moved in.

That month of August, in '95, was one of the hottest on record. I spent my time there in stifling heat, moving only from the milkman's house to the convent's tea-room, and back again, sometimes sitting by the fountain on the green along the esplanade to eat, and sometimes going to the nearby streets to scour shops for the cheapest food I could find, especially stale bread from the local bakery. Money was a problem; I didn't have much money left, and couldn't afford to eat; the milkman's wife reused to provide me with breakfast, though they gave me a kettle to make hot drinks. But I spent my time usefully, attending all the services and sitting in this tea-room to read endless religious books that I had in my back-pack; I also set myself the task of reading all the way though the gospels. The sour-faced old ladies who ran the tea-shop didn't like me; I overheard them telling the priest who came in, "What is she doing here? She looks suspicious." I once smiled when I heard them telling a funny story, and they snapped at me; "What are you laughing at!" "I was just amused by what you said," I replied. "Well you shouldn't be listening to our conversation!" They were very unkind to me! But the nuns themselves were kind enough, especially the "tertiaries" who were attached to the place; they told me their stories and had deep religious conversations with me. And I went to see the Mother Abbess, asking her if I could join the Benedictines. I was quite serious in this, as I had been a Benedictine nun for a short time in my youth; she told me I had to go home and write to her for several years, which wasn't a big help!

I took a trip to Glasgow, partly to get the Clopixol tablets from the prescription, which I needed to kick in when my injection was running low, and also partly to get hold of money, which I desperately needed if I was going to last out the month. I didn't want to try and get these things from Ruthwell, as they might be traceable on the computers. So I set off on the train, prescription and DSS Benefit book in hand. First I made my way to the main Post Office in Glasgow; imagine my horror when I presented my Benefit book, and the man said, "I'm sorry you can't cash that here, the only place you can cash it is in the Beechwood Rd Post Office in KirkMichaels." I went all red and panicky; "No, you must be wrong, you must be wrong!" I thought of getting into another queue, and asking someone else; at the last they got a supervisor to speak to me; "I'm sorry Madam, but you can only cash that DSS book in the designated place, which is KirkMichaels." My heart had fallen to the bottom of my boots; how was I going to survive for another two and a half weeks! I was "running scared" again as I pursued my way back to the train-station; I thought they would find out from their computers that I was a missing person. I went scared into the pharmacy attached to the station, presenting my prescription. The girl took this away, and brought back another lady who said, "Will you wait here a minute because there seems to be problem with this." I was petrified; I thought they had found out on computer that I was a missing person, and were busy reporting to the police that I was in their shop. I stood around, looking at the toiletries, in an agony of fear. *When they handed the tablets over, I ran out of there as if all hell were after me, and leapt on a train, in order to get back to the relative safety of Ruthwell.*

I wanted to stay in Ruthwell, but I didn't have the money; the milkman was demanding that I pay £50 a week which I didn't have. I remember I went one day to that dilapidated flat in Greenock, watching again the movement of the large yellow cranes out of the window, realising I could stay there for nothing, except for food, but I couldn't stomach it. I decided I would weave a story to the milkman, and get him to let me owe him money. He was a nice man, the milkman; I told him that my father who was a doctor was working down in Cornwall, and I couldn't get more money from him till he returned to Edinburgh; he trusted me. His wife didn't trust me; she kept yelling "If you trust that girl, you will never get your money back." It was good of him to trust me; when I left there, I owed him £150, having promised to send it on to him; and because he did trust me, I did send it on to him, sending a cheque off as soon as I returned to KirkMichaels, and phoning him to thank him for his kindness.

(NB. .It is obvious that if it weren't for this one man's kindness, I probably wouldn't have made it, and wouldn't have established my "stable mental health" away from the System that was so damaging to me. He was a kind stranger who helped me on my way.)

Hunger tormented me, as it had done in my other escape to Lytham-St.Annes. I used to watch people walk along the esplanade, eating tasty fish and chips, just longing for it. All I could afford was bread that was sold cheap at the end of the day; I had to make my money spin out. I can remember on the one occasion I decided I would buy some chips. And on the way back I ran across a busy road, too delighted at hot food to take notice, and I nearly got run over! And I met this guy, whilst I was upset; I explained, "I nearly got myself run over for the sake of some chips!" And as I walked along the shore talking with him, my eyes were opened to the light and the seagulls and the sunset; and it temporarily turned my feelings away from a life-denying monasticism. But he was only temporarily staying there as an oil-worker, and I never saw him again.

It was like a long "exile" there; I was filled with yearnings, filled with longings to see my son again, and to see my beloved Dr.James; and I was alone and sad; and the summer heat was oppressive and I was hungry. That month seemed to last a long long time. My mental health remained relatively good, but I realised on getting home that I was rather "depressed."

I was eager to travel home as soon as the section lapsed. I can remember phoning Dr.James from the phone-box on the sea-front, and I was blissful on hearing his voice. He knew I was coming back; he was expecting me. I went straight in again, throwing myself on his mercy, saying "Please don't let the police arrest me again." He said I was alright because the month was up, and he would see to it that the police wouldn't take me to the police-station. He phoned them saying "I have Mairi Colme here." After a short conversation with them he said "You have to stay here for a while; they insist on sending the sergeant down, to prove that it's you." I said "can't you just tell them it's me?" He said "they want to see you with their own eyes; don't worry I won't let them arrest you." So the police sergeant came to see me, and I was let free to go home, back to my own house.

In the few days following, I found myself in a terribly depressed state. I met Walter and Gabriel, and when they brought me home, sat miserably in the car, saying "I can't cope." In the few days following I said the same to Dr.James. My mind felt deadened and unresponsive,

436

and I just wasn't alive enough to deal with ordinary life; I repeated "I just can't cope." "It is unusual for you to so repeat yourself," he said, "there must be something wrong with you;" and he agreed to put me on Prozac. I said to him earnestly out of my misery, "I want to be well, happy and creative;" he said that was what he wanted for me too.

It was the end of August 1995, and finally I had broken the power that the Psychiatric System had over me, finally after a 7-year struggle! I had escaped over and over again until I had finally made it! It meant I was free; no longer pulled back and forth to Craigdene on a whim, and no longer forced to take medication that made me feel ill. I was finally liberated from Dr.McNeill's power.

Freedom gave me a new life, and I never looked back! There was no more endless Lithium, and no more high doses of Clopixol injection which left me "living in concrete." I was now free to choose my own medication regime, one by which I could control my own mind, the vagaries of my own brain. In the coming months I worked out together with Dr.James a regime that worked for me, and kept me well, happy and creative for many years; and he looked after me for another 7 years after '95.

It was by that single selfless act of love, when he gave me the Clopenthixol tablets during yet another of my hasty escape attempts, that he helped me to break the deathly grip the Psychiatric System had on me. And following that act of real "care," he spent the next 7 years being committed to keeping me out of that System, and keeping me safe. I owe him so much, not only for rescuing me from the System, but also for all those years he spent listening to me as my soul-friend; he created my stable mental health by his years of constant care.

Chapter 107
My Recovery.

Yesterday, - I write in January 2003,- I fortuitously met the Craigdene doctor who said to me back in 1994, "You have a serious mental disease, which is getting worse; we are thinking of keeping you locked up in hospital permanently." I said to him yesterday, earnestly: "Doesn't it prove a point that, after all that sectioning, locking up, injections, forcible medication, in hospital under your care for 7 years, now that I've been on my own, under my own steam, and self-medicating, I have stayed well and out of hospital for nearly 8 years! Doesn't it prove a point?!"

All that wasn't necessary!- the "raping" of my mind and being over and over again, the locking up, the forcible treatment by drugs, which made me ill and kept me ill. I was even re-sectioned for years under the Mental Health Act when I was at home on "trial leave," which is now considered a violation of human rights. And therefore I had to "escape" over and over again, in order to free myself from that Section, suffering terribly every time, trying to keep away for a month at a time without money, food, or any recourse, so that the section would lapse, and I could take charge of my own mind and life. *Finally I succeeded, in the Summer of 1995. And since then, by looking after myself, and through the care of one man, I have saved myself from any manic relapse.*

How did I do this? Partly it was by taking responsibility for managing my own medication -regime. I worked out together with Dr.James a regime that worked for me, and kept me well, happy and creative for many years; basically the Clopixol injection, though at one-sixth of the initial dose given to me, plus a peppering of daily tablets, of Carabamazine, Prozac and Procylidine, which seemed to balance out the side-effects. *But the point is, it had my freewill in it, my co-operation, my willingness to take care of my own "mental health problem." I wasn't forced by Dr.James to take medication against my will; it was an active and caring partnership.* "Recovery" as it is now being recognized today, is not about the patient's refusal to take psychiatric drugs and determination to do without them; it is rather a matter of learning to "manage" one's own mind with the aid of the drugs that are available. *Recovery is a state of wellness, well-being, the recovery of your own life for yourself, so you can achieve things the best that you are able, and live life to the fullest possible.*

And I never looked back after the summer of '95; I have been basically well and out of hospital ever since. Dr.James kept me well by looking after me, not only by allowing my co-operation and my freewill in the medication-regime, - and the incorporation of "freewill" is necessary for "recovery!" – *but also by teaching me how to watch my own mind, knowing and understanding its defects, and look after myself.* This careful watching of my own mind meant that I myself could pick up changes and alter the dosage of drugs accordingly. Dr.James' motto used to be, "Always be vigilant!"

This is a matter of "owing your own madness," knowing and understanding the vagaries of your own brain. And I would say this to anyone with a mental health problem: *The only road to wellness is to "own your own madness." Instead of relying on "them" to keep you well and medicate you, you must take responsibility for your own mind, your own brain, understanding its defect, observing it and knowing how to handle it, and keeping yourself well.*

The primary reason I kept well for those 7 years, whilst Dr.James was my soul-friend and like a father to me, - until he nearly died then left in April '02,- was that he provided a manner of Psychotherapy; I saw him every Friday for 7 years, pouring out my heart towards him every week. I knew I needed psychotherapy for years,- begged for it, to have in the place of all this sectioning and locking up, and forcible medication, - but I was told "there is no such thing anywhere in Kirkshire." And so I appealed and clung to this "one man," Dr.James, who by his own account was good at listening. *Psychotherapy worked!*
Through the death of both my mother and father, and through endless toils and tribulations with Walter, and through two gruelling court cases, in which I struggled to gain legal access-rights to my son, it kept me well.

For those with mental health problems Psychotherapy works! *It seems to me psychotherapy works because it channels the destructive manic energy away from the core of the mind, so that the mind doesn't harm itself. Manic depressives go mad because they cannot bear the pain of reality; come to terms with that reality through expressing it, and we don't go mad!*

The longer you go on being well, the more stable you become, and the more able you are to achieve things; in those 7 years I achieved a long list of qualifications from different colleges,- an HNC in communication and Organisation, an SVQ level 3 in Business Admin, an NC in Community Care, an ECDL in Computers, Higher Maths, and I'm presently halfway through a Maths degree. I could achieve nothing when my mental health was so precarious that I could have been stuffed back into a mental hospital at the drop of a hat! People came to trust me, I got a good relationship with my son, I created a life for myself "in the community." It took my own courage, but it also took the support of this "one man" to whom I owe it all. That soul-life of mine would have been lost, for I would have been permanently stuffed in the lock-up ward of a mental hospital, if it weren't for him!

Everbody had rubbished me, because I was accounted "mentally ill"; I was "existing in the prison of other people's minds"; I had no freedom and my voice was not heard; I was "dying daily" in that suffering. But in the end, because one man had faith in me, and showed compassionate attentiveness, and took care to "save me," I am now restored to a sense of self-worth!

As soon as I got myself "well" and out of the Psychiatric System in September '95, I started to battle through the courts for legal access rights to my son. My solicitor George McPherson, who had visited me several times in Craigdene, had told me *"you haven't got a hope whilst you are in the lock-up ward of a psychiatric hospital."* It was with this *"hope"* before me that I scrambled out of the deep well where the System and my own illness had put me.

We returned to the "old ways" where Walter and Gabriel were concerned when I came back from Ruthwell in the summer of '95. Walter claimed "you can see Gabriel whenever you like," but it was effactually controlled and supervised by himself. I could never take Gabriel anywhere myself; I always had to see him together with his Dad, usually at their house, and there was always this horrible sexually coercive thing coming from Walter. He made it plain that I always had to "please him" or else I wouldn't see my son any more. Saturdays were particularly bad, as he made it plain after we'd had a meal together and I'd put Gabriel to bed, that I had to please him sexually. By Christmas I'd had enough of it and couldn't stand it any more; I remember telling Ernest and Helen that I was determined to pursue it through the courts for proper Access rights; they told me I was stupid as I would never win more access time than Walter was already granting me; but they didn't know what I was going through.

Then I failed to "please" Walter on New Year's day, and he came round the next day shouting, "I'm finishing it, you get no more access; you're not behaving yourself; you never invited me to stay for a drink on New Year's day; if you don't apologise you can't have Gabriel." I did slavishly apologise, but he still said "you get no more access." A few days later I got a badly spelt and scribbled note through the letter box which read, "don't come down to my house today, as Gabriel doesn't want you to come today."

It was the event of 8th January which caused Walter to stop Access for a whole year. For Walter claimed that Gabriel was brought back "upset and hysterical" and said he didn't want to see his mummy any more. What happened was that I had asked Gabriel who "Hayley" was; I presume she was Walter's new girlfriend. And he said in Walter-like language "I'm not telling you my private business," and said he wanted to go home. When we got there the house was in darkness and Walter wasn't in; Gabriel became hysterical because there was no-one at home. *But Walter claimed from that day that Gabriel was "distressed at the prospect of seeing his mother," and didn't want to see me any more.*

A couple of days later on the 10th we had a meeting with Edward McBay, who was my mental health social worker and Robert Hardy, who was the social worker appointed to Gabriel. The latter had been trying to have talks with Gabriel, but Walter hated him and resisted his efforts. They together told Walter that he couldn't "make the leap" of stopping Access like that when it was "legally agreed." Walter claimed that I had been frightening Gabriel by saying "inappropriate things," especially about dying, and he claimed "Gabriel said he doesn't want to see his mummy any more." Robert Hardy objected "that's not true; what Gabriel said is that he wants everyone to stop arguing, and he can't bear any more rows."

But Walter was adamant, determined that Access should stop, and that I wouldn't be allowed to see "his son" any more. At my solicitor's behest, I went round and knocked on the door every Monday, Wednesday and Friday, for the long weary months of January, February, March, April; and he wouldn't let me in! And it wrung my heart to bits when occasionally I glimpsed them through the window, only to see Walter encouraging Gabriel to stick his finger up at me; or occasionally I encountered them outside, only for Walter to fold the child away from me and scurry away with him. For the whole of the calendar year of '96, the year he was 9, I never saw my son. I can remember attempting to give him a birthday present over the school-wall, only Gabriel crouched down saying "I'm not allowed to see you," before I was hounded away by the teachers. *That year screwed my heart up terribly!*

When I tried to take the matter to court, I hit a brick-wall; the legal aid board refused me legal aid; of course I didn't have the money to take to take it to court otherwise. It was June of that Summer that myself and Patricia sat in the miserable corridor of the LibDem offices in Kirkcraig, intending to appeal about the matter to our MP Ewan McDonald. When I sketched to him my tale, pleading for him to help me get legal aid, he was outraged; "What, not allow legal aid for a mother to get access to her young son!" And he called for telephone, pen and paper, and effected it right there and then. So it was thanks to him that I was able to take it to court.

It was finally called in court, being perpetually put off to later dates, as court cases are, on the 26th November. Walter had Dr.McSharry, the

442

child psychiatrist supporting him, and also the school-teachers. Dr.McSharry concurred that Gabriel didn't want to see me, and said I had a "fluctuating severe mental illness," and was "harmful" to Gabriel. I had the support of Dr.James of course, and he wrote a report to say that I had always looked after Gabriel as a baby "remarkably well," and had made sure he was put in a safe place if I were ever ill, and he called into question the veracity of asking Gabriel if he wanted to see his mummy in his Dad's presence, averring that, if I could have access to Gabriel without interference from his father, "things would go well." My social worker Edward McBay tried to be of help; in his letter he pointed out that I had been well since a medication change, and was going through "a sustained period of stability and improvement." The report from the school-teachers, though they said Gabriel had been "confused and withdrawn" since I'd stopped seeing him, was very nasty; they claimed that his "global difficulties" with his school-work were due to me, because he kept saying and writing that all the "trauma in his life," all his difficulties, miseries and problems, were thanks to his mother. And they claimed that when I once saw Gabriel at the bus-stop, he went "white-faced, shocked and terrified." There was a report made by a court reporter called Mary McGowan, and giving credence to Walter, she got all her facts wrong, and in addition wrote a pack of lies that were emanating from Walter's jaundiced view-point. *That was the hard thing about all this, - the lies; enduring the lies!*

On the 26th November I was awarded "interim Access," of two hours a week on a Tuesday at my house, supervised by a social worker. The social worker was to be Greta Christie. But Walter refused to co-operate. On Tuesday 3rd December we were at his house requesting Gabriel, but he argued with Greta, saying he wasn't going to let it happen. But Gabriel took over, took the lead, saying he wanted his mummy to stay. I sat down to let him know we would stay for a bit, and we had an hour with him in Walter's living room. It seemed to me that by virtue of the fact that I had an hour with him, "we won." And Gabriel at the end of it piped up that he "wanted to go to his mummy's house next week." The experience, of seeing my son for the first time in a year, put a warm glow inside of me.

But then Walter refused to let me see him again, refusing to comply with the court order. The social workers kept saying "we'll see if he complies next week." I asked the police for help, but they said it was a civil case rather than a criminal one. *Walter was in contempt of a court-order, and he was getting away with it! What was the point of making a court order if it couldn't be enforced!* I was becoming desperate as Christmas was approaching. I wrote to the MP Ewan

McDonald about it; he replied that the man had to be "brought before the court" to explain his refusal. Walter explained his refusal in a letter between the solicitors; he claimed that I had "whispered" to Gabriel about going to my house, tempting him with presents, that he had been "coerced and bribed." *It was absurd; he was claiming Gabriel was "coerced and bribed" whilst in the presence of the social worker!*

On the Wednesday before Christmas, the 18th December, he was indeed "brought before the court," to explain why he was, in official language, "obtempering the interlocutor." *He got a roasting from the sheriff, who said "you have to obey it, do you understand!"* Walter replied "Yes but, not when it goes against my son's express wishes." "How dare you answer me back!" said the sheriff, "there will be no buts!" Three times Walter went out with his solicitor, and three times came back with "Yes but." *Finally the sheriff said losing patience, "If you are unable to give me an unequivocal Yes, you won't be leaving this court under your own steam!" He was threatening to put him in jail there and then!* Walter backed down, and a few days later we received a letter "acknowledging that he had breached the order," and saying he would now comply with it.

So I first got that official Tuesday supervised Access on Christmas Eve. The experience was a joy, and Gabriel said it was "the best day of his whole life." After that Access progressed smoothly till the following Summer, at which time my solicitor said we should apply to the courts for the supervision aspect to be removed. Walter had admitted in a letter that Gabriel was "enjoying the Access." I went and asked Walter if he would let me see Gabriel unsupervised on a Saturday, as I had once allowed the same grace to him. He replied "you can see him whenever you want," but it had to be supervised by himself. I replied that I wasn't going to let it depend on his whim, it had to be "legally agreed;" but he said "I'm having nothing more to do with the solicitors and courts," and "I'm not having it unsupervised." So I walked out, saying I would take the matter back to my solicitor. George McPherson said to me on the phone, "a leopard doesn't change his spots; what he wants is you under his control again."

We had asked for a social work report, and it was good when it finally came out; it said I was "a devoted mother who shows genuine warmth and love for her son"; it said there was "no disturbed behaviour evident" from Gabriel; it said "due to her ability to provide care and control for him, we would have no concerns for his welfare if such visits were unsupervised." When it was called in court again on the 2nd July, I was concerned when the sheriff said he must find out Gabriel's point of view. I wrote a heartfelt letter to Walter saying "unless you give in about unsupervised access, Gabriel will be called to testify in court; we don't want that; so do the decent thing; I allowed Saturday access to you when Gabriel was just a baby." But he was adamant. I was distraught because I felt that Gabriel would say in court, due to Walter's long-term influence, "I don't want to see mummy on her own because she lies to me." But George McPherson told me, "Now is the time for holding your nerve."

It was called in court again on the 13th August, but we lost, as the order was not varied, and Access had to be continued supervised. However my solicitor asked for a proper "Proof," which was scheduled for 3rd-4th November. Shortly after I approached Walter again, begging him to be reasonable, but he spilt out a harangue of hatred and bitterness at me. I couldn't stand the way he twisted everything to his own sickened point of view. And after hard thinking I made a decision; "I don't want to get involved with him; I'd rather have the clean, clear, proper Access that the Courts award me."

In October I got a job, a proper 9to5 job with Kirkshire council as a clerical assistant, so I wrote a letter to Gabriel, explaining that I couldn't see him any more on Tuesday afternoons, saying "it is very important to me to continue seeing you; I do love you very much." Shortly after I had long deep talk to him, finding out that his Dad been telling him that, when I had left him at Maggie's when he was young, I'd "lied and broken his trust." I replied that it wasn't my fault that I couldn't come back for him, as I was locked up in hospital; but Gabriel said back "hospitals are for first aid, not prisons."

The "Proof" in court took place on 3rd-4th November'97. George McPherson encouraged me saying "at some point you are going to get Access on your own, and I think the time is right now." There were certain things I was determined to say; that I could give Gabriel a good education, and a good moral and religious upbringing, which were things he wasn't getting with Walter; that I was now well and counted as "fit for work"; that I wasn't doing this for myself, but for my child, as he would be emotionally damaged without a relationship with his mother; "I want to be there for him." George McPherson tried to prepare me by telling me to answer the questions simply and carefully, not going off at a tangent; he told me not to be cheeky or sarcastic, not to get angry, and not to dissolve into tears. *I was to be examined, cross-examined and re-examined in the witness-box; it was one of the greatest ordeals of my life.*

Before the recess for lunch it didn't go too well; the opposing solicitor, Ms.McWilliams flustered me by asking if Gabriel had ever called me "cow." I tried to explain that it was just a word he had picked up from school. Then when she asked if I had ever talked to Gabriel about "death," I elaborated on how we had seen a funeral, and I had explained to Gabriel how there was a body in the coffin. "Isn't it true, Ms.Colme," she retorted, "that you are obsessed with death!" George McPherson told me off at the lunch-break for "going off at a tangent," and not keeping to the question. In the afternoon I did better. Walter's solicitor claimed that I said "inappropriate things" to Gabriel, that I "whispered them in the toilet," out of the hearing of Greta Christie. I wrote on a piece of paper to my solicitor, "I was never allowed in the toilet with Gabriel; Greta Christie was with us all the time," and he made the point. Greta Christie was a witness, and it was made plain that I couldn't be saying "inappropriate things" as Walter claimed.

On the second day it was Walter's turn in the witness box, and he "shot himself in the foot" by saying Gabriel was happiest in his life when he had lots of Access with me. My solicitor made mincemeat of him, allowing his hatred to come out as he shouted, "in a hundred years I'll get peace, when she is dead." Walter claimed some nonsense about Gabriel having brought home a pair of my tights, which the sheriff dismissed as silly rubbish. And when it was made clear that he had "cut off his mother" because the child had just once said he didn't want to see me any more, the sheriff said he should have given guidance and this proved his "poor parenting." When the schoolteacher Ms.Rankine gave evidence, of Gabriel saying "my mummy is the cause of all the trauma in my life," and "mummy can't help me because she is poorly," the sheriff responded "What am I to make of that!"

And he said at the end; "this child is suffering, this child is being tortured; what am I to do to help this child!" *And so he came down on our side!* He said that the supervision aspect had to be gradually withdrawn, and that he would make an interim order of Tuesday and Friday nights 6-8pm, pending his written judgement. He said "I expect this to work for the benefit of the child."

Patricia and I were so gleeful after this that we were clapping our hands on the way back in the car. However it wasn't so simple, because again Walter obstructed the order, refusing to lift the supervision aspect. Christmas was approaching again, and again Walter wouldn't comply with a court-order. He shouted at me, "Nothing will ever move me, no court in the land will move me." George McPherson said "be strong; it's only two weeks in a battle of two years; we're going to get there." But Walter refused access over Christmas, saying that Gabriel had a cough, or was "weak," and that I could only see him supervised by himself. He wrote a nonsensical letter to the solicitors saying unsupervised Access wasn't acceptable to him, and that "lies are at the bottom of this problem; the truth didn't come out in court."

We were waiting for the Sheriffs written judgement to come out, and it did finally on 19th February '98. As George McPherson said it was "as good as we could ever have hoped for," granting me unsupervised Access 6-8pm Tuesday and Friday, and 12-8pm on Sundays. It was the substance of what it said which was the best thing, as it showed Walter's stance was untenable. It said beautiful lovely things about me, about my intelligence and care for my child; "a calm and thoughtful individual who loves the child very much and has his best interests at heart;" "a credible and reliable witness;" "her health has held up and her resolve to keep contact with her child has not waned." It said negative things about Walter; "a difficult man with stubborn views;" "I did not find him particularly truthful; he was often disingenuous." The sheriff said he believed the need for supervision had been firmly placed in the child's mind by the Respondent/Father; "the influence he exercises over the child is detrimental to the well-being of the child and harmful to the child's overall development." He said it was clearly the father who was upsetting the child, and putting unchildlike phrases in his mind, and that I myself had no opportunity to say anything to alarm or upset him. He concluded that the problem "emanates from inappropriate behaviour on the part of the Respondent/Father," not the mother, and "the fears are unwarranted." "I believe the Respondent/Father exaggerates the child's fears and that he himself has nurtured unwarranted concerns, which is surely to the child's detriment;" "the child's views are not necessarily his own but rather are those of the Respondent/Father which have been imposed on him over along period of time." This was brilliant stuff! *In effect it justified the agony of a two-year court-battle; we had won!*

Walter's fight collapsed after this; there was nowhere he could go with it after such a round condemnation. I had, following this, 4 years of good access-rights to Gabriel, from the age of 11 to 16, in which I dare to think we built up a good relationship and friendship, which will stand us in good stead for the future. George McPherson emphasised to me that, as regards Walter I should "remain suspicious of his motives for all time," never allowing myself to be manipulated by him again. I thanked my solicitor profusely for fighting the case, but chiefly, "thanks for having faith in me and for being willing to fight on my behalf when I didn't seem to have much going for me." It was good of him!

Chapter 110
2nd Court Case, – A Further Fight.

After winning that first Court case, on the 18th February '98, gaining Access every Tuesday and Friday night and the whole of Sunday afternoon, things proceeded satisfactorily for a while. I kept asking Walter for overnight Access during holiday times, because I wanted Gabriel to stay the night with me, but he steadfastly refused. We waited a whole year, until I went back to see my solicitor on 21st January; he wrote a letter to Walter which was badly received, so my solicitor initiated court proceedings again, asking the court to "vary the order" so as to grant me alternate weekends and time during the school holidays. *It was another long and gruelling procedure, which we in the end lost. So we won the first court-case, but lost the second.*

Before I went to see my solicitor I had a talk with Walter, asking if he would allow me overnight Access, but he was unreasonable. He threatened me with Gabriel's breakdown, shouting "if you put this on him now, he'll have a breakdown." He claimed Gabriel was "upset" because I had asked him about it; "you mean you were upset" I replied. This was borne out by a phone conversation when I heard Walter shouting to Gabriel "you were upset," and Gabriel replying "No I wasn't." I had been to the school to see the guidance teacher, as I was concerned that Walter was frequently not sending Gabriel to school; Mr Wilkinson said that the child was "emotionally damaged, but was now healing," thanks to me. My friend Harriet said I should try and gain more time with my son, as I was "a mother along the road," who could help his education.

With these things in mind I went along to see George McPherson on the 21st January, and he said it would be normal after a year of access to proceed to overnight Access, or what he called "residential contact." He said it would be considered "in the best interests of the child;" he said that any other itinerant sheriff would have the last judgement of Sheriff McEwan in front of him. *He said he would write a letter to Walter, officially requesting "residential contact," and if that failed to have an effect, would take the matter back to court.*

That letter didn't have a good effect. Walter yelled at me down the phone "from now on there will be no extra times nor nothing; there will be exactly as things official." When I went down to his house he ranted and raved and showed me he was putting George McPherson's letter in the bin. He said to Gabriel "you don't want overnight Access do you?" I said "he says what you want him to say because he doesn't want to upset you." I said that it is the adults who make the decision and it is presented to the child as an opportunity; if it were left to him, I'd never be seeing Gabriel. He yelled "you know what you yourself said, that he has been permanently emotionally damaged by your efforts to get hold of him through the courts." "You said that," I replied, "you can't tell the difference between the truth and your own emotions." "I know the truth," he started to rave.

I next saw George McPherson again on the 4th March. I told him first of all how Walter was saying nasty things about me to Gabriel, not only that I was "a witch," and "a liar," and he wanted to "dance on my grave," but that he had once come in to Gabriel late at night and given him terrible nightmares by saying, "when she realises what lies she's told, she'll hang herself." My solicitor responded that it was "scandalous" that he should say such things to a child. *He said this was a reason for going "flat out for Custody," in that Walter was obviously not acting in the child's best interests.* I had been thinking about the issue, and I told him my reasons for wanting increased Access rather than Custody; firstly out of kindness to Gabriel, as he was attached to his "little room," and also I had promised Gabriel I wouldn't go for Custody; also it was easier to control when I am the access parent, as I don't tug at Gabriel like Walter used to do; also I believed it would make a smaller quicker court case if I just applied for residential Access, as such a perfectly reasonable request would be granted. George McPherson argued against these points of mine, saying it would be best to "go in with our foot on the accelerator," and ask for Custody. He asked me why I was holding back, "Is it that you are afraid of having Gabriel?" I was put on the spot; I thought very hard, and answered, "it's not worth upsetting the balance between the three of us." I meant that at present the three of us were functioning without too much pain. He repeated "why are you hesitating, what are you afraid of?" After getting home and thinking for hours I had an adequate answer to that question; "I'm afraid of pain; the pain Walter can inflict."

I had a think about it during the following days; I tried to consider "what is the most loving thing to do"; and then wrote a letter back to George McPherson, explaining why I didn't want to go for Custody. "I believe Gabriel will cope with the difficult teenage years best if he continues to have the security of living with his Dad. If Walter were the Access parent he would tear the child apart with his possessive tugging of him; the pain between the three of us would increase, and would redound on Gabriel's head because he is the child in the middle; I believe the optimum working arrangement is as it is now, with myself as the Access parent. In addition, if I suddenly had custody of Gabriel it is likely to spoil the good but very fragile relationship I have built up with him."

Then I had an idea when in Safeways with my friend Louise; I thought I would go on a "Peace Mission" to Walter, suggesting that we solve it ourselves, that we do it amicably rather than going through the pain of taking it to court. I could say I was willing to make a legal agreement, perhaps with the help of the Kirkshire Family Conciliation Service; an agreement that I wouldn't go for Custody, if he would grant me increased Access. So I went round on the 17th March, bearing an olive branch, saying "we should do some give and take; surely if I give up on the idea of Custody, don't you think in return you could give me more Access?" It didn't work. He seemed to think I didn't want Custody anyway; he claimed Gabriel didn't want to stay at my house as he would feel "insecure"; he said he didn't want Gabriel feeling that my house was his "home." He was very aggressive, blaming everything on the estrangement between the two of us. So that was a failure; Walter just couldn't be "reasonable."

I was loathe to sign the legal aid papers; that was the point. Then an incident happened with Gabriel, which made me take the decision. Gabriel was at my house whilst his Dad was drinking at "Auntie Morag's." When Gabriel phoned him, wanting to go home to bed, his Dad said he'd come down "in a wee while." Gabriel became distressed at what was a long wait. When his Dad finally arrived, he shouted at Gabriel at my gate; "you are selfish; well I'm not letting you control my life." And Gabriel was quite clearly frightened of going with him. I said to myself, "poor lad, I wish I could rescue you from all this." My reaction was; "I am definitely going to court for increased Access." George McPherson said it was right that I should "bite the bullet"; as it was only natural and appropriate that Gabriel should sometime stay at my house, and if I didn't take it to court, I'd still be in the same situation in a year's time.

It was then a revelation to me when I went to see Catriona McVey, of the Kirkshire Family Conciliation service, in Inveroth. Gabriel had been expressing opinions to me which showed he was in two minds; he would say one day "it's up to me, I don't want overnight Access,"and the next, "my Dad unsettles me when he says these things about you, and it makes me feel I want to stay with you." But I knew he was coerced by the fact that Walter was impossible to live with once "upset." It was a real step forward for him when he said one day, "my Dad says you are knocking down my confidence, but somehow I feel that he is knocking my confidence; he is not allowing me my freedom."

451

When I told Catriona McVey the story, accompanied by Maggie, she said we had to ensure that Gabriel had a say. "Gabriel has rights"; there was apparently a new 1995 Act to protect his rights; the law says a 12-year-old child is old enough to give his own opinions in decisions affecting him; he could have his freedom not at the age of 16, but 12. Maggie concurred that I should say to Gabriel, "by the way you are allowed to do whatever you want, you can come and stay with me whenever you like."

It was the 10th May that I saw Catriona McVey again, and also my solicitor, and on the strength of that, I decided to go for Custody. Catriona McVey said that Gabriel's voice was not being heard, and what was going on amounted to "the emotional abuse of a 12-year-old boy." She said that for the sake of Gabriel's welfare, I must take the matter to the children's panel; alternatively going for a Custody order through a court would achieve the same end. George McPherson then told me "you have parental responsibility to act in his interests," and that means he should reside with me. "I want to set him free," I said earnestly. George McPherson said it had always been Walter's bullying against my softness and good nature; "he wants to bully and control you." I stated that I was now willing to go for Custody, as my arguments of a few months ago seemed no longer valid, and I wasn't afraid of "pain" any more, and I wasn't fearful any more, and, despite some of my friends negatively saying that I couldn't look after Gabriel, I was suddenly convinced that I would make a "cool teenager Mum." I expressed my concern that, when he found out, Walter would stop Access, but George McPherson said he would then be "shooting himself in the foot."

When I told Dr.James we had decided to go for Custody, he said "you might have done the right thing; we can only know in the future." And so it was decided that day.

Then there happened the fracas of the 17th May, the day after Gabriel had badly hurt his leg, going down a slide, and it was initially thought it was broken. Gabriel said it was still painful, and I had said I'd take him to see a doctor, because Walter refused to do so, shouting down the phone "there's nothing wrong with it; there's nothing you can do about it; I won't let you take him to the doctors." I went round to collect Gabriel, together with Patricia, but Walter said at the door "you are not taking him," pushing me down the steps. He threw into a rage, saying to Gabriel "I'm locking you in," and shutting him in the bedroom. Gabriel was hysterical looking at me from the window, and I assured him "he is not allowed to lock you in and shout at you." And I tried to calm him down, trying to get him to come out into the garden; somehow he managed it, and stood sobbing before I took him away to the doctors, his Dad yelling after us "you bring him straight back." Gabriel said to me on the way "I won't want to go back now, because I'm too frightened; my Dad's not kind to me." The doctor diagnosed that he had a sprained ankle and bruised bone, and shouldn't walk for a while. This incident made me say to the crying Gabriel, "I'm going to set you free from this; you'll be happier living with me."

The next day I arranged for Gabriel to speak to his own solicitor, because he said he wanted to speak to one; but he then said he daredn't go "because my dad will kill me." He had a word with this solicitor, Agnes Cowan on the phone, and she suggested that his Dad wouldn't find out; he replied "but he will find out, and then he'll kill me." He said he would suggest it to his Dad first, as this would be better than "deceiving" him. But on the way back to his Dad's house, he said he daredn't broach the subject, as his Dad would be too angry; "too bad!" he said. Agnes Cowan afterwards said that it was shame that a boy who was almost 13 should be too scared to speak to her.

The application for legal aid when it went in, said that the child was "fearful of his father" and "unreasonably influenced by his father." When it was his birthday at the beginning of June, when I suggested that he had a friend round at my house, he said his father had "forbidden it." I thought this was just not normal or natural, and that his Dad was being "the bane" of his life. There were other incidents when his Dad forbade him to go swimming with children of his own age. Then Gabriel told me that his Dad always left him late on Friday nights at his Auntie Morag's house whilst he went drinking, and sometimes he didn't come back for him till one in the morning. He said mournfully, "he doesn't look after me, he just forgets about me, and then he embarrasses me by calling me selfish." I replied that he wasn't selfish for wanting to go to his bed at one in the morning, and he was entitled to it.

It was after Walter and Gabriel came back from their Summer holidays at the end of July that they received notification about my legal aid. Walter seemed to panic, getting Gabriel to say to me on the phone, "my Dad says you can have overnight Access, if you admit a few things." George McPherson warned me not to agree to conditions as it was best to go to court. And what were these "things" they wanted me to admit? "You've got to admit you're sorry you lied about the tights." This was something Walter had in his bonnet about the last Court case, when Sheriff McEwan dismissed his assertion that Gabriel had come home with tights in his pocket! It was absurd. Gabriel went on, obviously distressed by his Dad, "my Dad says No and I say No; my Dad is not happy because of you; my dad is not happy; he's mad at you and he is mad at me as well; I want you to cancel this court." George McPherson said it was not appropriate for Gabriel to be involved in this way, arguing for the imposition of his father's will.

Then Gabriel came round and said "my Dad says you are a liar; my dad says No and I say No." I replied back, "I'm sick of all this nonsense that comes from your Dad; I'm not a liar, I'm your Mother; I don't tell lies." And I told George McPherson that "I'll plough straight ahead"; for I wanted to take Gabriel out of all this fear with his Dad, so that he could have a sense of freedom, and be able to grow up. It made me upset when Gabriel was left at my house several times when his Dad was out a the pub; I told Gabriel I wanted overnight Access "so that on nights like this, you can stay at my house." It was clear on such nights that Gabriel wasn't adequately cared for, and was frightened of his Dad. The child cried waiting for him, then asked if I could tell that he had been crying; "because if he knows I've been upset, he'll question me in that way he does." My friend Sadie told me to explain to Gabriel that having this right of overnight Access would "give him more freedom," and allow him to stay when he wanted, and that was the light in which I saw it.

The Minute lodged in court was served on Walter on 27th August; it stated that Walter was not acting in the child's best interests in failing to give me residential Contact. A couple of days later I was summoned to Walter's house to a meeting with "Auntie Fiona," another of Walter's sisters. She suggested, very reasonably, that we try overnight Access once a week on a Friday night. I tried to ascertain whether Walter was offering that, but he just ranted on like an emotional mess; "I want recognition that I didn't lie about the tights; the judge called me a liar, but the truth is going to come out; and that truth is going to destroy me and destroy everything." Auntie Fiona very reasonably said that this "wasn't important"; Gabriel was important. Walter went on about "all this hating of each other." I said back "I don't hate you, the emotion comes from you." I asked "are you offering this?" but could get no clear idea of what he was offering. Walter called Gabriel out in front of us, and the latter said in a quiet voice he didn't want overnight Access, at which his Dad said triumphantly "you see, I told you he doesn't want it." *When I subsequently took Gabriel home with me, he started shouting at me emotionally, "you are a liar, you tell lies, you lied about the tights." It was clear how Walter was putting all his own emotion onto Gabriel.*

Chapter 111
2nd Court Case, - A Failure.

On the 23rd September Gabriel first saw his own solicitor, a Mr.McNicol;
Walter took on this solicitor for him, and as Vivien said she could
imagine him "spouting poison in his ear all the way." The result was a
great bitterness and rage coming from Gabriel; he violently ripped the
TV times to bits, and said he had told Mr McNicol his mother was a liar;
"what's more my dad took my birth certificate, so that the court would
call me Gabriel McKay instead of Gabriel Colme"; he laughed bitterly,-
"so I've got you back!" I was upset by this, though Vivien told me he
lashed out at me because I was his mother, but I was also told to
demand respect. So I told Gabriel, "Don't you ever talk like that to me
again; I'm your mother, I'm not a liar." George McPherson told me to
simply say to him, "the court will decide the matter."

It was due to call in court on the 13th October. Walter had lodged
answers saying that he had never prevented residential Contact, but
had simply "acceded to the wishes of the child." It was agreed on the
13th October that residential Contact should take place on Friday 15th
October and Friday 29th October as an experiment; this was because
Gabriel expressed the view that he wanted to try "experimental
overnight access," and make up his mind afterwards. I was delighted
that Gabriel himself seemed to have worked it out, and delighted that
after 9 years, he was going to be sleeping at my house again! It was
continued to a Child Welfare Hearing on the 10th November, and
George McPherson warned me not to negotiate with Walter meantime.

The 10th November was an awful and horrible experience. The
solicitors spent hours "negotiating," whilst Vivien and I sat in the narrow
hallway being furiously eyed by Walter. At one point I happened to say
to him, about the Christmas arrangements, "do you realise what this
will mean," and he leapt up belligerently and started arguing; Vivien
intervened saying "stop it you two, you should not be talking to each
other." My solicitor told me of the "package" they had agreed, before
they took it into court; I pulled a face, because I saw that Walter was
offering it to suit him, so he could go out drinking on Xmas and New
Year's Eve. Moreover they were only offering alternate Friday nights,
and we had really thought I would get every Friday night and some
weekends. When the judge was reading out the court order proposal, I
got up and said "excuse me my Lord," because he was missing
something out. We came away feeling it was a horrible experience.

And afterwards Gabriel phoned me up saying he was upset that they hadn't included the next Friday, because he wanted it every Friday night. "Why didn't you tell them you wanted every Friday night?" I asked. He replied "Nobody asked me." *I thought what a shambles it was! They had talked to the child for hours and it was supposed to be a Child Welfare Hearing, and they had never asked him how often he wanted to see me!*

It was next due in court on the 26th January. Meantime Gabriel and I had a nice time together during several overnight stays over the Christmas holidays. It was particularly meaningful for me to have Gabriel stay during the night of the millennium celebrations; and on the 1st January 2000 he said "I don't want to go back to my Dad's house, I want to stay here longer." I went down with him and put it diplomatically to Walter, and so he did get to stay longer. Gabriel was still having problems with his Dad's behaviour when he was drinking; "he gets cross when I want to go home and threatens me; he says he'll leave me and things like that." I was appalled at this, but told him to arrange with his Dad that he should on these occasions "come to Mummy's house to sleep."

I put in proposals to my solicitor, to forward to the other solicitors about holiday Access. I suggested first of all that I have access every Friday night, but not alternate weekends as George McPherson suggested; this would then be perfectly fair, as it would split up the time each weekend, Saturday morning and Sunday afternoon with me, and the other afternoon and morning with this Dad. I then suggested a weekend in February, then a week in the Spring holiday, and two weeks during the Summer holiday, so then I could take Gabriel on holiday to Iona.

I found that Gabriel had received this proposal the weekend before it next called in court, when I saw him at his Dad's house, ill in his bed; and it caused him to be very negative and unkind toward me. He said "you are forcing me, you are persuading me"; and he said his Dad had helped him to write down what he wanted to say to his own solicitor. I told George McPherson how this showed he was being "unduly influenced by his father," and manipulated by him. *Gabriel also said, "I don't want a week with you; my Dad says you might snatch me away!"* I replied "don't be absurd; do you think I'm going to kidnap you or something!" I told George McPherson this showed how Walter was "putting unreasonable fears into the child's mind." I asked Gabriel why it was he said he didn't want more overnight Access with me, when manifestly he did; "so why are you saying that?" And he replied "I don't see enough of my Dad; he says he doesn't have time to take me out anywhere." I told George McPherson this was a "lame excuse coming from Walter," and it was his own fault if he didn't spend the time with him. *Walter was just being mean, depriving the child of quality time with his mother; "one night in 14 is not enough!"*

The day before it called in court on the 26th January, I knew Gabriel's solicitor was ensconced in their house all afternoon, so what the Mr. McNicol would say would be "all input from Walter." George McPherson replied to me when I told him this that I mustn't get upset or emotional, "and whatever you do, don't get ill." I told him it wasn't fair; "Walter has two solicitors speaking for him now." He said back that he "couldn't assault the integrity of Mr.McNicol." Then Gabriel phoned me and said in a high pitch of negativity, "my Dad's nice and you are evil; you are always persuading me, but it's a trick; you just want to win me, but I can't let you get away with anything; if you keep persuading me, I'll cut off those overnight stays." Given this bitter mood of mind the night before, it didn't bode well for the court.

We lost heavily that day in court. I had to just sit there and watch the lie being told; Mr.McNicol said "the child is adamant that he wants no change to the status quo." So we got no increase, and no iota, "not a sausage" for the holidays; out of all those weeks of school holidays Walter wouldn't even allow me a weekend! He said he would "generously propose" that I have Gabriel Tuesday and Friday afternoons as well as the evenings; but I got that anyway! My solicitor then proposed that a "curator" be appointed for Gabriel, who would "act in the best interests of the child," but the other two solicitors and the judge overruled him, saying that Gabriel at 14 was mature enough to be in the witness box. My solicitor then asked for a "full hearing," and the date was set for this. When I came out I remarked that it was "wicked," and George McPherson replied, "I know it's wicked, but he will be obstructive all he can."

My friends all told me after this that I should abandon all this hassle of a court case; what was the point of going through it all, and dedicating my life and all my time to being available for Gabriel, if at the end of the day he says "disagreeable things"! But I was determined to persevere, because I thought my relationship with my only son was worth fighting for; and so I struggled through to that date of the Full Hearing which, after a 13½ year struggle, comprised "my final day in court."

The date was now set for a "Full Hearing" on the 24th May 2000. My solicitor told me I would be in the witness-box and I would need witnesses; I chose Vivien and Sadie. He told me the Sheriff would proceed on a "non-interventionist rule"; it said courts should not make orders unless it was in the interests of the child to make the order. We needed to argue that it would be in the interests of Gabriel to give a structure to his life, so he is not caught in the middle, making decisions. It was really going to be a legal argument; whether or not there should be an order. The trouble was, Gabriel now being 14, was of an age when what he said would be accepted.

We got a letter from Walter's solicitor saying Gabriel didn't want to be "forced against his will." And we got a letter from Gabriel's solicitor, complaining bitterly all about the fire and the Sky Digital! Gabriel had complained that I wouldn't let him have the fire on, though this was because I couldn't afford the electric bar-fire; and that I "frequently blamed him for things that happen in the house;" though in actual fact he quite clearly did something deliberate to my Sky Digital out a sense of revenge, and had laughed when I had phoned him about it. It was absurd.

George McPherson at this point urged me to ask Walter myself for extra time during the school holidays, and there was a resulting fracas on the 28th March. I told Walter that he should offer me something "reasonable" during the holidays; if he wanted me to bend over backward to "babysit" for him on nights that he wanted to go out to the pub, he had to offer me something better. He was furious, yelled at me, and slammed the door on me with Gabriel on the inside, shouting "you are not going up there," whilst Gabriel was in tears. But he somehow escaped, and went off on his bike, whilst Walter shouted at me, "you are a wicked woman; you have hurt your son horribly, and everyone round here knows it." I was upset, and back at my house, Gabriel tore things up angrily shouting "Why did you do that!" I said back "I'll never do it again!" I had learnt my lesson; I would never again try to negotiate with Walter directly.

George McPherson when I told him of this was cross with me, saying "you as parents should be capable of negotiating it; you should be adult enough to do it." I then received a cross letter from Mr.McNicol, saying that Gabriel believed his parents were interested "solely in controlling his movements," and that his requests were "turned into a matter of conflict." He said that on such a day as the 4th April, when I had said he could stay if he liked, there was "pressure from both sides for him to make up his mind." George McPherson said of this, "I do not think it is right that Gabriel is put in a position where he is mediating between you and his father."

I went to see George McPherson on the 11th May, and when he asked if I was sure what I wanted, I said "Yes; I want you to go in with your horse galloping and your guns blazing." *He agreed, we agreed, that Gabriel is having to negotiate his own access rights, and he shouldn't have to do this. It is wrong in principle that he is used as negotiator, as the "peacemaker" between two parents. Therefore the court should give a structure and impose something. I told him emotionally, "I have Gabriel overnight one night in 14, and I never have him for more than 24 hours, and that is just not good enough; it is as if Gabriel and I are being punished by not having decent amounts of quality time with each other!"* My solicitor interrupted "Don't go down that route." I said how Gabriel is under pressure from his Dad, who is filling the child's mind with his own negative emotions. He challenged me, "Why not Residency? Why are you not going for Residency/ Custody?" I said I had my reasons which I would later try and outline to him. He said we would go through with it; "either we will win or we will lose."

A few days later I got a letter from him, explaining that the only thing challenged was whether there should be a court order fixing Access or not. In the joint minute of admissions Walter had admitted that residential Contact was "in Gabriel's best interests;" we were going to argue that it was therefore perverse of him not to allow it other than fortnightly in a Friday. He confirmed that we were asking for every Friday night, plus half the school holidays. He said hopefully Gabriel when giving evidence would repeat parrot-fashion what his father would tell him to say, and this would come out. He told me I had to be "consistent and reasoned" in my arguments of why I was seeking more Contact/Access rather than Residence/ Custody.

Accordingly I wrote to him my reasons. I did want the responsibility of being the Custody parent, and felt I would be a good teenager Mum, and idealistically wanted to set my son free, but was convinced that if I remained the Access parent it would be "kinder" to all concerned. Firstly, it would be kinder to Gabriel to leave things as they were; I didn't want to tear him away from the security of his bedroom, and of living with his Dad. Secondly, it would spoil the delicate relationship myself and Gabriel had built up, and it would be better if there were some space between us in the next few years. Thirdly, it would upset the balance between the three of us, leaving his Dad bitter and pained, and this would redound on Gabriel; as Access parent I didn't tug the child to bits, as Walter used to do. I also pointed out to George McPherson that Walter was a recluse who wasn't a fit father, who was frightening Gabriel, saying unkind things to him, filling him with his own negative emotion; and he was impossible to negotiate with, as I had tried over and over again.

The day of the Full Court Hearing was going to be the day that the whole "Court Case" of 13 ½ years duration, was going to be finally finished; for it was in effect, in legal terms, the same "Court Case" which when Gabriel was a 6-month-old baby had been initiated by Walter, demanding Access-rights to "his son." A few days before it was going to happen, Gabriel appealed to me to stop it from happening. And I replied, "It is better that we now go ahead and go through with it. It is definitely the last day of this dreadful court case forever! If we don't go out in this "blaze of glory," it will be cisted and hung over our head for ages!"

Chapter 112
The Final Court Judgement.

And so the "final day in court,"-which was in fact two days, the 24th and 25th May 2000 -finally happened. It didn't feel like a "blaze of glory," as the whole thing was horrific!

My solicitor wasn't very pleased with me. Sadie thought I answered the questions very well, and got over all the major points she said I should put across; - that Gabriel enjoyed his time with me, but he wouldn't ask for extra time because he is under the influence of his Dad, he was manipulated by his Dad; I had tried reasonable discussion with Walter, etc. And when cross-examined I answered very well I thought. They kept asking me about "Gabriel's view"; and I said that what he said was not his own view but his Dad's. Walter made a right fool of himself. Under cross-examination by my solicitor, he admitted that he'd never asked Gabriel for his "view," and hadn't realised till two weeks ago that we were asking for holiday Access. And he told downright deliberate lies which made me angry.

I kept whispering things to my solicitor, but he told me to stop doing it. He said at lunchtime, "answer the question; don't go off at a tangent." But I'm afraid I did so under cross-examination by Mr.McNicol as well; I just couldn't help it. At the end of it he said to me; "So Gabriel quite often gets hold of the wrong end of the stick!" I replied "he doesn't listen very well." He remarked "neither do you". And I added the quip, "Well he takes after his mother!" On the whole I couldn't take the questioning seriously. I mean it was said, as if I'd made a grave parental mistake, "did you tell Gabriel that this court-case might go on for two days?" I replied "So what!" I couldn't help but be flippant about it; I felt I could handle it. But George McPherson took me to task about it, and said I must be sombre, serious, reasonable. And then Mr.McNicol said "and did you say to Gabriel that if he said bad things about you, you could say bad things about him?" I cried out "for heaven's sake, that was a joke!" Well at least they didn't score any points off me; I wasn't bothered about it.

What bothered me was that it wasn't finished; but we had to go back for Gabriel's testimony the next afternoon. But given his hysterical state that day, and the fact that Walter said he wouldn't let him attend, I somehow doubted that it was ever going to happen. It was awful at the end there. We were told Gabriel was crying in the corridor; and then he came in, and yelled and wept and screamed. And when we were given permission, I went rushing out to comfort

461

him. But then his Dad got hold of him, and took him away from me as he always used to, saying he refused to let him come back the next day. I came back in and said earnestly, "It's best if it's finished with, it's best if it's over with." And then I said, "Walter is refusing to bring Gabriel back again tomorrow." *And then I think the worst thing, just as I was going out of there, was that Gabriel pointed his finger at me so viciously and said "I'll kill you, I hate you." That was what really shook me up; it wasn't all those hours of cross-examination; it was Gabriel's emotion at the end of the day.*

The next day was the day the Court-Case finally finished. Gabriel had his answers off pat, and my solicitor didn't break through them; "he had been schooled". There were some instances in which he said things to corroborate my evidence; such as, he didn't want to wait two weeks, and he wanted to stay longer, and his Dad said "you can't go up there ever again"; but these gave just brief glimpses of Walter's true character. I felt "I don't know why no-one can see through him". As I earnestly said to my solicitor afterwards, "what bothers me is that Walter's character never came out; it never came out that he is a liar and a manipulator."

Apart from that, Gabriel did quite well, being brave and trying to be truthful. The trouble was, he said he didn't want more time with me during the holidays. He said "No, definitely not." When my solicitor said "Why?" he replied "I need to build up my confidence." When asked "Why?" again, he replied "I don't trust my Mum." When asked "Why?" again, he replied "because I feel unsafe." When asked "Why?" again he said "because of things that have happened in the past." When asked "What things?" he said he preferred not to say. But these hateful fears and worries had been put into his mind by his Dad; and this was never brought out. I had said in my evidence the phrase "my Dad said you might snatch me away," but it wasn't corroborated.

I listened to the summing up, and decided we'd lost. "I think we've lost; I don't care." But I did care very much. I thought we had lost because their argument was more convincing than ours. I said earnestly to George McPherson in the foyer; "Why is it that I am a mother who cannot see her son for even a whole day! What have I done wrong! Why am I being punished!" George McPherson said I hadn't done anything wrong, and reassured me that we might still win the case; we would find out in about a month. I said "if I don't get any redress, then I think the whole System is rotten."

I went for comfort to my friend Maggie. She did my heart good the night before, saying "you are flowering from day to day; you are such a wonderful Mum; this is what you should have been like ten years ago; but they took that from under you feet." And she said this wonderful thing; "you had to struggle over rocks and broken ankles; but now your ankles are strong; and now you can go anywhere; you can go places they can't." I had watched a film that night, in which the children were taken away from the mother who was suspected of child abuse; and she had a loving husband and grandparents for the kids to stay with, and it was only for a couple of weeks, and yet her anguish was portrayed as the worst that a mother could possibly suffer! - - *What about me! I had my son taken away for seven years! No-one has a clue what anguish I went through! Maggie reminded me of how she had said ten years ago that I must either bend, or be broken by the System; "and they broke you to bits".*

But Maggie helped my feelings when I went to her house immediately afterwards on that final day. She said to me earnestly "At least Gabriel can never say you deserted him; at least you have fought all you can, you have done your very best." She said all that was left was that I should "enjoy the time you have with him, and get on with your own life, in the hope that he will want to come into your life." When I later talked to Dr.James I said so earnestly "Why is it that this has happened to me! What have I done wrong! I should write a book about it; it's time I told my story!"

I immediately afterwards got a letter from George McPherson, saying he knew I was "disappointed" that Gabriel was so adamant that he didn't want to see more of me, but I should take "the bare Contact," and stop phoning my son every night like I had been doing, and be "a bit more cold and matter of fact," so that he got the message that he couldn't "play with people's emotions" in the way he had done. He said we just had to "wait" for the Sheriff's written judgement, just "hoping" that he agreed with us. That judgement finally arrived on the 15th June, the day before I was due to set off to Iona.

And so on the 15th June 2000, came the final judgement in a Court Case which had in effect lasted 13 ½ years. And it was a terrible judgement, a terrible blow.

It said that the child "had settled views over the question of residential Contact to the Minuter/ Mother over the holidays that had been arrived at for his own reasons and without being imposed on him by the Respondent/ Father"; and he had "sufficient maturity and outlook for

463

decisive weight to be given to those views." It said of Walter that he was "prepared to go along with the wishes of the child," and painted him as whiter than white and everything he said as true. It said that clearly he didn't dominate over his son, or frighten him; it said clearly the child shouldn't be "bullied into anything," and that the mother should "let the child come to her rather than forcing him to do so." *I was appalled that the sheriff seemed to have accepted this position of Walter's "hook, line and sinker"! It took no cognizance of the fact that Walter had prevented me having Access for all those years, or of the earlier judgement of Sheriff McEwan, who had really had an insight into his character. What he finally "found in fact and in law" was that no Court Order should be made, and the child should be given the opportunity "to decide for himself" about residential Contact with his mother during the school holidays; "I have left that now entirely up to him."*

I was devastated. George McPherson said in his accompanying letter that the time had come to distance myself from Gabriel, and that now that the Court Case was finally finished, all I could do was leave him to make his own decisions. I phoned him up and said emotionally "but he has to beg his Dad." And he told me not to be negative; "just get it across to Gabriel that it's up to him." He said in a heartfelt way, "I'm sorry for you; it was a gamble going to court; and we lost."

And that was the end of the story. I had some Access rights to Gabriel until he was aged 16, in June of 2002, but it couldn't be said that I had "decent Access rights," such as any other Access parent should reasonably expect. For during school holidays I never had him for longer than a few extra overnight stays, which had to be begged and arranged. For a while I had him staying every Friday night, at his own request; but I never had him for so much as weekend, and in fact I believe I never saw him for more than a 24-hour stay! It was all due to the fact that we lost the second court case.

This grieved my heart; and I believe my lack of quality time with him, is the reason I never built up a sufficiently strong relationship with him, to bear the test of time, or the test of Walter pouring poison in his ear again after he passed his 16th Birthday, when of course the original Court Order no longer applied. Walter at this stage told him that he no longer needed to visit his mother, and "only a baby" would do so; with the result that for a whole year I hardly ever saw him. It has been slightly remedied now, but to what extent I as a mother have been able to forge a lasting "friendship" with my son, will only be discovered as a fruit in the mists of future-time!

Chapter 113
The Evil Psychiatric System.

Look at the perniciousness of the Psychiatric System! Look at what it did to me!

I was locked up and maltreated by the Psychiatrist Dr.McNeill, who kept stuffing me full of the Lithium that didn't work on me, permanently sectioned by him for 7 whole years ('88 to 95)! And since then, on my own and under the care of one man, my GP, who provided a manner of weekly Psychotherapy, I have been out of hospital and well for nearly 8 years now. Doesn't that prove a point?! Doesn't it prove the point that I didn't need to be locked up and maltreated in the first place!

I had good cause to go insane. I was a single mother with a baby son for 5 years, and then the father took the custody of the child off me through the law courts, claiming I was an unfit mother because mentally ill, with the collusion of the Psychiatric System. As an excuse for not championing my cause, himself afraid of this bully of a man, the psychiatrist years later said, "Well Walter was a very difficult man to deal with." This is pathetic as a reason for leaving me as a mother without Access to her son! I kept saying and writing in my manic anguish,- "I am insane with pain." Yet nobody asked me, "What is your pain? Can I take it from you, can you express it?" All they did was lock me up and give me forcible medication.

I kept escaping, over and over again, because I wanted to prove that I didn't need to be locked up and forcibly medicated against my will! I wanted to prove I could "own my own madness," be self-medicating, and make it on my own. It was a loop-hole in the Law that I exploited, but as I stayed months at a time in places like Lytham or Austria, I realised that to be able to do so, to be able to look after oneself without any recourse, and without arousing anyone's suspicions, it means that you must be strikingly mentally sane! And also I wrote poetry and I wrote whole books, so readily returning to a real and creative life when "put out there in the world"; *I was able to live a real, creative, meaningful life! So how could I deserve to be locked up? What justification was there for making me spend lost months of my life locked up! You can't heal a mind by locking it up!*

Recovery from mental illness is not easy; you have to accept the reality of what has happened to you. And what has happened to you is not so much the madness itself but the reaction of the Psychiatric System to it. *What is so disabling is not the madness itself so much as others attitude towards it; when this is in the form of your own psychiatrist's attitude, the result is crippling.*

Dr.McNeill connived with a pernicious legal system which took my tender young son away from me, due to the fact, not that I was an unfit mother which was manifestly untrue, but to the fact of the existence of prejudice and fear about mental illness in other people's minds. And then for years he scoffed at my efforts to maintain freedom of soul, and rubbed in the pain of my son's loss for year upon year; and when the pain resulted in emotion, he used to say, "there you are, you are emotional, you must be still ill." He forced me to take psychiatric medication, he robbed me of my freewill, he did his best to destroy my every effort at creating and maintaining a soul-life, always bringing my brave efforts into the dissolution of meaninglessness. *It was his psychiatrist hands which "signed away my meaning,"- gladly, exuberantly, violently! I couldn't begin to live and be free until I had broken these bonds, until I had gifted myself with the "voluntary essential impulse of will," of the freewill which signifies to us mortals that we have a soul.*

What does it do to us, when psychiatrists like Dr.Mc.Neill sign away our meaning, when they cripple us with their judging and condemning attitude? I'll tell you what it does; it destroys us! It leads to the destruction of our personality, and ultimately death. It is tragic that so many people I know, faces I remember whom I loved and cared for, have committed suicide. *And they took this as their only way out because they were "disabled" by a psychiatrist's mind and "trapped" by the System. It was never my illness that was disabling; it was Dr.McNeill's attitude toward it that was disabling!*

Suicide is thought of as a common problem of those with mental health problems. But it is not a self-imposed problem; it is a problem caused by our being "relegated to the cage-like walls" of other people's minds; *and we struggle and struggle against this "prison" of other people's making, until we reach the point of despair.* It is when you despair, when hope ceases and finally collapses in on itself, that you take that irrevocable and final act.

I was very upset a few years ago to hear that a young man I knew in the hospital called Steven had committed suicide. I had already been deeply shocked a few year's earlier to hear that the dear sweet young girl called Anne, with hair like a princess, had hung herself by her shoelaces in the bathroom. A multitude of my former friends have killed themselves in a multitude of different ways. But when I heard of

Steven's death, it really turned my stomach, for I was told that he jumped in front of a train, and that they were still "picking up his body parts" miles down the track! I mourned him for a while, because I remembered him as a "brave young man," with whom I shared a "comradeship" as fellow-prisoners in a harsh regime; he was always trying to "buck the System" and fight fiercely for his freedom just like me!

And now he had committed suicide, just like I had done! And in my sorrow I remembered vividly that suicide attempt, on that cold November night of '92, and I remembered why I had done it. You only get to that point of suicide when something happens, when after all your struggle to get up and fight over and over again, something happens to make you despair. Despair means the negation of hope. We need hope to live; "whilst I breathe I hope." In a sense, life is hope; without it we cannot live. With me it was that "Haldol Decanoate" depot injection which made me despair; it made me so incredible ill, so that I couldn't think or move or feel; I couldn't even brush my teeth and even my eyes were stiff. And seeing it was a long-term injection, before it wore off they were going to give me another one and then another one, and I would be like a zombie for all time! And I despaired! It was that dreadful mind-deadening depot injection which was my final defeat. I wondered what had made Steven despair, what had finally defeated him?

I once heard someone on a train pronounce, "Suicide is a coward's way out." I took issue with him; "it takes enormous guts to commit suicide." It does; even a Shakespearean hero hasn't enough courage to kill himself! Hamlet speaks of "the dread of something after death which puzzles the will." That is what it is like, in that moment,- the sheer dread that overcomes you paralyzes the will. It is like some great endless agonized moment in which you are suspended for all time. It is like the final confrontation with the ultimate meaning or meaninglessness of your life, the final nakedness of your soul standing there before all the worlds, - of time and eternity, of earth, heaven and hell. Time seems like a whirlpool about to suck you in, and you get the overwhelming sense that you are doing something dreadfully wrong that can never be put right; there will be no opportunity ever to amend it. It takes enormous guts to get beyond that moment, knowing that you are taking your own life! I shall never expunge from my memory the following moments when I felt that I was falling down and down forever, as if down an endless well, before the ice-cold water hit up my nostrils and shocked my body! You have to be so brave to jump into a dark and ice-cold sea, seeing it as a watery grave. So how brave do you have to be to jump in front of a train?

So Steven is yet another "voice that is not heard," another friend who has gone down to his suicide in silence! His outcry,- his outcry against the System which he battled, which must have trapped and defeated his spirit, and which finally overcame him,- will never now be heard. How many more have to die before someone, somewhere changes the System?

I have survived the System. Because I wasn't ordinary or normal and had some special gift, the sane people classified me as "insane." But I am a survivor. Thanks to Dr.James I have survived the assault upon me, and have now my creative gift intact. But many others have not been so lucky; many are dead, many are forever zombified and locked up.
My cry from the heart which is my purpose in writing this book is; Don't do this to us! We are not to be dismissed, we are not to be locked up! We are suffering and striving souls with our humanity to share!

Faced with someone who is "insane" there are two attitudes a doctor, someone who is supposed to "healing hands," can take; one is to judge, condemn, relegate into a prison of his own making; the other is to listen with compassionate attentiveness, thereby truly freeing that tormented soul. So, in my own story, just as by the one man, my psychiatrist Dr.McNeill, I was condemned and nearly destroyed, so by another man, my kind GP Dr.James, I was saved, rescued, redeemed! A doctor such as this can "save souls, save sanities!"

I want this book to condemn Dr.McNeill and all psychiatrists like him, for they increase the sum of human misery, and do all "manic" people a disservice by destroying the "glorious liberty" of free brethren, of us comrades who soldier forth to our destiny, - our destiny in the future of being free recognised citizens with a gift, with a story to share, with a meaningful and treasured life.

Chapter 114
The Psychiatrist Who Nearly Destroyed Me.

I was certified as "insane" for 7 years; I was sectioned under the Mental Health Act non-stop from '88 to '95; and all through the power of one man, one psychiatrist who gave me this dreadful label!

I escaped from the System; I made escape-attempts from the hospital over and over again, until I managed it; I consider that I proved myself "sane" by exploiting that loop-hole in the Mental Health Act which says that if you stay away from the hospital and are not found by the police for one month, then the section lapses; it presumes that if you can stay away in the middle of nowhere, with no money, no roof over your head, no food, and no help or recourse, with all the police of the country searching for you, for one month, *then you must be strikingly mentally sane!* This is what I did many times, till I finally broke the power that the mental health law and this one psychiatrist had over me.

The thing is, I know I have made a narrow escape, because a dire fate awaited me. I was told, "you have a serious mental disease which is getting worse; we are thinking of keeping you locked up in hospital permanently." I had long feared and dreaded the over-dose of drugs which, perpetually applied, could leave you a zombie. I only narrowly escaped being hospitalized and zombified forever; with no soul-life and no story to tell, it would have been a living death!

And just one psychiatrist did this to me! Because he labeled me as "mentally ill," I had no chance; all that time I had no choice, no freedom; when sectioned you are not even allowed to vote; you are a non-entity, condemned; what greater condemnation can there be than that society takes your child off you! I ask you; when someone labels you as "insane" how can you prove yourself sane?!

For 6 months at a stretch Dr.McNeill had me locked up in the "acute ward". Now if and when I got "manic," I'd come back down to earth in a week, but there was no way I could convince this man that I was simple "myself." I remember once lying on my bed, thinking I'd look relaxed and calm and this would convince him, perusing a book of the Dolomite mountains. I said to him "Look I was on that mountain-top; that's where I spent a week watching the sunset and sunrise." He said "as mad as ever, still hallucinating!" But I was on that mountain-top! That's where I got the book from, from the shop at the foot of the mountain!

He once said to me "Normal people don't go about scribbling on bits of paper!" "But that's what I do," I replied, "I'm a writer, I'm a writer!" So I'm mentally ill because I used to make notes during the day in order to do steadfast journal-writing every night? I'm mentally ill because I had a creative ability he didn't have?

He once said to me, "you must be ill because you're wearing glasses." The thing is, I was more aware sometimes of my need to wear them. "I need to wear them," I protested, "having pre-eclampsia when pregnant damaged my eyesight." "Huh, I don't see you walking into doors!" came his reply. So what sort of statement is that! Only people need glasses who go banging into doors?!

I used to dread getting back into the power of Dr.McNeill every time I was returned from one of my escape attempts. The first thing he would do was to increase all my medication and put me back on the dreadful Lithium, which is the drug he forced me to take for 7 years. Once when I was returned from a Newcastle hospital he increased my dose of Laragtil from 30 mg a day to 200 mg 4 times a day. So what-fold increase is that?! Does he really think I could have long have borne such an onslaught on my mind? The Lithium he forced me to take against my will for 7 years, made me feel incredibly ill, physically itchy and nauseated. He used to check up that I had taken it by means of blood tests. It is as if he had put me into a box, labeling me as "manic depressive," to which he had to apply that drug. But he kept telling me for 7 years that I was having relapses; was he really so stupid then as not to realize that it wasn't working?

He sectioned me non-stop for 7 years, simply signing yearly a piece of paper that renewed it; I didn't even have a right to a second opinion. I bewailed "the psychiatrist's hands that sign away my meaning." I begged and pleaded with him every time, "Look you will get a better response from me, and find me more positive, if you allow my freewill, instead of forcing me to do things against my will. Please don't section me!" His response was "well the law allows me to do this, and therefore I'll use my power to do it; I can, so I will!" So he is a megalomaniac miniature Hitler is he! No doubt Hitler said "Well I can slaughter 6 million Jews, so I will slaughter 6 million Jews!"

His coldness, narrow-mindedness and stupidity really come across! I was having intense mystical and spiritual experiences in my so-called madness; but because they didn't fit into his narrow scientific outlook, he rubbished me! I would say something to him about "the sea of God's love," and he would throw his eyes to heaven thinking "as mad

470

as ever!" *We who are considered "mentally ill" very much "exist in the prison of other people's minds." When that mind is your psychiatrist's, the result is crippling!*

I once said to him, because he had forced me to stay in my house where I didn't want to stay because it was full of pain, "You have turned my house into a prison-cell." His response was "Nonsense, prison-cells have bars at the window." Could he really be so stupid as not to see that what makes a prison is the robbing of your freedom, the violation of your inalienable right to be free? His lack of imaginative understanding of me, of what it was like to be me and to suffer what I suffered, was to the nth degree!

Doctors who are helpful and kind, who save and liberate with their "healing hands" are those who can pay compassionate attentiveness to another soul in their need and their pain. Did such a saving action come from my psychiatrist? On the contrary, he tormented me by cruelly probing me pain. Every week I was forced to go and see him, and every week he would ask "And how do you feel about the loss of your son?" I would get emotional, as any mother would, who was screaming to high heaven unable to see her young 5-year-old son. And then he judged and condemned me for that emotion. He would say "You are very emotional, so you must be still ill!" He condemned me because of the "life" in me; was that because he had no life in himself?

He used to say to me "you must be ill because you keep changing your mind." Now I never changed my mind with a kind of fluctuating, but because I was sincerely seeking a way forward. But look, not to be able to change and grow, and feel your way forward, to irrevocably make decisions which you never change, is to be "mentally ill" in the way that perhaps he himself was. Sane people are changeable; they allow change in themselves like clouds and sunlight; they are changeable as the weather is changeable! So was he labeling me as "ill" because I was not like him? To tell the truth I think I was more sane than he ever was!

I was seeking deep spiritual truths, which had too much energy to be contained by my own mind, and he rubbished them! Once when I returned from an escape to the Highlands, from where I brought back a really old and valuable rosary, made of semi-precious stone, which a wise priest had given me, I said when interviewed by him "at least I went all that way and came back with this!" And he said back scoffingly "it's just some cheap beads!" *It was so symbolic! The deep spiritual truths I had delved into madness to find, he rubbished! I looked back at* him and said silently; "you shall never break my spirit!" And he didn't. But then again it took me a further 7 years to recover from what he did to me in those 7 years when I was in his power; before I was able to forgive it and move on, and find a sense of self-worth!

This psychiatrist had enormous power over me, and he used that power wrongly. To have power over someone's life, and to abuse it, is to perpetrate evil. My cry from the heart is, "Don't do this to us! Don't rubbish us, because you fail to understand!" By his constant failure of imagination Dr.McNeill nearly destroyed my entire life!

I went every year to Iona, since I got "well" in the Summer of '95, gradually changing and mentally growing up, gradually able to take on my pain, until finally I realised it was time to transcend my pain. And I realised I could only do that, I could only transcend myself and move on, by forgiving.

I realised this as early as that holiday I took the day after the judgement arrived from the sheriff, which was so disappointing and painful, when it was plain we had lost that second court battle in which we had tried to obtain access rights more regularly at weekends and during school holidays. From the moment I arrived on the island I felt it was a place of "vision" and "wide horizons," and I felt the Abbey church was luke-warm and womb-like, as if I'd come home to that "place of grace." I felt healed and whole and "grown up at last."

My feeling for Gabriel occupied me at first, and it changed subtly. I suppose that deep down I was cross with him because of what he said in court, but I kept praying for him at every opportunity, and put a prayer in the intercessions box "for a 14-year-old boy, who needs to mature very quickly, and for his mother, who has gone through a lot of pain." Then one day when paddling on the beach I found a release and a melting of the heart toward him; "poor Gabriel, it's not his fault!" It was not his fault that he said what he did in court, or that he was born into such an emotional mess as existed between me and Walter. I was aware that I was trying to "solve the problem of forgiving Walter"; on Iona my life always "solved itself" very deeply.

Then I woke up one morning there feeling that I could forgive Dr.McNeill. "It's time I saw Dr.McNeill" I awoke saying; I could forgive him because it was past, and because he did what he did out of stupidity. He had lost seven years out of my life, but in contrast I thought of Walter, who had ruined my entire life and was still actively harming me; indeed, because he had spoilt my son's life too, he had "ruined my life beyond my own lifetime."

A woman called Janice tried to help me; she worked with abused children. I met her at a coffee-time, just after we were invited to write on a piece of paper something that had shattered our dreams, before symbolically tearing it up. I had written on my piece of paper that terrible thought I'd had when pregnant with Gabriel; "I wish I could tear this baby from my womb and leave it as a dead thing on your doorstep." I said to Janice after tearing it up "I wish it were as easy as that." She told me that if I could not forgive Walter, because he ruined my life, what I needed to do was see some good come out of it; I replied dolefully "no good will ever come of it." I said that as it could never be good that my life was ruined, I would never know the "letting loose" of forgiving Walter. The next day at coffee-time she said that if I couldn't forgive him, I should try and "bring him to God, and pray to God to forgive him." She said I should look at my hatred, "look at it and name it"; and then in the end "you might get to a stage when you don't want to hate any more." I burst into tears, hugging her and leaving the room.

I approached a wise old priest after Mass, and asked "How do you forgive a man who has ruined your life and is still actively harming you?" He explained to me that emotions can't be "bad" as they are mere human feelings; forgiveness is an act of the will. He explained that it took time for the "healing of the emotions." "Do you want to forgive him?" the priest asked. After that I went to the Abbey healing service and the prayer ended "and heal you of all that harms you"; and I realised that as long as I hated Walter it was harming me. The next day I was walking by a pebbly beach when what the priest said came home to me; *"Do I want to forgive him! I want him to roast in hell-fire for what he did to me! But for as long as I hate him, I am enthralled by him, enfettered by him!"* When I told Janice this, she said it was true that for as long as I couldn't forgive Walter, I was enchained by him and not free to live the rest of my life; if I could say "I want to want to forgive him" it was a big step forward.

When I got home I told Dr.James of my realisation on Iona; he said it was true that my hatred of Walter kept me enchained and enfettered; he had known it and seen it for ages. He told me a story of how a Jew who had all his family killed by the nazis couldn't forgive them; then one day he said "God forgive them," and from that moment he felt free. What I was aiming for now was some kind of "healing of the emotions"; I became convinced that a whole person should not have any bad memories; if you can give thanks for all your memories then you are healed. I can remember telling Helen earnestly that I didn't yet want to forgive Walter; but I could say I "want to want" to forgive him. As for Dr.McNeill, I found I was moving toward forgiving him.

In the next few weeks however Dr.James urged me not to go see Dr.McNeill, as I intended. He told me Dr.McNeill was "doing his best" but failed, "falling short of the mark" as in the Greek meaning of "sin," but he didn't intend to harm me. I replied adamantly "I must still go and

474

see him." My point was, "if I'm able to forgive him, I have to go tell him I forgive him." Dr.James pointed out that it would do no good, as Dr.McNeill would say he was unerringly right, prescribing Lithium once he had diagnosed me as manic depressive; he said that rather than considering himself wrong he would say I had changed my illness.

To help, whilst I was coming nearer to forgiving Dr.McNeill, I visited Craigdene, where I hadn't been for many years, and discussed the subject with the nurses who had been particularly kind to me, Geoffrey and Lorenzo. Geoffrey told me that the only way to forgive the man was to see him not as evil or as mean, but merely stupid; *it is easier to forgive as stupidity.* Lorenzo very earnestly talked to me in the kitchen with his own brand of wisdom; *"the past is past; there is no use regretting it, because it can't be changed; you must go forward and put it behind you; regret is no use!"* He also said to me earnestly, "his intentions were good; and how can anyone do better than have good intentions!"

Some of my other friends as well as Dr.James were telling me just to "forget it"; *but I replied that "forgetting it wasn't forgiving it," and I felt I had to confront the man, ask for an explanation, and tell him I forgave him.* As the date neared my friend Helen was suggesting how I should approach him; I shouldn't blame him or accuse him, but say "I have difficulty dealing with my feelings; I'm trying to let go of my anger, in order to move on and come to terms with the past; I need to understand it better." In particular I wanted to say, "Why didn't you listen to me, as I told you to stop forcing me, and let me have it in my control!" and "How can you justify not letting a mother see her 5-year-old son!"

Then the day I was due to see him, Dr.James came round; and he roundly told me to "forget it," himself giving an explanation of Dr.McNeill's behaviour. He repeated at me loudly; "he has done nothing to be forgiven for; he did the best he could in the situation; he did what he thought best at the time." He said that the reason why I was deprived of seeing my son for years was at the time in the early '90s there was a lot of concern about mentally ill mothers maltreating children. He said what he himself thought wrong was that Dr.McNeill had allowed me to make that decision of giving up custody of Gabriel when I wasn't well. "But the past is past," he said, "leave it behind, leave it alone, forget it!"

It was not this tirade that changed my attitude. It was the fact that he took me by the arm and I felt happily overcome. And this attainment of happiness let loose something in me, so that I then hastily set off to see Dr.McNeill saying to myself, "I am determined to forgive it and forget it!" Basically it was because I felt loved in the present, that I felt enabled to forgive, to "let go" of a sin that belonged to the past!

The meeting itself which happened on the 7th August wasn't the successful "letting loose" that I hoped it would be. For Dr.McNeill excused himself all the way along the line, said all the things Dr.James said he would say, and at the end of the day, never said he was sorry. He stated "I have nothing to reproach myself for; I did the best I could for you in the circumstances." He made the points that he had himself started me on the depot injection that had made me well, that I had apparently suddenly become "better,"that he had to force me because I was a "difficult patient to treat," that I had "run rings round the mental health act," that he hadn't let me see my son when I was "manifestly ill." And he said that he had made the careful decision to let me lose custody of Gabriel because "you can't have it both ways; you can't want control of your own life and then blame other people when you do." I said something about the "great wound" this had left in my life; he said he had done the best in the circumstances, and I "wasn't fit" to look after Gabriel at the time.

I looked out of the window at the pouring rain. At least he had tried to give an explanation. I stood up saying "I am determined to forgive it and forget it." He uttered a long explanatory sentence, and I put out my hand and shook his, saying "I'm trying to forgive you." It struck me immediately afterwards, going out into the rain, that seeing forgiveness is an act of the will, I should have said "I do forgive you"; but the thing is, I never felt that release of the heart. This was because, as I realised afterwards, he had never apologised; he hadn't shown one ounce of sorriness! I saw that forgiveness is not unilateral, but a two-way thing; even God requires that we be sorry and repent before we are forgiven.

But it was done; in a true way I had forgiven him; in a sense I had the "letting loose" of forgiving him before setting off to see him! After that, hatred of him didn't bother me any more.

Chapter 116
Finally Forgiving, – Walter.

It remained for me then to try and forgive Walter.

I happened to see Walter the day after I forgave Dr.McNeill; this was by the dodgems at the Lammas Fair which was taking place in the town. I happened to find him just next to me, and amid all the noise, overcome by a sudden feeling, *I leaned forward and said in his ear; "I think it's time we forgave each other, don't you?"* He replied *"Yes, for Gabriel's sake."* A while after that I happened to encounter him in the supermarket; we conversed a minute and parted; then I rushed back to him saying earnestly "thankyou for being so nice to me." It seemed a warm rush of the heart, like "an impulse of the holy spirit."

What enabled me to finally grasp the pain and transcend it, was the talks I was having with Dr.James. Again he was telling me to "let it go, forget it"; he told me to "push bad memories out of my mind" by counting to ten. I said back to him that I was "doing this healing of memories thing" which the priest on Iona had told me of, convinced that you can "give thanks for all your memories and be healed." It was Dr.James who helped me to explore my own wound. He said to me, "If you had a choice between not having a child at all and having Gabriel, which would you choose?" I said I wanted a "love-child" and felt Gabriel was "ruined," but to answer the question, I would say it was good for me to be a mother. He spoke of "the qualities I had learnt by being a mother," and so I could thank Walter for giving me Gabriel. I said how I felt Walter had "ruined my life" in that he had "ruined the best part of me,"- my sexuality, my purity and integrity. But in saying it to him I realised this wasn't really true in that I had "grown intact again," thanks in fact to my relationship with himself.

It was our next talk, on the 21st September, which really cracked it! I was telling him of that memory I had which epitomised all my pain; when I was going up that hill with Gabriel in the pushchair, and we encountered Walter, who said "If it weren't for me, you wouldn't have a son." I tried to explain how I went crazy with pain, feeling that Walter had "ruined the potential of all my life," because he had left me "burdened with a baby" who was "born outside of wedlock, outside of love." I said Walter had "sullied my soul," and I "didn't have choice," wasting my life trying to make good the mistake. He earnestly asked me if I knew when early man first realised when intercourse led to child-birth; it wasn't till they had domesticated animals; apparently up until then birth was looked upon as a gift of the earth-goddess. I said I didn't know what he meant, so he spelt it out; *"look at your child as a gift from God, a gift from your own body, of your own fertility; it doesn't matter where the sperm came from."* Something deep within me cried out *"Yes!"* He said I should look on Walter as an "external accident" who happened to be there, a mere annoyance like the rain when I wanted to cross the road. I repeated forlornly "but Gabriel was born outside of wedlock and outside of love," but he pointed out that King Solomon was born in such a way, and "you can't say it's not God's law; God doesn't see things in that way."

I went home, feeling this cry of "Yes" inside of me, and that night, taking off from this "mysticism" of Dr.James', *I was filled with memories of my own mysticism at the time of Gabriel's birth. For I too was seeing my child as "a gift from God" in this way when I was bearing him and when I gave birth. I saw him as born "wholly and solely out of my love," because it was my love that was keeping him alive in my womb.*

For I used to think like this; - *I have jealously guarded the pulse-point of my being from being known by anybody else; it is because I never said Yes to Walter, because he never knew me or touched this "pulse-point," that I have always maintained that he is not the father of my child It is because I never said Yes to Walter, but did in the depths of my suffering say "Yes" to God, that I have always maintained that Gabriel is God's love-child. Thus Walter is not Gabriel's father. I have always believed that even if a test of paternity were taken, it would not show Walter as the father. For I have always maintained that I could only conceive a child when I could say a complete "Yes" to God, and without that true union which is "knowing," I don't believe that you can conceive a child! A doctor may not believe in such mysticism, but I shall never be convinced otherwise! He is my child, and not Walter's. For I was loving God in his conception, and in the further creation of his being, and Walter wasn't there at all! Walter wasn't there at that pulse-point where I was saying Yes to God!*

This was why I used to claim "Walter McKay is not the father"; it's the way I used to look at it when I was mad, believing the child was born out of my love alone, rather like in the case of the Virgin Mary. It was helped by the fact that the day I conceived him was a day it was theoretically impossible to conceive. And at the birth I cried out "it is all true." And then when I was so-called well, everyone told me to come down to earth, and see that he was conceived in a particular place and time by a particular man; I had to recognise that Walter McKay was the father, and give him rights. *But this mysticism of Dr.James', which was also my mysticism, made me leap at a truth I wanted to believe, and cry "Yes!"*

It germinated a seed; a seed of a changed attitude toward my son and his father; I seemed to grasp the pain and transcend it! Encountering them at the supermarket a few times, I was invited to a slide-show, of photos at their house, and then to a Halloween celebration, when we all drank wine together; we talked in a civilised way and Gabriel seemed to take comfort in having his two parents together. Then I was invited to a cup of tea with them in Safeways, and Gabriel was beaming with happiness. *A "letting loose" seemed to have happened in me! I realised the truth of what Dr.James was saying, "he is a pathetic little man, who isn't worth hating." I thanked him, because apparently he had "probed my wound and healed me."*

Soon we were having lunch together in "Safeways" every Saturday; and we started going places together in the Spring; we got on well for a while. But soon in May Walter started getting amorous with me, saying "I feel for you, and always have," kissing me along the Willow Braes. I tried to say "I don't want any physical contact," but I felt bullied and coerced, as he was demanding I should "keep him happy" and I was afraid of offending him. The problem went from bad to worse; he started putting his arm round me, saying "do you still have feelings?" As well as being sexually demanding, he was intrusive, always trying to get inside my house; and he never let me have Gabriel except when it was suitable and convenient for him. *The nub of the problem lay in that I had forgiven Walter whilst not liking him; "he is a man who hurt and harmed me, whom I have forgiven; I don't have to expend myself trying to keep him happy."*

Pater Leo said to me in his letters "it is enough that you have forgiven him," and it was "unrealistic to think he will change." I explained that it was "difficult to get it right with him," in that I was trying to be kind to him without liking him. *Pater Leo pointed out what was wrong, as he could see it clearly; I had made a "spiritual experience," he said, but Walter hadn't. For me it was an act of forgiveness; for me it was "selfless, benevolent and clear." But Walter had made no such act of forgiveness; he just wanted to go back to what he felt before. He hadn't taken it on board, he hadn't moved on. He just thought he could go back to the sexually coercive relationship he had with me before Gabriel was ever born.*

The problem persisted and made my life a misery. I tried to hold out this "unconquerable benevolence and invincible goodwill," but it was a "sexually coercive relationship" which I could do without. It was a re-run of the horrid relationship we had had before Gabriel was born. He was insisting on my kissing him, saying "make me feel wanted"; and when I said I didn't want these kisses and "didn't need physical warmth," he said I should do it to please him. I was in a pickle with all this sexual bullying; then he started falling out all the time saying "I'm not wasting my time with you," walking out, and then trying to make up again with kisses the next week. *I said forlornly to Dr.James "I was struggling with him in '85, and I'm still struggling with him."*

I gave up with it in the end. I told him in November '02 that I was "ceasing to relate to him"; the only way I could put paid to these sexual games he was playing, was to stop relating to him altogether. This was a great success, and I have been happier since not seeing him at all. The point is, not that we couldn't establish a good and right relationship, but that I did basically forgive him for what he had done to me! And that was my "letting loose," my setting free from the fetters of hatred which were harming me, and preventing me from walking on.

So that is everything forgiven! I have even been able to fully forgive Dr.James, for the pain he caused me that I held against him. So now I am like a bird, able to fly on its own and truly free! And I have my stable mental health, and a bagful of qualifications, and the world at my feet. So I can pursue my own way, free of the past, and unafraid.

Chapter 117
The Doctor who Saved Me.

I regard Dr.James as the doctor who, by his compassionate attentiveness and healing hands, saved my soul-life; he saved both my soul and my sanity at one swift swoop!

He rescued me singlehandedly; for after my liberation from the psychiatric system in '95, because of my traumatic experiences, I refused to have any dealings with anyone to do with the psychiatric services, and so it fell upon him as my GP to look after me in every way. And he created my stable mental health by his years of constant care; he helped build in me a basic stability and sanity, so that I could really get somewhere and achieve things! He not only supervised my medication and gave me this healing weekly psychotherapy, he watched me and taught me to watch myself, so that I came to understand my brain's defect and manage it myself. He taught me to truly "own my own madness," which I'd had struggled in vain to do for years. He was always there for me, and made himself available to me whenever I was in need. I needed someone to have the guts to believe in me, and be committed to me, and he did that! He was committed to keeping me out of hospital; and it was that commitment that saved me.

However I found myself left so pained and angry, when the relationship came to an end, when after extreme illness he left his job and the area in April '02, because I felt abandoned and left with "nothing." *And at the end of the day, he seemingly "abandoned" me into a loneliness of grief and loss. Indeed I felt "all washed up, like a mariner who had a ship, abandoned on a solitary shore!"*

Now in the light of that grief, the Psychotherapy seemed shot through with fallibility. I came to see it as a kind of bondage or enthralment; I was waiting and yearning every week for just some sign of affection. And this was because we had such a deep relationship in '93 that it meant all my affections and emotions were bound up in him, in his being and in his presence. I felt that by fastening all of my emotions and affections around him, and then subsuming to himself the whole of me for those "good 7 years," he not only ended the abuse of those "bad 7 years," for which I owe him my gratitude, he also left me with nothing.

That was the point; I was "left with nothing"! I ended up blaming him for "curtailing" my life, for closing down life's potential for me; for he took me from my ability to respond to three offers of marriage, which at least offered me "something real,"- a family life at the end of the day, which is the one thing I really craved and needed. It seemed to me he knew I was offering my complete heart's love for all those years, yet never let me loose from its demands, but "dangled me" on an emotional string. So I was left struggling to face the reality of this relationship, and reconcile the opposite extremes; although on the one hand he was my "creator," saving and rescuing me, gifting me with a soul-life, on the other hand he seemed to have harmed me and wasted that soul-life. What a quandary I was in, feeling that the same man to whom I was so grateful had seemingly "ruined the life he gave me!"

From that position of pain, I "looked back in anger" at the whole story I had written, and it seemed to me that this "one deep beautiful friendship" of my entire life was wrong and abusive. I struggled in the night-time hours with awarenesses about it. For it seemed to me that I was "vulnerable" at that time when he "took me up and cared for me," when my young son had just been taken off me, and when I was "childish and mystical." And it seemed to me that he very cruelly tried to break up with me that summer of '94, leaving me "walking on the edge;" the pain and ravages to my mental health caused by it, still remained with me!

The point is, he involved all of my soul-life in my total self-giving, and then pulled out of it to my destruction! I felt he had himself so deep into my relationship with God, that I couldn't get him out again! He even demanded of me that I tear and destroy my journals, which are offerings to God; and then he told me to "go love someone else," failing to see that I could never really love anyone else again like that! I was left incapable of loving anyone afterwards really, and it had taken me a decade to recover! Because I couldn't "let go"of him on that trip to Iona, I resolved to "hold onto a belief in that love" for the rest of my life. The result was that I was left "dangling," emotionally dependant on him, because all my affections were centred on him. And that was a waste of my life; I was focused on him as if there were no-one else in the universe, not able to open my heart or love again. And so I felt basically that as well as helping me and saving me, he had harmed me and wronged me.

Whilst I was lost in the pain and anger of it all, there came a day, at the end of April '03, - when due to my other experiences of "forgiving" both Walter and Dr.McNeill, thereby knowing in my heart what such "forgiveness" is like, - I realised, "I can only move on by forgiving him." And that very day I made this "act" of forgiveness, - and it was an act, as forgiveness is in the will, - and it suddenly brought a great release of the heart. And after that I could see in gratitude how much he had really done for me. And I knew also how much I really loved him!

Once my anger was gone, as it was instantaneously, my whole perception of the relationship was changed. I saw that it was indeed complex and emotionally charged, a mixture of intense pain and bliss, but the thing was, we mended it and walked on with it; we did "bear one another's burdens like Abelard and Eloise." What that relationship did, for all its intense highs and lows, was to forge between us a deep intellectual and spiritual friendship. We were indeed "best friends" for all those years. I shared with him, and told him everything, and he listened with care and love, and reflected it back to me with wisdom. I couldn't have become who I am without him!

It was true that in a sense I was "in bondage" to him, in that I needed him so badly and couldn't do without my dependency on him all those years. But if he did "dangle me" emotionally, that was because I myself couldn't let go of him. And I made my choice to love him, which was a true and soul-deep choice. He couldn't be blamed for taking me up and loving me when I was vulnerable; the important thing, look, was that he did love me when I was "childish and mystical," because in that state I was "most myself," without the inhibitions and wads of reality that we put around ourselves. He saw the core of me, the mystical heart of me, and loved it. He loved me; we loved each other. *When no-one else cared about me, when no-one else loved me or believed in me, when everyone else had written me off as incurably mad, he took me up and loved me. And this is precious, and it is what made the ensuing friendship soul-deep and lasting!*

I believe it was because we had such a deep relationship, because "we did some giving and taking at so deep a level," that I now have a sane mind and a creative soul-life! For perhaps the intensity of what we shared caused him to "care" about me so deeply, as to expend a lot of his time and energy keeping me safe; he kept me "safe" from the System in the same way as you would put a treasured object into a hidden place! And also perhaps what he saw in me during that time, of the valid mysticism which hid behind my madness, led him to have faith in me. *And that faith saved me; he had faith in me during the years when I couldn't have faith in myself! Perhaps it is always true in such cases that we are saved by someone else's faith!*

In effect he "created me" rather in the way Professor Higgins creates Eliza in "My Fair Lady"; he took me from the gutter where I was poor, unstable and ill, and made me rich in my mature and stable mental health. He's given me back myself; he's given me the world at my feet. And so even though I've gone through all the pain and anger caused by my loss of him, yet with my bird's wings fluttering and able to fly alone and truly free, I know I need to thank him for creating me who I am!

Chapter 118
Transcending.

I have always known that my creativity is linked with my madness. And it has always seemed to me that because other "sane" people cannot understand this creativity, they label it as "insanity." The story of "Erehwon" has always impressed me; a seeing man arrives in the land of the blind, and because he has eyes that they don't have, they gouge his eyes out, believing it is a disease he needs to be cured of!

The division into "sane" and "insane" is all in the perception. Because Dr.McNeill couldn't see me as the fixed and recognisable persona that he wanted to see, he classified me as "insane." "You are changeable," he said, meaning that if I were changeable I was ill; it is a trick that psychiatrists employ. But now having mastered my "insanity," I am more "sane" than the sane people are!

The trouble is, "people like me" are condemned; we don't get a look-in; as a group we are indeed "the poor of the earth." I have felt that wherever I go "I can't stop people locking me up;" it is a shame that I have to see the world, not as a place where I can find the fulfilment of my potential, but as a place where others, seeing me as non-acceptable, look for opportunities of locking me up! I may be "proud of my madness" before God, but I can't be in front of other people, as I would be stigmatised and ostracised. Because of my "madness" I had my child taken from me; what greater condemnation could there be from society than that!

But manic depression should not be treated as a negative "illness" which we should be ashamed of; rather it is a positive creative gift! All manner of artists, poets, musicians down the ages have been manic depressives, and the insight it has given them has informed their work. *I am proud of my madness, and not ashamed of it; I am proud of its connection with my creativity; I am proud of how brave I am in facing it, how I re-create life in the face of it all. Madness is knowledge; I am proud of my madness and of my knowledge.*

And so I say honestly that I do not regret this "madness." I live precariously, but as long as I live creatively, I don't care. It is part of my character; the precariousness and creativity of my existence belong together in my nature. I wouldn't have it any other way! *I don't mind the madness because I see it as the price I pay for living an intense creative life; it is the "defect" that matches my gift; the "dark side" of my creativity. It is the people with defects who have the gifts!*

Dr.James once said to me, because I apparently had such a raw deal from life, "I have always felt so sorry for you." And I replied with passionate energy, with a look of rapture on my face which he said he could never forget; "Don't feel sorry for me! I have seen and known things you couldn't possibly even imagine! I have experienced the naked Glory of God!" *And so I will honestly say, I do not regret any of the experiences contained in this book, any of this "madness," these wide extremes, this capacity for ecstasy, because it has brought me a life of drama and passionate intensity, and a knowledge of things and truths which otherwise I would not have had, and an insight into God's love. I wouldn't want to be without that "madness" as it has given me a unique knowledge of that love! I do not regret it!*

When I was on Iona in the year 2000, I met the same old wise priest, who had told me that the only solution, to enable myself to be free and walk on, was "forgiveness." And on this occasion, he told me whilst I was sorrowing that I should "live for today, live in the present moment." He said "the past is binding you in chains; let it go." And I realised that I had to "write my story" before I could achieve that wisdom of old age; "writing a book would help me let it go." *And it was as if I heard a voice echoing from the abbey's stones; "Write this book!" And I committed myself to doing so. My final act of transcending and forgiving could only be achieved by writing this "one book."*

So I have completed this book now, and told my story, and the past is washed away and forgiven, and I am able to move on, to live the little life left to myself, with the grace of the days God may give me!